I0055285

Animal Health and Welfare:
An Issue of Veterinary Clinics

Animal Health and Welfare: An Issue of Veterinary Clinics

Edited by Lauren Boyle

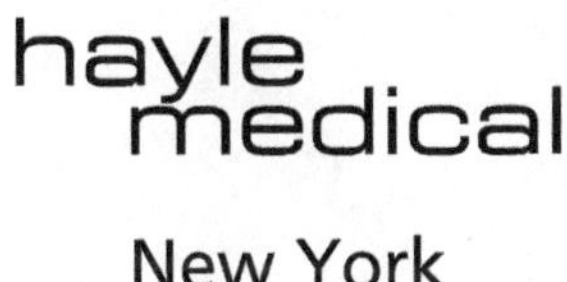

New York

Hayle Medical,
750 Third Avenue, 9th Floor,
New York, NY 10017, USA

Visit us on the World Wide Web at:
www.haylemedical.com

ISBN: 978-1-63241-824-1

Cataloging-in-Publication Data

Animal health and welfare : an issue of veterinary clinics / edited by Lauren Boyle.
p. cm.
Includes bibliographical references and index.
ISBN 978-1-63241-824-1
1. Veterinary medicine. 2. Animal health. 3. Animals--Diseases. 4. Animal welfare.
5. Veterinary hospitals. I. Boyle, Lauren.
SF745 .A55 2020
636.089--dc23

Table of Contents

Preface

The main aim of this book is to educate learners and enhance their research focus by presenting diverse topics covering this vast field. This is an advanced book which compiles significant studies by distinguished experts in the area of analysis. This book addresses successive solutions to the challenges arising in the area of application, along with it; the book provides scope for future developments.

Veterinary science is the field of medicine, which is concerned with animal health and welfare. Food production and safety, zoonosis control, animal disease control and animal welfare are some of the key focuses of this field. Animals suffer from a number of diseases, such as biliary fever, leucosis, pneumonia, bladder stones, blain, filariasis, epilepsy, fasciolosis, etc. Animal welfare involves considerations of disease, longevity, immunosuppression, physiology, behavior and reproduction. It is based on the belief that animals are sentient, and experience pain and suffering. It also addresses the aspects of animal cruelty, poaching, animal testing, behavioral enrichment, blood sport, etc. This book is compiled in such a manner, that it will provide in-depth knowledge about animal health and welfare. From theories to research to practical applications, case studies related to all contemporary topics of relevance to veterinary medicine have been included herein. This book, with its detailed analyses and data, will prove immensely beneficial to professionals and students involved in veterinary science and medicine at various levels.

It was a great honour to edit this book, though there were challenges, as it involved a lot of communication and networking between me and the editorial team. However, the end result was this all-inclusive book covering diverse themes in the field.

Finally, it is important to acknowledge the efforts of the contributors for their excellent chapters, through which a wide variety of issues have been addressed. I would also like to thank my colleagues for their valuable feedback during the making of this book.

Editor

1

Anatomical distribution and gross pathology of wounds in necropsied farmed mink (*Neovison vison*) from June and October

Anna Jespersen[1,2*], Jens Frederik Agger[3], Tove Clausen[2], Stine Bertelsen[1], Henrik Elvang Jensen[1] and Anne Sofie Hammer[1]

Abstract

Background: Wounds are regarded as an indicator of reduced welfare in mink production; however, information on the occurrence and significance of wounds is sparse. To provide a basis for assessment and classification of wounds in farmed mink, the distribution pattern and characteristics of wounds in farmed mink in June and October, respectively, is described. A total of 791 and 660 mink from 6 to 12 Danish mink farms, respectively, were examined. The mink were either found dead or were euthanized due to injury or other disease. Mink included from June were kits in the pre-weaning and weaning period (1–2 months old). Mink included from October were juveniles in the late growth period (approximately 5–6 months old) or older. Macroscopic pathology and wound location was systematically recorded.

Results: There was considerable variation in morphology as well as location of wounds between June and October. Wounds were primarily located on the front parts of the body and in the head in June (1–2 month old kits) and mainly on the rear parts of the body and on the tail in October (5–6 month old kits and older). Moreover, there were significantly more females than males with wounds for most wound types, and significant differences in occurrence of ear and tail base wounds between certain colour types.

Conclusions: Wounds varied significantly from June to October with respect to morphology and anatomical location. Wounds in June were primarily located on the front parts of the body and in the head, while wounds in October were mainly present on the hind parts of the body and on the tail. The majority of the wounds were found in specific well defined skin areas and could therefore be grouped into categories according to anatomical location.

Keywords: Mink, *Neovison vison*, Pathoanatomy, Season, Skin, Wound

Background

In Denmark and other mink producing countries, the impact of skin wounds and injuries on the welfare of mink has been in focus through resent years. Wounds are believed to be an indicator of reduced welfare in mink production due to pain and social stress [1]. Knowledge on the occurrence and significance of wounds in mink is sparse; however, Danish studies indicate, that around 10 % of mortality among mink kits is caused by bite wounds [2, 3]. The occurrence of wounds seem to increase in early and late growth season, respectively, and there may be differences in the causal mechanism between wounds in the early growth season and wounds occurring after weaning [3–5]. Due to the lack of knowledge about wounds in mink, management of wounds is carried out on a non-scientific background subjected to convenience and individual preferences. In other species, wounds are often characterized according to type, aetiology and degree of contamination [6]. Furthermore, for some species, specific assessment criteria have been defined for certain wound types or injuries, enhancing clinical handling of these lesions, e.g., shoulder wounds in sows [7] and hock lesions in cattle [8]. To provide a

*Correspondence: ajes@sund.ku.dk
[1] Department of Veterinary Disease Biology, Faculty of Health and Medical Sciences, University of Copenhagen, Ridebanevej 3, 1870 Frederiksberg C, Denmark

basis for wound assessment in mink, we have characterized wounds macroscopically according to anatomical distribution in dead farmed mink collected during two periods of the mink production cycle, i.e., the early and late growth season, i.e., June and October, respectively.

Methods

The study was designed as a cross sectional study of dead mink collected continuously from 6 to 12 Danish mink farms over the months of June and October, respectively. The mink were either euthanized for welfare reasons or were found dead and stored in freezers until subsequent necropsy. Mink collected in June were all kits (1–2 months old) whereas mink from October included both juveniles and adults (5–6 months and older). The mink had been managed according to standard procedures following general legislation and guidelines for mink production. They were kept in standard cages with inserted kit wire mesh floors during the month of June, where the dam and kits were still together. From weaning until pelting in November the mink were kept in pairs or in groups of up to four mink in the same cage. A full necropsy was performed on all animals after thawing [9], specifically including registration of skin wounds. Registration of individual data including fur colour and sex was done for all animals. Wounds were examined macroscopically including registration of wound location, size (length × width measured in cases where the wound was not too irregular for correct wound area calculation), scab formation, granulation tissue formation, contraction, oedema, degree of infection, exudation/exudate type and condition of surrounding skin areas and wound edges including undermining of intact skin. Based on the location, wounds were categorized as: ear wounds, scalp wounds, neck wounds, shoulder wounds, thigh wounds, tail base wounds and tail tip wounds. Furthermore, there was a category of other wounds, i.e., less common wound locations that could not be placed in the before mentioned categories. A total of 791 mink from June and 1186 mink from October were examined. Of these, 526 pelted mink (without skin) from October were excluded from the dataset due to limited ability to identify wounds. The proportion of mink with different wound types in June and October and the distribution of wound types between sexes and colour types was calculated and presented graphically and in table form, respectively. If a mink had more than one wound, it might count for more wound types. Mink with injuries characterized as only post mortal due to the lack of tissue reaction (June: n = 216, October: n = 55) were solely included as part of the total number of mink for the calculation of proportions. Logistic regression was performed in SAS version 9.4 (SAS Institute, Cary, North Carolina, USA) using proc genmod for estimating significance of associations between wound type and sex and between wound type and colour using maximum likelihood parameter estimates for multiple comparisons of colour types. A p value of 0.05 was considered statistically significant.

Results

In total, one or more wounds were found in 244 (244/791 = 30.8 %) mink from June and 291 (291/660 = 44.1 %) mink from October. The seasonal distribution of lesion types (pathoanatomical) is illustrated in Fig. 1 which shows that most wounds in June were located on the front parts of the body and in the head,

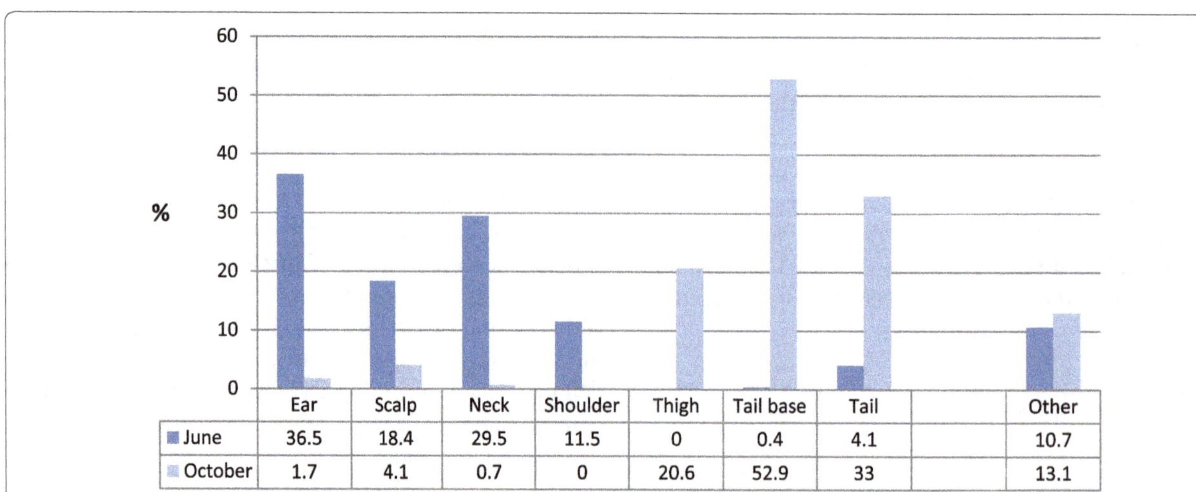

	Ear	Scalp	Neck	Shoulder	Thigh	Tail base	Tail		Other
June	36.5	18.4	29.5	11.5	0	0.4	4.1		10.7
October	1.7	4.1	0.7	0	20.6	52.9	33		13.1

Fig. 1 Distribution of wound types. Proportion of wound types (pathoanatomical) found in dead or euthanized mink with wounds on 6 farms (June, n = 244) and 12 farms (October, n = 291), respectively. Since mink may have more than one wound type, the percentages add up to more than 100 %

and that most wounds in October were located on the rear parts of the body and on the tail. Most wounds in June occurred in the second half of the month. In October the occurrence was more even over the entire month. Ear wounds (36.5 %) and neck wounds (29.1 %) were the most frequent location in June, whereas wounds at the base of the tail (37.3 %) and on the tail (23.2 %) were the most frequent location in October. Scalp wounds in June also include kits that were presumably killed by the dam by crushing of the skull (seven kits). Of animals with wounds, a total of 91.8 % and 94.8 % in June and October, respectively, had wounds categorized as ear, scalp, neck, shoulder, thigh, tail base or tail wounds. The distribution of the most common wound types (at least one wound per animal) in males and females, different colour types as well as mean wound size is given in Table 1. There were significantly more females with wounds than males for neck, shoulder, thigh, tail base and tail wounds, and significantly more ear wounds among males than females. There were significantly more black mink with ear wounds than both brown and white/light mink. White/light mink had also significantly fewer tail base wounds than both brown and blue/grey mink (Table 1).

Pathologically, wounds varied according to anatomical location. In general, most wounds were not covered by a scab except for certain small wounds located on the neck or shoulders of mink kits which were covered by a thick semi-moist or greasy layer of exudate and debris. Signs of a reparative process like granulation tissue formation, wound contraction and epithelialization were seldom distinguishable, but oedema was usually present along the wound margins which were often irregular or frayed. The wounds were often contaminated and some showed signs of infection as defined by the presence of thick purulent exudate. Typical pathomorphological appearances of most frequent wound types are presented in Figs. 2 and

Table 1 Distribution of sex and colour type and mean wound size for common mink wounds

Wound type (June)	**Sex**		**Colour type**					**Mean wound size (cm^2)**
	♂ n = 320	**♀ n = 325**	**Black n = 60**	**Brown n = 562**	**Blue/grey n = 18**	**White/light n = 102**	**Other n = 41**	
Ear	46 (14.4 %)	20 (6.2 %)	12[a,b] (20.0 %)	46[a] (8.2 %)	2 (11.1 %)	3[b] (2.9 %)	4 (9.8 %)	7.8 n = 53
	P = 0.001		P = 0.01					
Scalp	21 (6.6 %)	22 (6.8 %)	7 (11.7 %)	31 (5.5 %)	0 (0.0 %)	3 (2.9 %)	2 (4.9 %)	8.2 n = 34
	P = 0.916		P = 0.137					
Neck	15 (4.7 %)	52 (16.0 %)	4 (6.7 %)	55 (9.8 %)	2 (11.1 %)	7 (6.9 %)	4 (9.8 %)	8.7 n = 66
	P = 0.0001		P = 0.818					
Shoulder	3 (0.9 %)	25 (7.7 %)	1 (1.7 %)	20 (3.6 %)	0 (0.0 %)	3 (2.9 %)	4 (9.8 %)	7.8 n = 20
	P = 0.0001		P = 0.253					
Wound type (October)	**Sex**		**Colour type**					**Mean wound size (cm^2)**
	♂ n = 283	**♀ n = 355**	**Black n = 49**	**Brown n = 476**	**Blue/grey n = 25**	**White/light n = 81**	**Other n = 25**	
Thigh	8 (2.8 %)	49 (13.8 %)	4 (8.2 %)	42 (8.8 %)	2 (8.0 %)	9 (11.1 %)	3 (12.0 %)	9.5 n = 80
	P = 0.0001		P = 0.946					
Tail base	19 (6.7 %)	131 (36.9 %)	8 (16.3 %)	118[a] (24.8 %)	9[b] (36.0 %)	10[a,b] (12.3 %)	7 (28.0 %)	19.2 n = 141
	P = 0.0001		P = 0.031					
Tail	31 (11.0 %)	63 (17.7 %)	5 (10.2 %)	71 (14.9 %)	3 (12.0 %)	11 (13.6 %)	6 (24.0 %)	6.2 n = 22
	P = 0.015		P = 0.624					

Number and proportion of dead or euthanized mink presenting wounds on ear, scalp, neck and shoulder (June), or thigh, tail base and tail (October). The results are stratified according to sex and colour type. Mean wound size is given for each location. Due to occasional more wound types on the same mink and due to inability to determine the sex of all animals, the numbers may not be the same as the total proportions given in the text

[a,b] Estimates with the same letter are significantly different in multiple comparisons

Wound type	*Description*	*Example of gross appearance*
Ear wounds	Wounds involving the ear, varying from minor lacerations of the pinna to large wounds with absence of the entire external ear and surrounding skin.	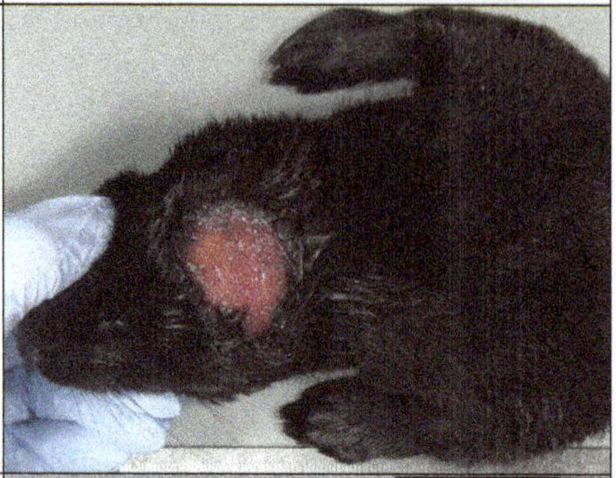
Scalp wounds	Wounds on the scalp or the dorsocranial part of the neck, varying from small bite marks (tooth marks) to larger wounds comprising the entire scalp.	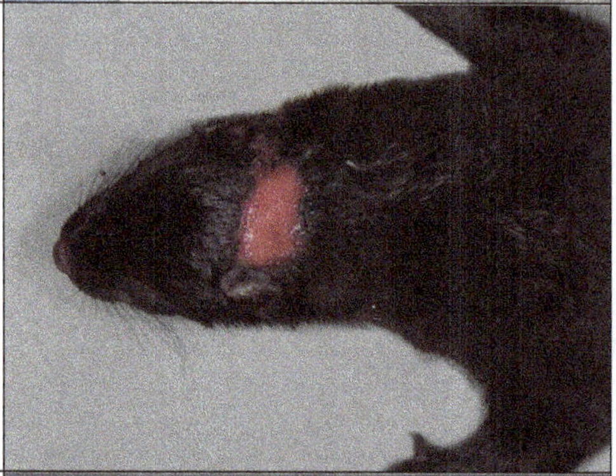
Neck and shoulder wounds	Wounds of varying sizes located on the side of the neck or over the shoulder area. Varying from small crust covered lesions to larger wounds without crusts.	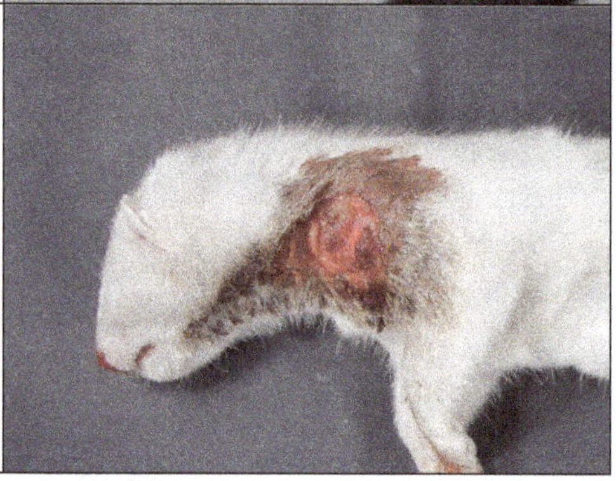

Fig. 2 Pathoanatomical characteristics of wounds. Most common wounds seen in farmed mink in June

3. Due to the general lack of discernible reparative tissue, exact wound age could not be determined on macroscopic basis.

Discussion

The development of a systematic basis for classification and clinical assessment of wounds in mink is necessary for the investigative efforts targeting control and prevention of wounds in this species. Though some mink with wounds may have died from other causes, the results are an indication of the proportion of mink that died or were euthanized due to skin lesions as opposed to other causes. Post mortal injuries may have erased signs of wounds occurring prior to death, contributing to an underestimation of frequencies. Moreover, pelted mink were excluded from the dataset which may have also led to a slight underestimation of the true proportion of dead wounded mink. The results are presented as frequencies and relative numbers and do not relate to the total number of mink on the farms.

Mink breed once each year and the kits are born late April or early May. The age of the majority of the mink present on the farm is therefore roughly the same throughout the year. The months June and October were

Wound type	*Description*	*Example of gross appearance*
Thigh wounds	Wounds located in the area between the base of the tail and the tarsal joint. Varies from minor bite marks (tooth marks) to large open wounds. Often characterized by undermining of skin under the wound edge (registered in 33/60 mink with one or two thigh wounds).	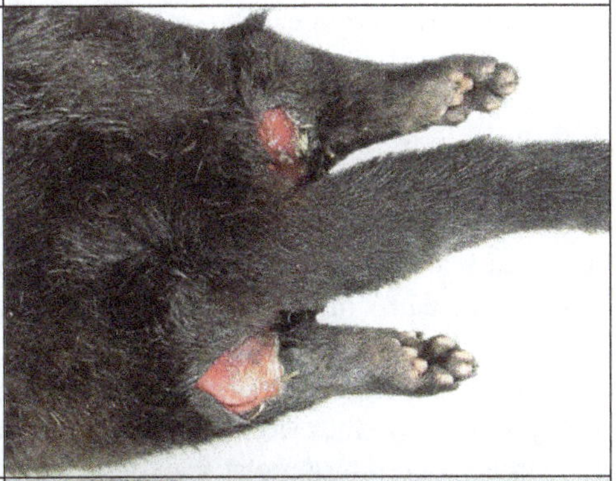
Tail base wounds	Wounds on the base/root of the tail, frequently reaching considerable dimensions (Table 2) with undermining of skin (registered in 93/154 mink with tail base wounds). Occasional presence of abscess.	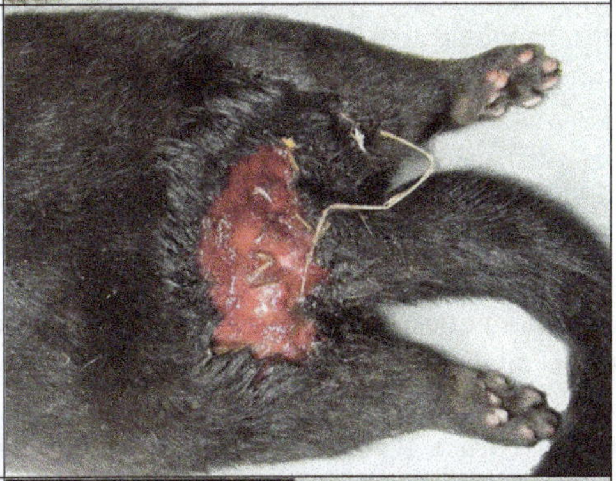
Tail wounds	Wounds located on the tail, often on the tail tip. Occasionally characterized by amputation of parts of the tail with exposed bone (rarely the entire tail).	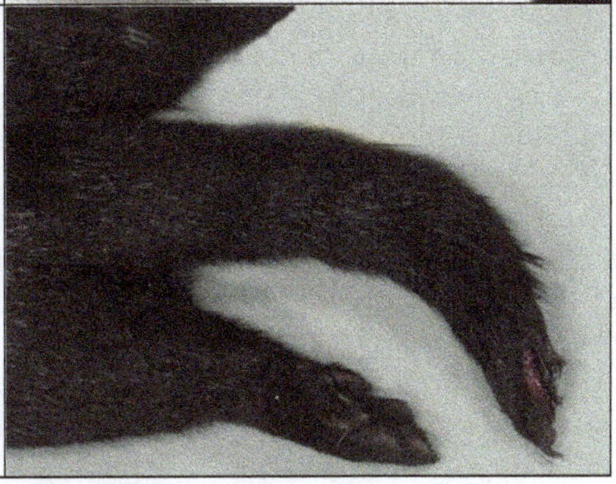

Fig. 3 Pathoanatomical characteristics of wounds. Most common wounds seen in farmed mink in October

selected for the study due to a report of increased frequency of wounds in these months compared to other periods in the mink production cycle [3]. This may be related to the age and developmental stage of the mink and management conditions related to the beginning and end of the growth season (i.e., weaning time and the period prior to pelting). As seen from Fig. 1, wounds were primarily located on the front parts of the body or in the head in June, while wounds in October were mostly located on the hind parts of the body and the tail. This likely represents the different behavioural mechanisms of the two age groups, leading to the formation of wounds during the two periods [4, 5]. Although some wound types may have overlapping morphological appearance, the distinct pathoanatomical distribution of wounds may reflect underlying risk or causal factors, similar to e.g., shoulder wounds in pigs [10] and breast/keel lesions in poultry [11]. Until further knowledge is at hand about the wound causal mechanisms in mink, it seems reasonable to maintain the proposed categories, and it is recommended that the classification of pathoanatomical location is included in future studies.

In June, the increasing occurrence of wounds through the end of the suckling period may be explained by the increased nutritional demands of the kits combined with a decline in the dam's milk output and an increased competition for resources [12]. From early to mid-June, there will be increasing risk of bite wounds resulting from fights between siblings as part of this resource competition [4, 12]. In June, most wounds occurred from midmonth (6 weeks of age), which is in accordance with findings in other studies [12–14]. Dehydration or thirst may cause the well-known licking behaviour, where the kits lick or suck on the dam's mouth [4, 15]. If this behaviour is directed towards the ears and other body parts of their siblings, it may lead to small lacerations or a moist dermatitis that may develop into wounds of varying size. The smaller wounds covered by a moist scab described in the neck and shoulder area may be such "lick-induced" lesions. A specific type of wound, rarely seen in the early growth period, is the characteristic crushing of the skull and tooth marks penetrating the scalp. They are inflicted to kits by the dam, presumably due to the dam's frustration or stress from not being able to escape her kits demanding presence [16, 17].

Many of the wounds seen after weaning and until pelting, where the mink are housed in pairs (typically one male and one female) or in groups of up to four, are bite wounds resulting from aggression between cage mates [18]. The location of wounds on the mink's hind parts may be interpreted as a flight/chase situation, where the bitten mink tries to escape the biting mink. The large size of wounds (Table 1) may be due to continuous biting since the submissive mink cannot escape. The submissive mink will likely be the smaller of the pair/group, which is supported by the findings of a larger proportion of wounds in females than in males (Table 1). Previous studies have demonstrated a similar ratio of lesions in females compared to males [3, 12, 17]. Similarly, the dominance of ear wounds in males has been demonstrated previously [12]. For ear wounds white/light and brown mink had significantly fewer wounds than black mink. For tail base wounds, white/light mink had significantly fewer wounds than both brown and blue/grey mink (Table 1). The reason for this is unknown, but may reflect behavioural and temperamental differences between the colour types [19]. Apart from the specific location, wounds found during October were often associated with undermining of skin which may result from ruptured abscesses, i.e., similar to what is often seen in cats [20]. This may also explain the large mean size of wounds, especially on the base of the tail. In areas where skin is not firmly adhered to the underlying tissues, initially the tension and resilience of the skin causes the wounds to widen once inflicted.

Accurate assessment of wound age was not possible based on gross pathology and would require histological examination. Although wound healing in mink is expected to include the same phases as in other mammals, no detailed studies of mink wound pathology have been published so far. It was considered out of the scope of this report to present histopathological results. The general failure to identify signs of reparation may be explained by quick discovery and euthanasia of wounded mink by farm personnel or that mink often die from their wounds in the acute stage.

In conclusion, we found a significant seasonal variation in location of wounds in farmed mink. Wounds in June were mainly situated on the front parts of the body and in the head, while wounds in October were mainly present on the hind parts of the body and on the tail. There were significant differences in occurrence between males and females, and for some wound types differences between certain colour types. The results may provide a basis for further studies of the cause and mechanisms behind different wound types as well as for developing guidelines for wound assessment in mink. Furthermore, the pathoanatomical wound distribution may define which wound types to focus on in future studies of prevention and management of wounds in farmed mink.

Authors' contributions

AJ participated in data collection and analysis and drafted the manuscript as well as participated in coordination of the study. JFA carried out the statistical analysis. TC and SB participated in collection of data. HEJ and ASH conceived the study and participated in its design. ASH furthermore participated in data collection and coordination of the study. All authors read and approved the final manuscript.

Author details

[1] Department of Veterinary Disease Biology, Faculty of Health and Medical Sciences, University of Copenhagen, Ridebanevej 3, 1870 Frederiksberg C, Denmark. [2] Kopenhagen Fur, Langagervej 60, 2600 Glostrup, Denmark. [3] Department of Large Animal Sciences, Faculty of Health and Medical Sciences, University of Copenhagen, Groennegaardsvej 8, 1870 Frederiksberg C, Denmark.

Acknowledgements

We would like to thank the participating farmers for help and cooperation during the project. Special thanks are also given to our former master students Nanna Bonde-Jensen and Maria Lassus as well as to Susanne Sommerlund for participating in necropsies.

Competing interests

The authors declare that they have no competing interests.

References

1. The Scientific Committee on Animal Health and Animal Welfare. (2001) The welfare of animals kept for fur production. Report of the European Commission, Health & Consumer Protection Directorate-general. 2001. http://ec.europa.eu/food/fs/sc/scah/out67_en.pdf. Accessed 20 Jul 2015.
2. Clausen T. Hvad dør minken af gennem et produktionsår. In: Møller SH editor. Store mink—store udfordringer, Produktion af højtydende mink uden uønskede følgevirkninger, internal report of Danmarks Jordbrugs-Forskning. Husdyrbrug. 2006;2:68–78. **(In Danish)**.

3. Hansen MU, Weiss V, Clausen T, Mundbjerg B, Lassén M. Investigations in causes of death among mink kits from June to October. Danish fur breeders research center, Holstebro. Annual Report. 2008;2007:99–107.
4. Brink A-L, Jeppesen LL. Behaviour of mink kits and dams (*Mustela vison*) in the lactation period. Can J Anim Sci. 2005;85:7–12.
5. Hansen SW, Møller SH, Damgaard BM. Bite marks in mink—induced experimentally and as reflection of aggressive encounters between mink. Appl Anim Behav Sci. 2014;158:76–85.
6. Dernell WS. Initial wound management. Vet Clin Small Anim. 2006;36:713–38.
7. Jensen HE, Bonde MK, Baadsgaard NP, Dahl-Pedersen K, Andersen PH, Herskin MS, et al. A simple and valid scale for clinical assessment of shoulder wounds. Dansk Veterinærtidsskrift. 2011;09:6–12 **(In Danish)**.
8. Kester E, Holzhauer M, Frankena K. A descriptive review of the prevalence and risk factors of hock lesions in dairy cows. Vet J. 2014;202:222–8.
9. Hammer AS, Dietz HH. Necropsy of the mink. In: Jensen HE, editor. Necropsy: a handbook and atlas. Frederiksberg: Biofolia; 2011. p. 231–50.
10. Jensen HE. Investigation into the pathology of shoulder ulcerations in sows. Vet Rec. 2009;165:171–4.
11. Allain V, Mirabito L, Arnould C, Colas M, Le Bouquin S, Lupo C, et al. Skin lesions in broiler chickens measured at the slaughterhouse: relationships between lesions and between their prevalence and rearing factors. Br Poult Sci. 2009;50:407–17.
12. Clausen TN, Larsen PF. Partial weaning at six weeks of age reduces biting among mink kits (*Neovison vison*). Open J Anim Sci. 2015;5:71–6.
13. Clausen TN, Larsen PF. Dividing big litters at 6 weeks of age reduces number of bites among mink kits. In: Kopenhagen Research, Aarhus N, editors. Annual Report 2012. 2013. p. 173–6.
14. Clausen, TN. Impact of weaning time on mink kits day 49 or day 56. In: Kopenhagen research, Aarhus N, editors. Annual Report 2011. 2012. p. 162–7.
15. Brink A-L, Jeppesen LL, Heller KE. Behaviour in suckling mink kits under farm conditions: effects of accessibility of drinking water. Appl Anim Behav Sci. 2004;89:131–7.
16. Clausen TN. Kit death from birth to August the first. Danish fur breeders research center, Holstebro. Annual Report. 2010;2009:97–103.
17. Clausen TN, Larsen PF. Impact of weaning age on kit performance. In: Proceedings of the Xth International Scientific Congress in fur animal production, Copenhagen; 2012. p. 336–40.
18. Hanse SW, Møller SH, Damgaard BM. Bite marks in mink—induced experimentally and as reflection of aggressive encounters between mink. Appl Anim Behav Sci. 2014;158:76–85.
19. Trapezov OV, Trapezova LI, Sergeev EG. Effect of coat color mutations on behavioral polymorphism in farm populations of American minks (*Mustela vison* Schreber, 1777) and sables (*Martes zibellina* Linnaeus, 1758). Russ J Genet. 2008;44:444–50.
20. Miller WH, Griffin CE, Campbell KL. Bacterial skin diseases. In: Miller WH, Griffin CE, Campbell KL, editors. Muller and Kirk's small animal dermatology. 7th ed. St. Louis: Elsevier; 2013. p. 184–222.

2

Is transport distance correlated with animal welfare and carcass quality of reindeer (*Rangifer tarandus tarandus*)?

Sauli Laaksonen[1*], Pikka Jokelainen[2,3,4], Jyrki Pusenius[5] and Antti Oksanen[6]

Abstract

Background: Slaughter reindeer are exposed to stress caused by gathering, handling, loading and unloading, and by conditions in vehicles during transport. These stress factors can lead to compromised welfare and trauma such as bruises or fractures, aspiration of rumen content, and abnormal odour in carcasses, and causing condemnations in meat inspection and lower meat quality. We investigated the statistical association of slaughter transport distance with these indices using meat inspection data from years 2004–2016, including inspection of 669,738 reindeer originating from Finnish reindeer herding areas.

Results: Increased stress and decreased welfare of reindeer, as indicated by higher incidence of carcass condemnation due to bruises or fractures, aspiration of rumen content, or abnormal odour, were positively associated with systems involving shorter transport distances to abattoirs. Significant differences in incidence of condemnations were also detected between abattoirs and reindeer herding cooperatives.

Conclusions: This study indicates that in particular the short-distance transports of reindeer merit more attention. While the results suggest that factors associated with long distance transport, such as driver education, truck design, veterinary supervision, and specialist equipment, may be favourable to reducing pre-slaughter stress in reindeer when compared with short distance transport systems, which occur in a variety of vehicle types and may be done by untrained handlers. Further work is required to elucidate the causal factors to the current results.

Keywords: Reindeer, Meat inspection, Stress, Handling, Transport, Trauma, Aspiration of rumen content, Abnormal odour, Welfare

Background

In Fennoscandia, semi-domesticated reindeer are grazing most of the year freely on natural pastures. Traditionally, reindeer were slaughtered on the field during round-ups, and no transportation to slaughter houses was needed. Field slaughter facilities were erected ad hoc until the 1980s, at which time slaughtering moved to more developed and modern export abattoirs. Nowadays, most of the reindeer in Finland are slaughtered in officially approved abattoirs. The development of a network of regional abattoirs created the need for intensive transportation of live reindeer and led to the evolution of reindeer transportation [1].

Most of the transportation of live reindeer by motor vehicles takes place for slaughter in autumn and early winter [1]. The vehicles include vans and trailers, and for longer distances, special reindeer transport trucks. In addition to transporting to slaughter, vehicle transportation is occasionally used when reindeer are moved between pastures, or to supplementary feeding sites or corrals for winter months. Motor vehicles, helicopters, snow mobiles and quad bikes (ATVs) are used as aids when herding and gathering reindeer for summer or autumn (slaughter) round-ups.

In Finland, all animal transportation is regulated by the Finnish Animal Transport Act (1429/2006) and the

*Correspondence: hirvi54@gmail.com
[1] Department of Veterinary Biosciences, Faculty of Veterinary Medicine, University of Helsinki, P.O. Box 66, 00014 Helsinki, Finland

Council Regulation (EC) No 1/2005 on the protection of animals during transport and related operations. There is no specific act for reindeer and thus these regulations are also valid for the transportation of reindeer.

Any external stimulus that challenges homeostasis can be viewed as a stressor to animals [2]. Emotional stimuli are the most common and important stressors in animals with a highly developed nervous system [3–6]. Animals react differently when they are captured, restrained, or immobilized. Even animals that seem to adapt to the situation may suffer from stress and be vulnerable to related damaging changes [7, 8]. Transportation is known to cause substantial stress in domesticated animals [9, 10] and it likely provokes an even more severe stress response in semi-domesticated animals.

The transportation and its impact on the welfare of semi-domesticated reindeer has been an issue of concern in Fennoscandia. The transportation to slaughter includes pre-slaughter handling of the animals; rounding up, herding, holding in enclosures, manual handling, loading, road transport, and unloading. After the transport of reindeer, traumas are commonly found [11–13]. Trauma may be caused by a physical impact by antlers, hooves, metal or wooden projections, or animals falling and being trampled on by others. Such trauma can take place any time during handling, transport, holding, or stunning. Bruises can vary in size, and be superficial or severe and may be seen in different parts of the carcass or even over the entire carcass.

Reindeer, like wild animals, are susceptible to stress caused by human presence, handling, capturing, and transportation. Manual handling and restraint have been found to be one of the major stress factors for reindeer [12–15]. There are indications of a cumulative effect of repeated stress events. In herded reindeer, stress associated lesions, such as abomasal haemorrhage, as well as myocardial and muscular degeneration have been described [11, 13–15]. Physical trauma also cause stress, but as they are often the result of aggression by other animals in the crate, they may also be considered a result of stress behaviour [12].

The detrimental effects of pre-slaughter handling on blood chemistry (aspartate transaminase (ASAT), urea, cortisol) and muscle glycogen stores can cause increased pH values resulting in lower meat quality; these effects have been demonstrated in several Fennoscandian studies [12–22]. Management and handling stress are also reflected by an increase in numbers of both immature and mature neutrophils and a decrease in lymphocyte count, which is correlated to the degree of stress to which the animals have been exposed. Prolonged exposure to stress results in a decrease in the number of eosinophils in peripheral blood [12].

Rehbinder et al. [12], Rehbinder [13] and Wiklund et al. and [14, 20] demonstrated that the use of a lasso to capture reindeer for slaughter was the most stressful handling procedure among those studied. In these studies, lorry transport, helicopter herding, and fixation of animals by hand without the use of a lasso resulted in lower stress responses as measured by meat pH values, blood metabolites used as stress markers i.e. ASAT, urea and cortisol, and abomasal lesions, compared to the lasso capture procedure. The calves have been reported to have higher muscle pH [19] and plasma urea [12, 13] values after herding and handling stress than adults. The authors concluded that calves are more susceptible to stress than adult animals due to more vigorous physical exertion depleting their energy stores more rapidly. Exhausted animals were in general found to have extremely high meat pH values, with 31.1% of the carcasses being classified as intermediate Dark, Firm and Dry meat (DFD) ($5.8 < pH < 6.2$) and 31.2% as DFD ($pH > 6.2$) [19].

Natural long-duration stress, such as harsh weather and snow conditions especially in winter time, can also cause poorer meat quality; glycogen stores are used before slaughter and the pH-value remains high [14, 23]. In addition, the animals' physical condition and nutritional status have a considerable effect on their ability to tolerate various stress factors, such as lorry transport and holding [20].

Hyvärinen et al. [16] found elevated serum urea values associated with reindeer gatherings. Furthermore, the levels were correlated with the distance of the drive and time spent in the corral. The study by Wiklund et al. [15] confirmed the finding that a "stress-flavour" could develop in reindeer meat after intensive pre-slaughter handling of the animals. The animals captured by use of lasso or herded by helicopter for prolonged three days had the highest scores of an unpleasant, strong, even acrid smell, which was described by a trained expert panel as a pungent odour, sickeningly sweet odour, sharp flavour, and sickeningly sweet flavour [15]. It is common knowledge among reindeer herders that animals that have been exposed to stressful pre-slaughter handling give meat with an unfavourable odour [15] which is sometimes referred to as "urine smell" [1, 13]. Several studies have tried to correlate the concentrations of substances such as putrescine, spermidine, spermine, creatine, creatinine, and dimethylamine in reindeer meat and plasma with the presence of 'stress-flavour' in the meat, but the issue is still unresolved, as reviewed by Wiklund [15]. According to Rehbinder [13], depletion of muscular glycogen stores, increased catabolism of muscular protein, muscular degeneration, and increased blood-urea levels cannot be excluded as a cause of an altered and bad taste of the meat.

In Sweden, lorry transport did not affect the ultimate pH of the muscles of bulls and calves and the incidence of high pH and intermediate DFD in reindeer hinds was greater only after transport of more than 500 km [19]. In Finland, Nieminen et al. studied the impact of transportation of reindeer in 1993 [24] and in 2000 [25]. In these studies, the transportation distances varied from 30 to 400 km and transportation times from 1 to 5.5 h. The reindeer were reported to be peaceful and in good shape after transportation and only minor bruises were detected.

Aspiration of rumen content during stunning is a common finding during slaughter in production ruminants, leading to the condemnation of lungs at meat inspection [26]. There is, however, apparently, no published data of the causes or incidence of this phenomenon. Aspiration of rumen content is also often seen during reindeer meat inspection. Hanssen et al. [27] reported the transportation of reindeer on lorries to result in more liquid rumen content. In addition, a marked stress response with abomasal erosions or ulcers will affect the digestive tract and its utilization of fodder [13, 15]. It is also common that digestive disorders occur amongst reindeer after supplementary feeding [1, 28]. Reindeer are usually supplementary fed with silage and pellets [1], which often leads to fullness and distension of the rumen. These feeds are medium or high protein rich, which greatly increases their water requirements. For example, adult female reindeer eating pellets have been reported to drink 3.2–3.5 l of water per day, while reindeer fed lichens drank only 0.1 l per day [29]. More liquid rumen content may perhaps predispose to regurgitation and aspiration of rumen content during stunning.

There has been a lot of public debate concerning the long-distance transportation of reindeer by motor vehicles; in particular, with regards to the effect of transportation on the wellbeing of the reindeer. The aim of this study was to partially respond to these concerns by exploring whether the distance of the transportation of live reindeer to abattoirs is associated with higher rates of meat condemnations. We focused on injuries, bruises and fractures, but stress-related abnormal odour and aspiration of rumen content were also surveyed. The outcomes investigated are not only indicators of compromised welfare but also relevant for the brand and reputation of reindeer meat production.

Methods

The reindeer population data were obtained from database of the Reindeer Herders' Association. The reindeer meat inspection data were collected from official documents from meat inspection veterinarians (see Additional file 1) at all the approved reindeer abattoirs of Finland, from the slaughter seasons (autumn and early winter) 2004–2005 to 2015–2016. The meat inspection and hygiene control in abattoirs was conducted by veterinarians who work under the control of Regional State Administrative Agencies of Lapland. For this study, the number of bruises and fractures and stress-related abnormal odour and aspiration of rumen content, which lead to partly or total carcass condemnations for human consumption, were included. We recorded the number of inspected reindeer originating from Finnish reindeer herding areas (669,738 reindeer from 4208 slaughter batches), the number and the percentage of condemnations due to bruises or fractures, aspiration of rumen content during stunning, and organoleptic evaluations of abnormal odour.

Statistical analyses

For statistical analyses, the transportation distances were classified into five categories: 0 = 0 km, reindeer walk from the round-up corral to abattoir; (1) 1–60 km; (2) 61–150 km; (3) 151–300 km; (4) >300 km. The transport distances for each slaughter batch were defined to be the shortest distance along the road from the geographical centre of the reindeer herding cooperative to the abattoir. In addition, the reindeer were classified according to their region of origin: The Finnish reindeer herding area was divided into the area specifically intended for reindeer herding (Area 2, northern part) (Finnish Reindeer Husbandry Act, 14.9.1990/848) and the remainder (Area 1, southern part) (Fig. 1).

We analysed the association between the occurrence of bruises or fractures, abnormal odour, and aspiration of rumen content leading to condemnations and the transport distance of reindeer to abattoirs using Spearman's rank correlation coefficient. The relationship between the regional origin of reindeer and the proportion of condemnations was analysed using two by two contingency tables and Chi squared tests.

The comparison of proportion of condemnations between abattoirs and 56 reindeer herding cooperatives was made by using non-parametric Kruskal–Wallis test using slaughter batch as a unit of observation. In one abattoir, animals were bled in the horizontal position (as opposed to vertical position). To determine if the proportion of animals aspirating rumen contents differed in this abattoir compared to the others, we used a post hoc multiple comparison analysis identifying homogenous subsets (significance level 0.05).

All statistical analyses were conducted using SPSS 19 software.

Results

The reindeer population in Finland during the study period was on average 197,807 (190,776–209,365) individuals, of which an average of 102,778 (71,580–124,152)

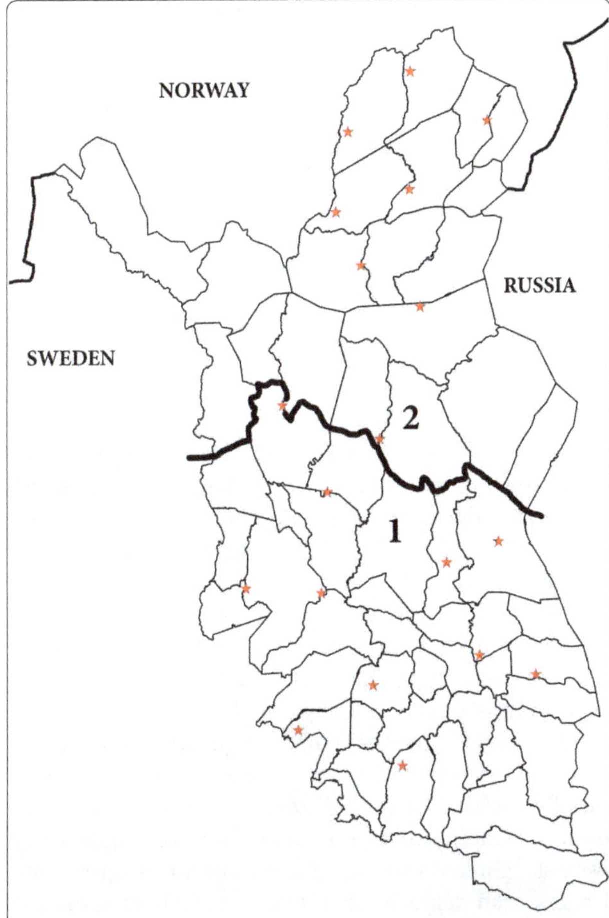

Fig. 1 Finnish reindeer herding area indicating the area specifically intended for reindeer herding (Area 2, northern part) and the remainder (Area 1, southern part). *Fine lines* are the borders of reindeer herding cooperatives and the *red stars* are official reindeer abattoirs

were slaughtered annually. Of the slaughtered reindeer, 77% were calves (6–8 months old). Approximately 74% of the reindeer were slaughtered in 19 EU-approved reindeer abattoirs; the rest were slaughtered in the field for private consumption and direct marketing (Regional State Administrative Agencies of Lapland).

The inspection data of 669,738 reindeer (Area 1, 234,821; Area 2, 434,917) from 4208 slaughter batches (Area 1, 2318; Area 2, 1890) were included in the study; data from 333 slaughter batches were excluded because of missing information. Eighty-three percent of the reindeer were slaughtered during October–December. The average distance that animals were transported to slaughter was 87 km (range: 0–450 km) in the whole area, 62 km (10–390 km) in the southern area (Area 1), and 117 km (0–450 km) in the northern area (Area 2).

The meat inspection findings associated with part or whole carcass condemnation from 2004 to 2016 are presented by region in Table 1, (Fig. 1). Bruises and fractures, and aspiration of rumen content, were more common in Area 1 compared to Area 2 (Table 1; $\chi^2 = 50.58$, df = 1, $P < 0.001$; $\chi^2 = 2212.93$, df = 1, $P < 0.001$; respectively).

The transport distance to the abattoir was negatively correlated with the number of condemnations due to bruises/fractures (Spearman's rank correlation $r_s = -0.20$, N = 4208, $P < 0.0005$), aspiration of rumen content ($r_s = -0.04$, N = 4208, P = 0.005), and abnormal odour ($r_s = -0.04$, N = 4208, P = 0.011). The correlations of aspiration of rumen content and abnormal odour with travel distance were however weak, whereas the negative correlation between the condemnations due to bruises and fractures and transport distance indicated a definite and strong relationship.

The number of bruises and fractures leading to condemnations during reindeer meat inspections are presented by the five transport distance categories in Table 2. Multiple comparison after Kruskal–Wallis ANOVA indicated that the incidence of bruises and fractures was lower in the transportation distance category 0 (no transport) than in the transportation distance category 1 (1–60 km) ($P < 0.05$). The slaughter batches were smaller in the categories of short transport than in the category of no vehicle transport (280 and 123 reindeer respectively).

There were significant differences between abattoirs in the incidence of bruises and fractures (range 0.20–2.02%,

Table 1 Indicators of compromised welfare of reindeer leading to meat inspection condemnations in Finland (2004–2016)

Origin of reindeer[a]	No of reindeer	Mean transportation distance (km)	Bruises and fractures (n, %)	Aspiration of rumen content (n, %)	Abnormal odour (n, %)
Area 1	234,821	62	1533 0.6%	1265 0.54%	65 0.03%
Area 2	434,917	117	2246 0.5%	36 0.008%	126 0.03%
Whole area	669,738	87	3779 0.6%	1301 0.2%	191 0.03%

[a] The map showing the areas: Fig. 1

Table 2 Bruises and fractures leading to condemnations during reindeer meat inspections, by transport distance categories

Transport distance		Inspected reindeer (n)	Inspections (n)	Reindeer in inspections (mean)	Bruises and fractures (n)	Bruises and fractures (%)
km	Category					
0	0	129,521	464	280	590	0.45
1–60	1	260,688	2123	123	1970	0.75
61–150	2	124,402	1038	120	743	0.60
151–300	3	89,124	328	272	386	0.43
≥301	4	66,005	255	259	90	0.13
Total		669,740	4208	159	3779	0.56

mean 0.71%, SD 2.93%; Kruskal–Wallis test, $H = 564.73$, $df = 19$, $P < 0.0005$), rumen content aspirations (range 0.00–2.47, 0.50%, SD 3.02%; Kruskal–Wallis test, $H = 660.94$, $df = 19$, $P < 0.0005$) and abnormal odour (range 0.00–0.74%, 0.08%, SD 1.77%; Kruskal–Wallis test, $H = 109.54$, $df = 19$, $P < 0.0005$) as well as between all 56 reindeer herding cooperatives (range 0.00–7.69%, 0.74%, SD 3.07%; Kruskal–Wallis test, $H = 523.07$, $df = 55$, $P < 0.0005$), (range 0.00–3.22%, 0.53%, SD 3.15%; Kruskal–Wallis test, $H = 612.35$, $df = 55$, $P < 0.0005$), (range 0.00–0.68%, 0.08%, SD 1.85%; Kruskal–Wallis test, $H = 91.81$, $df = 55$, $P = 0.001$), respectively.

Multiple comparisons identifying homogenous subsets (significance level 0.05) indicated that condemnation caused by aspiration of rumen content was on average higher in the abattoir in which the bleeding after stunning was done on animals that were lying horizontally (2.4%), compared to those in which the animals were bled while hanging vertically (0.2%).

Discussion

Our results indicate that the studied indicators of compromised physical welfare of slaughter reindeer are associated with the distance of transportation for slaughter: short transport distances were associated with more compromised reindeer welfare and carcass quality. In addition, we found that the incidence of these indicators varied significantly among reindeer herding cooperatives and abattoirs.

Bruises and factures were negatively associated with transport distance. This perhaps unexpected finding could be explained by the fact that most long-distance transport of slaughter reindeer is done with trucks that are specifically designed for the transportation of reindeer. These trucks must be inspected and approved by authorities and the driver must be specifically educated to be qualified and licenced for long-range animal transportation. The trucks have specially designed ramps for loading and unloading reindeer with minimal manual handling and they are sectioned into several pens that allow separation of calves from adult animals, which markedly reduces bruising and other injuries [11]. Conversely, transportation of reindeer for short (under 65 km) distances does not require any qualifications or approvals for the drivers nor the vehicles. Vans or trailers, which may in some cases be unfit, are used for the short-distance transportation, and the loading and unloading is done manually, reindeer by reindeer. Our results, therefore, suggest that the quality of the method of transportation more than compensates the potential negative effects of long-distance transportation. However, the finding that lower proportion of reindeer that were slaughtered without vehicle transport had traumatic lesions than reindeer that underwent short transport, indicates the impact of manual loading, unloading and the suitability of the transport vehicle on the injuries.

Our result that the proportion of reindeer having bruises/fractures detectable in meat inspection did not increase with the distance of transportation to abattoir is in accordance with former studies on the effects of transportation. In line with our conclusions, previous studies [19, 20, 24, 25], reported that lorry transport did not significantly impair reindeer meat quality indices. In addition, the historical meat inspection data from years 1980–1986 [33] indicated that bruises and fractures were common and were detected in 5.3% of the reindeer. This was in spite of the fact that only 11.5% of the reindeer were transported to the approved regional abattoirs and the rest were slaughtered in the field in connection to, or very near the round-up places, practically with no need of vehicle transport [33].

The significant differences in the appearance of bruises and fractures between individual cooperatives and abattoirs may be due to the different handling practises. For example, round-ups and their timing, maintenance of enclosures, transport corridors and ramps, routines for loading and unloading the animals, waiting times in corrals and in abattoirs, and understanding the natural behaviour, as highlighted in literature [12–15, 34], as well as the degree of tameness of reindeer [13], may differ. There are no stunning pens in Finnish reindeer abattoirs to support the animal, but the restraint is done manually, so bruising is also possible during the stunning and could occur also after stunning when the animal collapses on the floor [35].

In total, the current slaughter welfare conditions in Finland can be considered relatively good, with 0.6% of slaughter reindeer having detectable injuries, in particular when comparing with the situation in period 1980–1986, when bruises and fractures were reported in 5.6% of reindeer [33]. The situation has evolved in the same way also in Sweden: during 2000–2007, the proportion of injuries was 1% [36] and during 2006–2013, trauma or fractures were registered in 0.13% of reindeer carcasses and in 0.88% of the heads [37]. It must be noted that our data do not include the traumas in the head, which are typically seen in antlers, because such trauma do not usually lead to condemnations.

The apparently reduced incidence of bruises and fractures is likely due to the increased information and education delivered by the Reindeer Herders' Association and related organizations and authorities which has led to improved handling methods and transports. One contributing factor can also be the fact that in Finland, especially in the northern reindeer herding area, veterinarians are present practically in every bigger slaughter round-up, administrating anti-parasitic treatment and at the same time doing animal welfare work, for example inspecting the fitness of animals for transportation.

Rumen content can become more liquid because of handling stress [13, 15], transportation [27] and supplementary feeding [28, 29]. This may predispose animals to aspiration of liquid rumen contents during or after stunning. In our study, aspiration of rumen content was reported in 0.2% of Finnish slaughter reindeer. The negative correlation to the distance of slaughter transport was not as clear as in bruises and fractures, while there were significant differences between individual cooperatives and abattoirs. In addition, aspiration of rumen content was a significantly more common finding in the reindeer from Area 1 compared to Area 2, reflecting decreased welfare and supporting that it could be associated with handling, transport, behavioural and feeding stress. In the southern area, reindeer are often held in lairage, waiting for the herd to grow big enough for the slaughter batch, sometimes several days. During that time, they are supplementary fed, usually with silage and pellets, which often leads to the fullness and distension of the rumen (unpublished observations).

During stunning, especially if the bolting accuracy or cartridge strength are not ideal, the unconsciousness is not immediate and reindeer continue to breathe which can result in regurgitation and aspiration of rumen content. It is known that slaughter without stunning (ritual slaughter) increases the possibility of aspiration of blood and, in the case of ruminants, rumen content [30]. All Finnish reindeer abattoirs use penetrating captive bolt pistols to stun reindeer. It is concluded that an animal effectively stunned with a penetrating captive bolt pistol, as indicated by the presence of certain signs and the absence of others, like failure to collapse, rhythmic breathing, eyeball rotation and, positive corneal reflex, has little possibility of a reversal of the brain function [31]. However, in cattle, the prevalence of shallow depth of concussion following captive bolt shooting was 8% for all cattle and 15% for young bulls, and 2.7% of animals maintained spontaneous breathing [32]. It is likely that this happens also during reindeer slaughter.

The finding that aspiration of rumen content was more common if the bleeding was done when the reindeer were in horizontal position compared to those abattoirs where reindeer were in a hanging position, was not surprising. It is logical that the regurgitation can reach lungs more easily if the animal is in horizontal position during commonly occurring reflexive gasping [32]. Aspiration of rumen content is also a concern for meat hygiene, since potential pathogens are transported to the clean side of the abattoir and can contaminate other carcasses and organs [38, 39].

"Stress flavour" occurs in reindeer meat after intensive handling of the animals prior to slaughter [15, 18, 20]. In our study, the finding registered was abnormal odour, which may include also other odours diagnosed by meat inspectors. A strong abnormal odour which lead to condemnations was diagnosed in 0.03% of reindeer. The real incidence of abnormal flavour is likely much higher, for example, Hanssen and Skei [40] detected moderate ammonia-like taint in two and a weak taint in seven samples of 29 reindeer which had been transported in lorries before slaughter. Nevertheless, our results show that the same trend as for bruises, fractures and rumen content aspiration was also detected in abnormal odour, having a negative correlation with transport distance and with significant differences between abattoirs and cooperatives. These patterns are in accordance with the published views that detecting abnormal odour is related to stress [15, 18, 20, 27, 40].

There are many more factors associated with transport and connected operations that could contribute to the observed effect of transport distance and that were not covered in this work. These include handling, holding, habituation, sex effect, socialisation, stunning, and the slaughter process. The differences in incidence between abattoirs and herding cooperatives reinforce this further.

Our study was based on the observations and meat inspection findings made by several veterinarians, which may cause bias on the results. All the reindeer meat inspectors have participated in education for meat inspection and harmonizing meat inspection decisions, and the reporting is simple. The strengths of the study include a long study period (>10 years) and a large number of observations, and the data were collected from official meat inspection decisions of condemnations. Because minor lesions and deep bruises, are not always detectable in the meat inspection, the true incidence of these indicators is likely higher.

Conclusions

Long distance transport of reindeer in approved reindeer trucks and conducted by educated drivers was associated with less stress and trauma to the animals than transport for short distances, the latter requiring more manual handling, being conducted in a variety of vehicle types, and by untrained handlers. Although the welfare of reindeer during transportations and connected activities has improved, significant differences in incidence of bruises or fractures, aspiration of rumen content, and abnormal odour were detected between abattoirs and between reindeer herding cooperatives, emphasizing that there still is room for improvement. Although further research is required to elucidate the impact of all factors that are involved in transportation and that may be associated with stress and welfare of reindeer, the results of this study indicate that in particular the short-distance transports and related operations merit more attention. This is likely not limited to slaughter transport, but rather relevant to all transportation of reindeer e.g. to a feeding corral or to a different pasture area.

Authors' contributions

SL designed the study. JP performed the statistical analyses. The results were interpreted by SL, PJ and JP. SL and PJ drafted the manuscript. All authors participated in writing and editing of the manuscript. All authors read and approved the final manuscript.

Author details

[1] Department of Veterinary Biosciences, Faculty of Veterinary Medicine, University of Helsinki, P.O. Box 66, 00014 Helsinki, Finland. [2] Estonian University of Life Sciences, Kreutzwaldi 62, 51014 Tartu, Estonia. [3] Faculty of Veterinary Medicine, University of Helsinki, P.O. Box 66, 00014 Helsinki, Finland. [4] Statens Serum Institut, Artillerivej 5, 2300, Copenhagen S, Denmark. [5] Natural Resources Institute Finland, Yliopistokatu 6, 80100 Joensuu, Finland. [6] Production Animal and Wildlife Health Research Unit, Finnish Food Safety Authority Evira, Elektroniikkatie 3, 90590 Oulu, Finland.

Acknowledgements

We thank the reindeer herders and reindeer veterinarians in Finland and the crew of Regional State Administrative Agencies of Lapland for their cooperation in data collection. Special thanks goes to Juho Tahkola. We also thank Anniina Holma-Suutari who was involved in planning and drafting of this work and Susan Kutz for revising the English of the manuscript. This work was done in the project "Reindeer health in the changing environment 2015–2018" funded by the Finnish Ministry of Agriculture and Forestry (MAKERA).

Competing interests

The authors declare that they have no competing interests.

Funding

The study was partly funded by the Finnish Ministry of Agriculture and Forestry (MAKERA).

References

1. Laaksonen S. Tunne poro–poron sairaudet ja terveydenhuolto [Know the reindeer–diseases and health care of reindeer]. Riga: Livonia Print; 2016.
2. Moberg GP. Biological response to stress: Key to assessment of animal well-being. In: Moberg GP, editor. Animal stress. Baltimore: Waverly Press; 1985. p. 27–49.
3. Levi L. Emotional stress. Proceedings of an international symposium arranged by the Swedish delegation for applied medical defense research, Stockholm, February 5–6, 1965. Forsvars-medicin. 1967;3:Suppl 2.
4. Selye H. Stress without distress. New York: Lippincott Williams & Wilkins; 1974.
5. Stephens DB. Stress and its measurement in domestic animals: a review of behavioral and physiological studies under field and laboratory situations. In: Brandly CA, Cornelius CCE, editors. Advances in veterinary science and comparative medicine. New York: Academic Press; 1980. p. 179–210.
6. Becker BA. The phenomena of stress: concepts and mechanisms associated with stress-induced responses of the neuro-endocrine system. Vet Res Commun. 1987;11:444–56.
7. Harthoorn AM. Problems related to capture. Anim Regul Stud. 1997;l:23–46.
8. Bartsch R, Connell EE, Imes GD, Schmidt JM. A review of exertional rhabdomyolysis in wild and domestic animals and man. Vet Pathol. 1977;14:314–24.
9. Dvorak M. Adrenocortical activity of young calves in relation to transport and traumatic stress. Docum Vet (Brno). 1975;8:119–26.
10. Simensen E, Laksesvela B, Blom AK, Sjaastad OV. Effects of transportations, a high lactose diet and ACTH injections on the white blood cell count, serum cortisol and immunoglobulin G in young calves. Acta Vet Scand. 1980;21:278–90.
11. Andersen G. Transportskader på rein ved ulike transportmidler [Transport damage to reindeer by different means of transport]. Norsk VetTidskr. 1978;90:543–53.
12. Rehbinder C, Edqvist L-E, Lundstrom K, Villafane F. A field study of management stress in reindeer (*Rangifer tarandus* L.). Rangifer. 1982;2:2–21.
13. Rehbinder C. Management stress in reindeer. Rangifer. 1990;3:267–88.
14. Wiklund E, Andersson A, Malmfors G, Lundström K. Muscle glycogen levels and blood metabolites in reindeer (*Rangifer tarandus tarandus* L.) after transport and lairage. Meat Sci. 1996;42:133–44.
15. Wiklund E, Malmfors G, Lundström K, Rehbinder C. Pre-slaughter handling of reindeer bulls (*Rangifer tarandus tarandus* L.)-effects on technological and sensory meat quality, blood metabolites and muscular and abomasal lesions. Rangifer. 1996;3:109–17.
16. Hyvärinen H, Helle T, Nieminen M, Väyrynen P, Väyrynen R. Some effects of handling reindeer during gatherings on the composition of their blood. Anim Prod. 1976;22:105–14.
17. Nieminen M. The composition of reindeer blood in respect to age, season, calving and nutrition. Oulu: Dept. of Zoology and Dept. of Physiology, University of Oulu; 1980.

18. Essén-Gustavsson B, Rehbinder C. The influence of stress on substrate utilization in skeletal muscle fibres of reindeer (*Rangifer tarandus* L.). Rangifer. 1984;4:2–8.
19. Wiklund E, Andersson A, Malmfors G, Lundstrom K, Danell Ö. Ultimate pH values in reindeer meat with particular regard to animal sex and age, muscle and transport distance. Rangifer. 1995;15:47–54.
20. Wiklund E. Pre-slaughter handling of reindeer (*Rangifer tarandus tarandus* L.) effects on meat quality. Uppsala: Department of Food Science, Swedish University of Agricultural Sciences; 1996.
21. Wiklund E, Rehbinder C, Malmfors G, Hansson I, Danielsson-Tham M-L. Ultimate pH values and bacteriological condition of meat and stress metabolites in blood of transported reindeer bulls. Rangifer. 2001;21:3–12.
22. Wiklund E, Malmfors G, Finstad G. Renkött- är det alltid mört, gott och nyttigt? [Reindeer meat- it is always tender, tasty and healthy?]. Rangifer Report. 2007;12:71–7 **(in Swedish with English abstract)**.
23. Petajä E. DFD meat in reindeer meat. Proceedings: 29th european congress of meat research workers. Italy: Salsomaggiore; 1983. p. 117–24.
24. Nieminen M, Kumpula J, Soppela P, Heiskari U, Risto A, Kantola P. Teurasporojen elävänäkuljetus, kuljetuskokeilu ja tutkimusprojekti [Transport of living reindeer to slaughterhouse]. Rovaniemi: Porotutkimus; 1993.
25. Nieminen M. Teurasporojen elävänä kuljetus–käsittelyn ja ruokinnan vaikutukset poroon sekä lihan kemialliseen koostumukseen ja laatuun [Transport of living reindeer to slaughterhouse–the impact of handling and transport to the composition and quality of reindeer meat]. Finland: Riista- ja kalatalouden tutkimuslaitos; 2000.
26. Gil JI, Durão JC. A colour atlas of meat inspection. Boca Raton: Taylor & Francis; 1990.
27. Hanssen I, Kyrkjebø A, Opstad PK, Prøsch R. Physiological responses and effect on meat quality in reindeer (*Rangifer tarandus*) transported on lorries. Acta Vet Scand. 1984;25:128–38.
28. Nilsson A, Olsson I, Lingvall P. Comparison between grass-silage of different dry matter content fed to reindeer during winter. Rangifer. 1996;16:21–30.
29. Soppela P, Nieminen M, Saarela S. Water requirements of captive reindeer hinds with artificial feeding. Rangifer Special Issue. 1988;1988(2):74–5.
30. Zoethout CM. Ritual slaughter and the freedom of religion: some reflections on a stunning matter. Human Rights Q. 2013;3:651–72.
31. Gregory N, Shaw F. Penetrating captive bolt stunning and exsanguination of cattle in abattoirs. J Appl Anim Welf Sci. 2000;3:215–30.
32. Gregory NG, Lee CJ, Widdicombe JP. Depth of concussion in cattle shot by penetrating captive bolt. Meat Sci. 2007;77:499–503.
33. Rahkio M. Poron, hirven ja valkohäntäpeuran lihantarkastustiedot Suomessa vuosina 1980–1986 [The meat inspection data of reindeer, moose and white-tailed deer in Finland in 1980–1986]. Helsinki: Eläinlääketieteellinen korkeakoulu; 1988.
34. Mejdell CM, Heggstad E, Hagen A, Grøndahl AM. Håndtering og transport av tamrein ved slakting – dyrevelferdsmessige utfordringer [Handling and transport of reindeer at slaughter - animal welfare problems]. Norsk VetTidskr. 2014;2:126.
35. Belk KE, Scanga JA, Smith GC, Grandin T. The relationship between good handling/stunning and meat quality in beef, pork, and lamb. Proceedings of the International Congress Animal Handling and Stunning Conference on February 21–22, 2002 at the American Meat Institute Foundation. 2002. http://www.grandin.com/meat/hand.stun.relate.quality.html. Accessed Dec 2016.
36. Mossing T. Sammanställning av besiktningsresultat vid renslakt 2000–2007 [Summary of inspection results of reindeer slaughter in 2000–2007]. Umeå universitet. Gård & Djurhälsan. 2007. http://www.gardochdjurhalsan.se/upload/documents/Dokument/Startsida_Andra_djurslag/Ren/101020_ren_rapport_renslakt.pdf. Accessed Dec 2016.
37. Statistik fyndregistrering vid slakt 2006–2013 [Statistics of findings registration at slaughter 2006–2013]. Gård & Djurhälsan. http://www.gardochdjurhalsan.se/upload/documents/Dokument/Startsida_Andra_djurslag/Ren/Statistik_fyndregistrering_vid_slakt_2006-2013.pdf. Accessed Dec 2016.
38. Laaksonen S, Oksanen A, Julmi J, Zweifel C, Fredriksson-Ahomaa M, Stephan R. Presence of foodborne pathogens, extended-spectrum β-lactamase -producing Enterobacteriaceae, and methicillin-resistant *Staphylococcus aureus* in slaughtered reindeer in northern Finland and Norway. Acta Vet Scand. 2017;59:2. doi:10.1186/s13028-016-0272-x.
39. Zweifel C, Fierz L, Cernela N, Laaksonen S, Fredriksson-Ahomaa M, Stephan R. Characteristics of Shiga toxin-producing *E. coli* O157 in slaughtered reindeer from northern Finland. J Food Prot. 2017;3:454–8.
40. Hanssen I, Skei T. Lack of correlation between ammonia-like taint and polyamine levels in reindeer meat. Vet Rec. 1990;127:622–3.

Structural changes in femoral bone microstructure of female rabbits after intramuscular administration of quercetin

Ramona Babosova[1], Hana Duranova[1], Radoslav Omelka[2], Veronika Kovacova[1], Maria Adamkovicova[2], Birgit Grosskopf[3*], Marcela Capcarova[4] and Monika Martiniakova[1]

Abstract

Background: Quercetin is one of the best known flavonoids being present in a variety of fruits and vegetables. It has cardioprotective, anticarcinogenic, antioxidant, anti-inflammatory and antiapoptotic properties. Some studies suggest that quercetin has protective effects on bone. However, its influence on qualitative and quantitative histological characteristics of compact bone is still unknown. In our study, 12 clinically healthy five-month-old female rabbits were divided into four groups of three animals each. Quercetin was applied intramuscularly in various concentrations; 10 µg/kg body weight (bw) in the E1 group, 100 µg/kg bw in the E2 group, and 1000 µg/kg bw in the E3 group for 90 days, 3 times per week. Three rabbits without exposure to quercetin served as a control (C) group. Differences in femoral bone microstructure among groups were evaluated.

Results: Qualitative histological characteristics of compact bone differed between rabbits from the E1 and E2 groups. Primary vascular longitudinal bone tissue was not found in some areas near the endosteal surface due to increased endocortical bone resorption. In addition, periosteal border of rabbits from the E1 group was composed of a thicker layer of primary vascular longitudinal bone tissue than in the other groups. In all groups of rabbits administered quercetin, a lower density of secondary osteons was observed. Histomorphometrical evaluations showed significantly decreased sizes of the primary osteons' vascular canals in individuals from the E1 and E2 groups. Secondary osteons were significantly smaller in rabbits from the E1, E2, E3 groups when compared to the C group. Cortical bone thickness was significantly increased in females from the E1 and E2 groups.

Conclusions: The results indicate that quercetin has not only a positive dose–response on qualitative and quantitative histological characteristics of the compact bone of female rabbits as it would be expected.

Keywords: Bone microstructure, Histomorphometry, Quercetin, Rabbit, Intramuscular administration

Background

Flavonoids belong to the group of polyphenolic secondary herbal substances that have beneficial effects on human health [1]. Quercetin (2-(3,4-dihydroxyphenyl)-3,5,7-trihydroxy-4H-1-benzopyran-4-one; 3,3′,4′,5,7-pentahydroxyflavone) is one of the best characterized flavonoids present in fruits and vegetables [2]. It has cardioprotective [3], anticarcinogenic [4], antioxidant [5], anti-inflammatory [6] and antiapoptotic properties [7]. It also protects against reactive oxygen species (ROS) and reactive nitrogen species (RNS) [8, 9]. Some studies [10, 11] suggest that quercetin also has protective effects on bone as it inhibits bone loss by affecting osteoclastogenesis. Horcajada–Molteni et al. [12] and Tsuji et al. [13] state that quercetin and its dietary analogue rutin inhibit osteopenia in ovariectomized rats. On the other hand, quercetin stimulates differentiation of osteoblasts and MG-63 osteoblast-like cells in rats [14]. Besides its beneficial health effects, potentially toxic actions of quercetin related to mutagenicity, prooxidant activity, mitochondrial toxicity, and inhibition of key

*Correspondence: birgit.grosskopf@biologie.uni-goettingen.de
[3] Institute of Zoology and Anthropology, Georg-August University, 37 073 Göttingen, Germany

enzymes involve in hormone metabolism have been demonstrated [15, 16]. However, the impact of quercetin on qualitative and quantitative histological characteristics of the compact bone is still unknown. Therefore, the aim of this study was to investigate femoral bone microstructure of adult female rabbits after intramuscular application of quercetin.

Methods

Animals

The study was conducted on 12 clinically healthy adult female rabbits of meat line M91, maternal albinotic line (crossbreed New Zealand White, Buskat rabbit, French Silver) and paternal acromalictic line (crossbreed Nitra's rabbit, Californian rabbit, Big Light Silver) of approximately 5 months of age, with a body weight (bw) of 4.00 ± 0.5 kg. Animals were obtained from an experimental farm of the Animal Production Research Centre in Nitra (Slovak Republic) and were housed in individual flat-deck wire cages under a constant photoperiod of 12 h of daylight, temperature 20–24 °C and humidity 55 ± 10 %, with an access to food (feed mixture) and drinking water ad libitum. Adult female rabbits were randomly divided into four groups of three animals each: E1, E2, E3 and C. The rabbits from the E1, E2 and E3 groups were intramuscularly injected with quercetin (Sigma-Aldrich, Germany) at doses of 10, 100 and 1000 μg/kg bw, respectively for 90 days, 3 times per week. The doses of quercetin (reflecting the natural exposure of animals to quercetin in rabbit feed) were chosen based on literature data [17–19]. Rabbits from the C group (controls) were injected by a saline solution at the same time for 90 days. In general, the rabbits were kept for other investigations (e.g. histological and biochemical analyses) at the Animal Production Research Centre in Nitra. The present study was performed as an additional investigation focused on compact bone microstructure.

Procedures

At the end of experimental period (i.e. after 90 days), all the rabbits were killed and their femurs were used for analyses. For histological evaluation, the right femurs were sectioned at the diaphyseal midshaft and the segments were fixed in HistoChoice fixative (Amresco, USA). The segments were then dehydrated in increasing grades (40–100 %) of ethanol and embedded in Biodur epoxy resin (Günter von Hagens, Heidelberg, Germany) as previously described [20]. Transverse sections (70–80 μm) were prepared with a sawing microtome (Leitz 1600, Leica, Wetzlar, Germany) and fixed onto glass slides by Eukitt (Merck, Darmstadt, Germany) [21]. The qualitative histological characteristics of the compact bone were determined according to the internationally accepted classification systems of Enlow and Brown [22] and de Ricqlés et al. [23], who classify bone tissue into three main categories: primary vascular tissue, non-vascular tissue and Haversian bone tissue. Various patterns of vascularization occur in primary vascular bone tissue: longitudinal, radial, reticular, plexiform, laminar, lepidosteoid, acellular, fibriform and protohaversian. Three subcategories in Haversian bone tissue are known: irregular, endosteal and dense. The quantitative (histomorphometrical) variables were assessed using the software Motic Images Plus 2.0 ML (Motic China Group Co., Ltd.). We measured area, perimeter, minimum and maximum diameters of primary osteons' vascular canals, Haversian canals, and secondary osteons in the four cross-sectional quadrants (i.e. anterior, posterior, medial and lateral) to minimize inter-animal differences. The diaphyseal cortical bone thickness was also measured by Motic Images Plus 2.0 ML software. Twenty random areas were selected and average thickness was calculated for each femur.

Statistics

Statistical analysis was performed using SPSS 8.0 software. All data were expressed as mean ± standard deviation (SD). The unpaired Games-Howell's test was used for establishing statistical significance between all groups.

Results

Qualitative histological analysis

The periosteal and endosteal surfaces of femurs in rabbits from the C group were formed by primary vascular longitudinal bone tissue. This tissue included vascular canals, which ran in a direction essentially parallel to the long axis of the bone. Near endosteal surfaces, primary vascular radial bone tissue (formed by branching or non-branching vascular canals radiating from the marrow cavity) and/or Haversian bone tissues were also found. Haversian bone tissue was characterized by the presence of isolated and scattered secondary osteons (irregular Haversian bone tissue) or by a large density of the osteons (dense Haversian bone tissue). The middle part of the *substantia compacta* was formed by a layer of irregular and/or dense Haversian bone tissues (Fig. 1a).

Rabbits exposed to quercetin displayed differences in compact bone microstructure compared to the C group. In rabbits from the E1 (Fig. 1b) and E2 (Fig. 1c) groups, primary vascular longitudinal bone tissue was not observed in some areas (in anterior and posterior views) near endosteal surfaces. These areas were created by primary vascular radial and/or Haversian bone tissues. The middle part of *substantia compacta* was formed not only by Haversian bone tissue but also by primary vascular longitudinal bone tissue. In rabbits from the E1 group, the

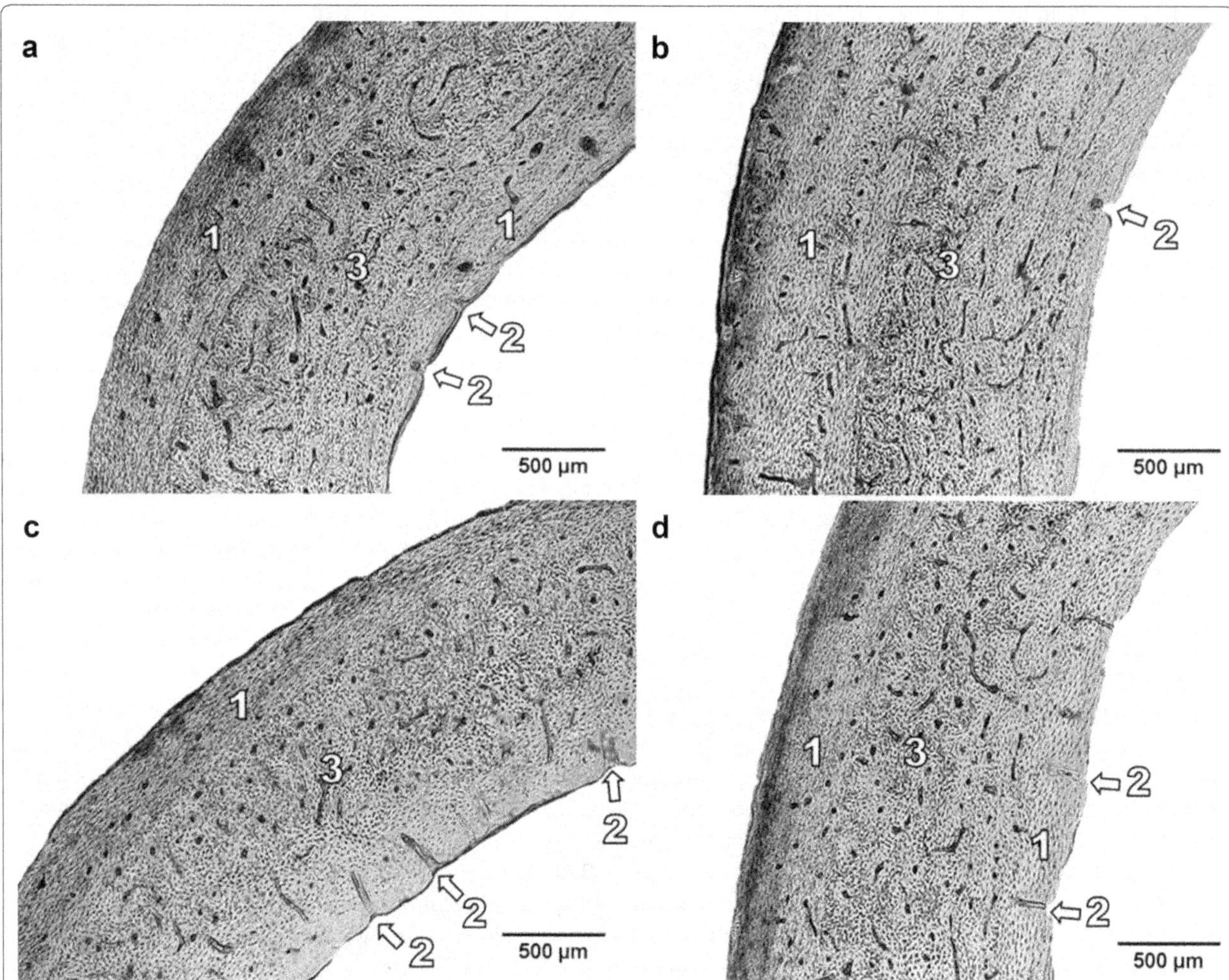

Fig. 1 **a, d** Photomicrographs showing the structure of the compact bone of rabbits from the C and E3 groups. *1* Primary vascular longitudinal bone tissue. *2* Primary vascular radial bone tissue. *3* Dense Haversian bone tissue. **b, c** Photomicrographs showing the structure of the compact bone in rabbits from the E1 and E2 groups. *1* Primary vascular longitudinal bone tissue. *2* Primary vascular radial bone tissue. *3* Irregular Haversian bone tissue

periosteal border consisted of a thicker layer of primary vascular longitudinal bone tissue when compared to the other groups. The animals from the E3 (Fig. 1d) group had a compact bone microstructure similar to rabbits from the C group although the number of secondary osteons was lower as found in rabbits from the E1 and E2 groups.

Quantitative histological analysis

In total, 480 vascular canals of primary osteons, 480 Haversian canals and 480 secondary osteons were measured. The results are summarized in Table 1. All variables (area, perimeter, maximum and minimum diameters) of the primary osteons' vascular canals were significantly decreased in groups E2 and E3 when compared to the C group. Significant differences were also found between E1 and E2, and E1 and E3 groups (except for minimum diameter). Haversian canals' values did not differ significantly between groups. On the other hand, secondary osteon values were significantly lower in rabbits from the E1, E2 and E3 groups compared to the C group. Significant differences were also demonstrated between the E1 and E2 groups.

Cortical bone thickness of rabbits from the E1 and E2 groups was significantly increased compared to the C group. In addition, statistically significant differences were also identified between the groups E1 and E2, and the groups E1 and E3 (Table 2).

Discussion

The results of qualitative histological analysis are in accordance to those of others [24–26]. Primary vascular longitudinal, primary vascular radial, irregular

Table 1 Data of the primary osteons' vascular canals, Haversian canals and secondary osteons in adult rabbits from the E1, E2, E3 and C groups

	Rabbits group		N	Area (μm^2)	Perimeter (μm)	Max. diameter (μm)	Min. diameter (μm)
Vascular canals of primary osteons	E1	(1)	120	399.27 ± 63.02	71.83 ± 5.84	12.57 ± 1.39	10.15 ± 1.02
	E2	(2)	120	358.42 ± 52.11	67.82 ± 4.88	11.77 ± 1.02	9.73 ± 1.00
	E3	(3)	120	359.38 ± 62.33	67.90 ± 5.66	11.75 ± 1.18	9.77 ± 1.14
	C	(4)	120	408.30 ± 79.95	72.22 ± 7.21	12.43 ± 1.45	10.45 ± 1.34
	Games–Howell's test			1:2**; 1:3**; 2:4**; 3:4**	1:2**; 1:3**; 2:4**; 3:4**	1:2**; 1:3**; 2:4**; 3:4**	1:2*; 1:3**; 2:4**
Haversian canals	E1	(1)	120	329.56 ± 57.64	65.15 ± 5.51	11.33 ± 1.16	9.30 ± 1.17
	E2	(2)	120	317.14 ± 54.53	63.84 ± 5.67	11.08 ± 1.27	9.15 ± 1.04
	E3	(3)	120	318.62 ± 56.46	64.02 ± 5.63	11.18 ± 1.16	9.10 ± 1.07
	C	(4)	120	334.86 ± 69.49	65.47 ± 6.67	11.37 ± 1.35	9.38 ± 1.18
	Games–Howell's test			*NS*	*NS*	*NS*	*NS*
Secondary osteons	E1	(1)	120	5976.51 ± 2236.50	276.00 ± 51.00	48.79 ± 9.85	38.04 ± 8.15
	E2	(2)	120	4945.24 ± 1691.32	252.24 ± 44.01	44.93 ± 8.60	34.31 ± 7.17
	E3	(3)	120	5355.22 ± 2046.25	262.10 ± 48.34	46.37 ± 9.67	35.97 ± 7.77
	C	(4)	120	6982.93 ± 2773.93	299.10 ± 55.97	53.13 ± 10.65	40.80 ± 9.44
	Games–Howell's test			1:2**; 1:4*; 2:4**; 3:4**	1:2**; 1:4*; 2:4**; 3:4**	1:2**; 1:4*; 2:4**; 3:4**	1:2**; 2:4**; 3:4**

N number of measured structures; *NS* non-significant differences

$P < 0.05$ (*); $P < 0.01$ (**)

Table 2 Cortical bone thickness in adult rabbits from the E1, E2, E3 and C groups

Rabbits group		N	Cortical bone thickness (μm)
E1	(1)	120	1224.78 ± 160.09
E2	(2)	120	1104.79 ± 127.29
E3	(3)	120	1059.01 ± 151.78
C	(4)	120	1055.53 ± 112.34
Games–Howell's test			1:2**; 1:3**; 1:4**; 2:4*

N number of measurements

$P < 0.05$ (*); $P < 0.01$ (**)

Haversian and/or dense Haversian bone tissues were found in all groups of rabbits. However, exposure to quercetin at levels of 10, 100, and 1000 μg/kg bw three times per week through 90 days leads to changes such as increased bone resorption, lower number of secondary osteons in the compact bone microstructure. These lesions were the most significant in rabbits exposed to the lowest dose of quercetin (10 μg/kg bw; E1 group), although they were also present in the E2 group given a dose of 100 μg/kg bw. The absence of primary vascular longitudinal bone tissue in some areas near the endosteal border and a lower density of secondary osteons in the middle part of the *substantia compacta* in these animals influences accelerated bone resorption at the endosteal surface.

Despite an increasing knowledge of quercetin's beneficial activities as high potential free radical scavenger in vitro, it may also have prooxidant effects under certain conditions [27, 28]. This prooxidant activity can contribute to the generation of ROS [29, 30] which have been shown to stimulate osteoclastic bone resorption [31].

According to Ahlborg et al. [32], excessive bone loss from the endocortical surface induces a mechanical stress on bone tissue, resulting in stimulation of periosteal bone apposition. Deposition of bone tissue onto the periosteal surface is considered to be an adaptive bone response to maintain resistance to bone loss and fractures. In our study, the predominance of periosteal bone apposition over endocortical bone resorption was associated with the thickest layer of primary vascular longitudinal bone tissue (E1 group) and increased thickness of cortical bone in rabbits from the E1 and E2 groups [33, 34]. The lower density of secondary osteons in the middle part of *substantia compacta* in rabbits from the E1, E2 and E3 groups could lead to weakness of biomechanical properties of their bones due to increased formation of microcracks [35].

The results also revealed significantly decreased sizes of the primary osteons' vascular canals in rabbits from the E2 and E3 groups. Primary osteons' vascular canals contain blood vessels which provide nutrition for the bone [36]. Pries et al. [37] showed that blood vessels can adapt its structure (vascular remodeling) in response to continuous functional changes. The results of several in vitro studies [38–41] documented the suppressive effect of quercetin on the expression of enzyme nitric oxide synthase (eNOS), which catalyzes a release of nitric oxide (NO), and endothelial cell proliferation. NO acts as a potential vasodilator and decreased production leads to vasoconstriction of blood vessels [42]. Therefore, the reduced size of primary osteons' vascular canals may be associated with structural changes of blood vessels present in primary osteons due to a negative effect of higher doses of quercetin on the eNOS expression. In addition, vascular endothelial growth factor (VEGF) is considered to play a central role in angiogenesis under pathological conditions [43, 44]. Several studies [45–47] have demonstrated an inhibitory effect of quercetin on the expression of VEGF. Furthermore, the inhibitory effect of quercetin on proliferation, migration and differentiation of endothelial cells during angiogenesis was observed [48, 49]. For this reason, quercetin-induced changes during angiogenesis could contribute to the smaller primary osteons' vascular canals in rabbits from the E2 and E3 groups. Interestingly, the size of the vascular canals of primary osteons did not change in rabbits from the E1 group. This indicates a dose-dependent effect of quercetin on their size. On the other hand, significantly decreased sizes of the secondary osteons were observed in all groups exposed to quercetin. We assume that evident alterations in the size of secondary osteons in these animals could be related to the destruction of collagen fibers present in the secondary osteons [50]. Kang et al. [51] found that quercetin (6.25–50 μmol/l) inhibited collagen synthesis on keloid-derived fibroblasts in vitro. The negative effect of various concentrations of quercetin (20, 40, and 80 μmol/l) on collagen reduction (more than 50 % in case of the highest dose) in human fibroblasts was also confirmed by Stipcevic et al. [52].

Conclusions

The study demonstrates that prolonged intramuscular application of quercetin has a significant effect on both qualitative and quantitative histological characteristics of the compact bone in adult female rabbits at doses of 10, 100, and 1000 μg/kg bw. A positive dose–response of quercetin has been identified for the sizes of primary osteons' vascular canals and secondary osteons. On the contrary, quercetin had a negative dose–response on qualitative histological characteristics of the compact bone and cortical bone thickness. Our study provides initial information related to quercetin's impact on femoral bone microstructure in rabbits. These findings may be useful for future insights into bone microstructural changes after the application of various nutrients.

Authors' contributions

RB was responsible for quantitative histological analysis of bones and writing the article. HD was responsible for qualitative histological analysis of bones. RO was responsible for the statistical analysis. VK was responsible for cortical bone thickness analysis. MA was responsible for photodocumentation of histological sections. BG was responsible for preparation of histological sections and corresponds with co-authors. MC was responsible for animal care and sampling of femora. MM conceived and designed the research and helped with writing an article. All authors read and approved the final manuscript.

Author details

[1] Department of Zoology and Anthropology, Constantine the Philosopher University, 949 74 Nitra, Slovakia. [2] Department of Botany and Genetics, Constantine the Philosopher University, 949 74 Nitra, Slovakia. [3] Institute of Zoology and Anthropology, Georg-August University, 37 073 Göttingen, Germany. [4] Department of Animal Physiology, Slovak University of Agriculture, 949 76 Nitra, Slovakia.

Competing interests

All authors declare that they have no competing interests.

Funding

This study was supported by the Grants VEGA 1/0653/16 and KEGA 031 UKF-4/2016. This work was supported by Research Centre AgroBioTech built in accordance with the project Building Research Centre "AgroBioTech" ITMS 26220220180.

References

1. Middleton E Jr, Kandaswami C, Theoharides TC. The effects of plant flavonoids on mammalian cells: implications for inflammation, heart disease, and cancer. Pharmacol Rev. 2000;52:673–751.
2. Chen C, Zhou J, Ji C. Quercetin: a potential drug to reverse multidrug resistance. Life Sci. 2010;87:333–8.
3. Nordeen SK, Bona BJ, Jones DN, Lambert JR, Jackson TA. Endocrine disrupting activities of the flavonoid nutraceuticals luteolin and quercetin. Horm Cancer. 2013;4:293–300.
4. Zhang F, Cui Y, Cao P. Effect of quercetin on proliferation and apoptosis of human nasopharyngeal carcinoma HEN1 cells. J Huazhong Univ Sci Technol Med Sci. 2008;28:369–72.
5. Wein S, Behm N, Petersen RK, Kristiansen K, Wolffram S. Quercetin enhances adiponectin secretion by a PPAR-gamma independent mechanism. Eur J Pharm Sci. 2010;41:16–22.
6. Wein S, Schrader E, Rimbach G, Wolffram S. Oral quercetin supplementation lowers plasma sICAM-1 concentrations in female db/db mice. Pharmacol Pharm. 2013;4:77–83.
7. Csokay B, Prajda N, Weber G, Olah E. Molecular mechanisms in the antiproliferative action of quercetin. Life Sci. 1997;60:2157–63.
8. Nickel T, Hanssen H, Sisic Z, Pfeiler S, Summo C, Schmauss D, Hoster E, Weis M. Immunoregulatory effects of the flavonol quercetin in vitro and in vivo. Eur J Nutr. 2011;50:163–72.
9. Dehghan G, Khoshkam Z. Tin (II)—quercetin complex: synthesis, spectral characterization and antioxidant activity. Food Chem. 2012;131:422–6.
10. Boots AW, Li H, Schins RP, Duffin R, Heemskerk JW, Bast A, Haenen GR. The quercetin paradox. Toxicol Appl Pharmacol. 2007;222:89–96.
11. Sharan K, Mishra JS, Swarnkar G, Siddiqui JA, Khan K, Kumari R, Rawat P, Maurya R, Sanyal S, Chattopadhyay N. A novel quercetin analogue from a medicinal plant promotes peak bone mass achievement and bone healing after injury and exerts an anabolic effect on osteoporotic bone: the role of aryl hydrocarbon receptor as a mediator of osteogenic action. J Bone Miner Res. 2011;26:2096–111.
12. Horcajada-Molteni MN, Crespy V, Coxam V, Davicco MJ, Remesy C, Barlet JP. Rutin inhibits ovariectomy-induced osteopenia in rats. J Bone Miner Res. 2000;15:2251–8.
13. Tsuji M, Yamamoto H, Sato T, Mizuha Y, Kawai Y, Taketani Y, Kato S, Terao J, Inakuma T, Takeda E. Dietary quercetin inhibits bone loss without

effect on the uterus in ovariectomized mice. J Bone Miner Metab. 2009;27:673–81.
14. Prouillet C, Maziereb JC, Maziereb C. Stimultatory effect of naturally occurring flavonols quercetin and kaempferol on alkaline phosphatase activity in MG-63 human osteoblasts through EKR and estrogen receptor pathway. Biochem Pharmacol. 2004;67:1307–13.
15. Okamoto T. Safety of quercetin for clinical application. Int J Mol Med. 2005;16:275–8.
16. Zhang Q, Zhao XH, Wang ZJ. Cytotoxicity of flavones and flavonols to a human esophageal squamous cell carcinoma cell line (KYSE-510) by induction of G2/M arrest and apoptosis. Toxicol In Vitro. 2009;23:797–807.
17. Choi JS, Li X. Enhanced diltiazem bioavailability after oral administration of diltiazem with quercetin to rabbits. Int J Pharm. 2005;297:1–8.
18. Knab AM, Shanely RA, Jin F, Austin MD, Sha W, Nieman DC. Quercetin with vitamin C and niacin does not affect body mass or composition. Appl Physiol Nutr Metab. 2011;36:331–8.
19. Lesniak AW, Kolesarova A, Medvedova M, Maruniakova N, Capcarova M, Kalafova A, Hrabia A, Sirotkin AV. Proliferation and apoptosis in the rabbit ovary after administration of T-2 toxin and quercetin. J Anim Feed Sci. 2013;22:264–71.
20. Martiniakova M, Omelka R, Grosskopf B, Sirotkin AV, Chrenek P. Sex-related variation in compact bone microstructure of the femoral diaphysis in juvenile rabbits. Acta Vet Scand. 2008;50:15.
21. Martiniakova M, Omelka R, Jancova A, Stawarz R, Formicki G. Heavy metal content in the femora of yellow-necked mouse (*Apodemus flavicollis*) and wood mouse (*Apodemus sylvaticus*) from different types of polluted environment in Slovakia. Environ Monit Assess. 2010;171:651–60.
22. Enlow DH, Brown SO. A comparative histological study of fossil and recent bone tissues. Part I. Texas J Sci. 1956;8:405–12.
23. de Ricqles AJ, Meunier FJ, Castanet J, Francillon-Vieillot H. Comparative microstructure of bone. In: Hall BK, editor. Bone 3, bone matrix and bone specific products. Boca Raton: CRC Press; 1991. p. 1–78.
24. Enlow DH, Brown SO. A comparative histological study of fossil and recent bone tissues. Part III. Texas J Sci. 1958;10:187–230.
25. Martiniaková M, Vondráková M, Fabiš M. Investigation of the microscopic structure of rabbit compact bone tissue. Scripta Medica (Brno). 2003;76:215–20.
26. Martiniakova M, Omelka R, Chrenek P, Vondrakova M, Bauerova M. Age-related changes in histological structure of the femur in juvenile and adult rabbits: a pilot study. Bull Vet Inst Pulawy. 2005;49:227–30.
27. Wattel A, Kamel S, Mentaverri R, Lorget F, Prouillet C, Petit JP, Ferdelonne P, Brazier M. Potent inhibitory effect of naturally occurring flavonoids quercetin and kaempferol on in vitro osteoclastic bone resorption. Biochem Pharmacol. 2003;65:35–42.
28. Woo JT, Nakagawa H, Notoya M. Quercetin suppresses bone resorption by inhibiting the differentiation and activation of osteoclasts. Biol Pharm Bull. 2004;4:504–9.
29. Metodiewa D, Jaiswal AK, Cenas N, Dickancaite E, Sequra-Aquilar J. Quercetin may act a cytotoxic prooxidant after its metabolic activation to semiquinone and quinoidal product. Free Radic Biol Med. 1999;26:107–16.
30. Harwood M, Danielewska-Nikiel B, Borzelleca JF, Flamm GW, Williams GM, Lines TC. A critical review of the data related to the safety of quercetin and lack of evidence of in vivo toxicity, including lack of genotoxic/carcinogenic properties. Food Chem Toxicol. 2007;45:2179–205.
31. Garret IR, Boyce BF, Oreffo ROC, Bonewald L, Poser J, Mundy GR. Oxygen-derived free radicals stimulate osteoclastic bone resorption in rodent bone in vitro and in vivo. J Clin Invest. 1990;85:632–9.
32. Ahlborg HG, Johnell O, Turner CH, Rannevik G, Karlsson MK. Bone loss and bone size after menopause. N Engl J Med. 2003;349:327–34.
33. Seeman E. The periosteum—a surface for all seasons. Osteoporos Int. 2007;18:123–8.
34. Seeman E. Bone quality: the material and structural basis of bone strength. J Bone Miner Metab. 2008;26:1–8.
35. O'Brien FJ, Taylor D, Lee TC. The effect of bone microstructure on the initiation and growth of microcracks. J Orthop Res. 2005;23:475–80.
36. Greenlee DM, Dunnell RC. Identification of fragmentary bone from the Pacific. J Archaeol Sci. 2010;37:957–70.
37. Pries AR, Reglin B, Secomb TW. Remodeling of blood vessels: responses of diameter and wall thickness to hemodynamic and metabolic stimuli. Hypertension. 2005;46:725–31.
38. Leikert JF, Rathel TR, Wohlfart P, Cheynier V, Vollmar AM, Dirsch VM. Red wine polyphenols enhance endothelial nitric oxide synthase expression and subsequent nitric oxide release from endothelial cells. Circulation. 2002;106:1614–7.
39. Huisman A, Van De Wiel A, Rabelink TJ, Van Faassen EE. Wine polyphenols and ethanol do not significantly scavenge superoxide nor affect endothelial nitric oxide production. J Nutr Biochem. 2004;15:426–32.
40. Wallerath T, Li H, Godtel-Ambrust U, Schwarz PM, Forstermann U. A blend of polyphenolic compounds explains the stimulatory effect of red wine on human endothelial NO synthase. Nitric Oxide. 2005;12:97–104.
41. Jackson SJ, Venema RC. Quercetin inhibits eNOS, microtubule polymerization, and mitotic progression in bovine aortic endothelial cells. J Nutr. 2006;136:1178–84.
42. Martynowicz H, Skoczyńska A, Wojakowska A, Turczyn B. Serum vasoactive agents in rats poisoned with cadmium. Int J Occup Med Environ Health. 2004;17:479–85.
43. Adair TH, Montani JP. Angiogenesis. San Rafael: Morgan & Claypool Life Sciences; 2010.
44. Kim J, Lim W, Ko Y, Kwon H, Kim S, Kim O, Park G, Choi H, Kim O. The effect of cadmium on VEGF-mediated angiogenesis in HUVECs. J Appl Toxicol. 2012;32:342–9.
45. Zhong L, Chen FY, Wang HR, Ten Y, Wang C, Ouyang RR. Effects of quercetin on morphology and VEGF secretion of leukemia cells NB4 in vitro. Zhonghua Zhong Liu Za Zhi. 2006;28:25–7.
46. Hung H. Dietary quercetin inhibits proliferation of lung carcinoma cells. Forum Nutr. 2007;60:146–57.
47. Santini SE, Basini G, Bussolati S, Graselli F. The phytoestrogen quercetin impairs steroidogenesis and angiogenesis in swine granulosa cells in vitro. J Biomed Biotechnol. 2009;2009:1–8.
48. Igura K, Ohta T, Kuroda Y, Kaji K. Resveratrol and quercetin inhibit angiogenesis in vitro. Cancer Lett. 2001;171:11–6.
49. Songo I, Vannini N, Lorusso G, Cammarota R, Noonan DM, Generoso L, Sporn MB, Albini A. Anti-angiogenic activity of a novel class of chemopreventive compounds: oleanic acid terpenoids. Recent Results Cancer Res. 2009;181:209–12.
50. Dylevsky I. Obecná kineziologie (in Czech). Praha: Grada Publishing; 2007.
51. Kang LP, Qi LH, Zhang JP, Shi N, Zhang M, Wu TM, Chen J. Effect of genistein and quercetin on proliferation, collagen synthesis, and type I procollagen mRNA levels of rat hepatic stellate cells. Acta Pharmacol Sin. 2001;22:793–6.
52. Stipcevic T, Piljac J, Vanden Berghe D. Effect of different flavonoids on collagen synthesis in human fibroblasts. Plant Foods Hum Nutr. 2006;61:29–34.

4

Serological patterns of *Actinobacillus pleuropneumoniae*, *Mycoplasma hyopneumoniae*, *Pasteurella multocida* and *Streptococcus suis* in pig herds affected by pleuritis

Per Wallgren[1,2*], Erik Nörregård[3], Benedicta Molander[3], Maria Persson[1] and Carl-Johan Ehlorsson[3]

Abstract

Background: Respiratory illness is traditionally regarded as the disease of the growing pig, and has historically mainly been associated to bacterial infections with focus on *Mycoplasma hyopneumoniae* and *Actinobacillus pleuropneumoniae*. These bacteria still are of great importance, but continuously increasing herd sizes have complicated the scenario and the influence of secondary invaders may have been increased. The aim of this study was to evaluate the presence of *A. pleuropneumoniae* and *M. hyopneumoniae*, as well as that of the secondary invaders *Pasteurella multocida* and *Streptococcus suis* by serology in four pig herds (A–D) using age segregated rearing systems with high incidences of pleuritic lesions at slaughter.

Results: Pleuritic lesions registered at slaughter ranged from 20.5 to 33.1 % in the four herds. In herd A, the levels of serum antibodies to *A. pleuropneumoniae* exceeded $A_{450} > 1.5$, but not to any other microbe searched for. The seroconversion took place early during the fattening period. Similar levels of serum antibodies to *A. pleuropneumoniae* were also recorded in herd B, with a subsequent increase in levels of antibodies to *P. multocida*. Pigs seroconverted to both agents during the early phase of the fattening period. In herd C, pigs seroconverted to *P. multocida* during the early phase of the fattening period and thereafter to *A. pleuropneumoniae*. In herd D, the levels of antibodies to *P. multocida* exceeded $A_{450} > 1.0$ in absence ($A_{450} < 0.5$) of antibodies to *A. pleuropneumoniae*. The levels of serum antibodies to *M. hyopneumoniae* and to *S. suis* remained below $A_{450} < 1.0$ in all four herds. Pigs seroconverted to *M. hyopneumoniae* late during the rearing period (herd B–D), or not at all (herd A).

Conclusion: Different serological patterns were found in the four herds with high levels of serum antibodies to *A. pleuropneumoniae* and *P. multocida*, either alone or in combination with each other. Seroconversion to *M. hyopneumoniae* late during the rearing period or not at all, confirmed the positive effect of age segregated rearing in preventing or delaying infections with *M. hyopneumoniae*. The results obtained highlight the necessity of diagnostic investigations to define the true disease pattern in herds with a high incidence of pleuritic lesions.

Keywords: Pig, Respiratory disease, Pleuritis, Antibodies, Disease pattern

*Correspondence: Per.Wallgren@sva.se
[1] National Veterinary Institute, SVA, 751 89 Uppsala, Sweden
Full list of author information is available at the end of the article

Background

Respiratory illness is traditionally regarded as the disease of the growing pig, and has historically been associated with bacterial infections such as *Mycoplasma hyopneumoniae* [1–3] and *Actinobacillus pleuropneumoniae* [4–6]. These bacteria still are of great importance, but the continuously increasing herd sizes have complicated the clinical picture. As the number of transmission events between pigs in a population is equal to the number of pigs multiplied with the number of pigs minus one [$x = n * (n - 1)$], they will escalate as the herd size increase [7]. Thus, the number of transmission events between pigs will increase with a factor of around four if a population is doubled and with a factor of around 100 if a population is enlarged ten times.

The increased number of transmissions between pigs may increase the influence of other microbes. *M. hyopneumoniae* and *A. pleuropneumoniae* are important pathogenic microbes, but co-infections may intensify or prolong clinical signs of respiratory disease [8–11]. It has also been observed that the incidence of respiratory illness may vary with season [12]. Therefore, infections in the respiratory tract of grower pigs have become regarded as a syndrome rather than linked to single microorganisms [11, 13, 14]. This syndrome is referred to as the porcine respiratory disease complex (PRDC). As stated above PRDC is regarded to be dominated by bacterial species, and important primarily pathogenic bacterial species include *M. hyopneumoniae* [1–3] and *A. pleuropneumoniae* [4–6]. The frequent demonstration of interferon-α in serum in growers during the first week after arrival to fattening herds [15, 16] suggest that PRDC can be associated with viral infections, and that PRDC can also include the influence of secondary invaders such as *Pasteurella* spp [17, 18].

When Sweden in 1986 as the first country in the world banned the use of low dose antibiotics in animal feed for growth promotion, some introductory health disturbances were recorded. As a consequence, a strict age segregated rearing from birth to slaughter was implemented in a large scale, which improved health as well as productivity [19, 20]. As seen in Fig. 1, the incidence of recorded pathogenic lesions in the respiratory tract at slaughter decreased during the last decade of the twentieth century [21]. The registrations of pneumonia at slaughter has remained stable at that level since then. In contrast, the incidence of recorded pleuritis at slaughter has continuously increased since the year 2000, as has the clinical evidence of actinobacillosis [22]. Discussions concerning the reason for this increase has included suggestions of introduction of new strains, or mutation of existing strains of *A. pleuropneumoniae*. However, acute actinobacillosis has in Sweden historically been dominated by serotype 2, and is still dominated by that serotype [22]. Further, Pulse Field Gel Electrophoreses has revealed that strains isolated in the twenty-first century were identical to strains isolated in the 1970s and 1980s [23]. As a consequence, the increase of actinobacillosis and pleuritic recordings at slaughter has merely been linked to the continuously increasing herd sizes with increasing number of transmissions of microbes between pigs, within and between units [22].

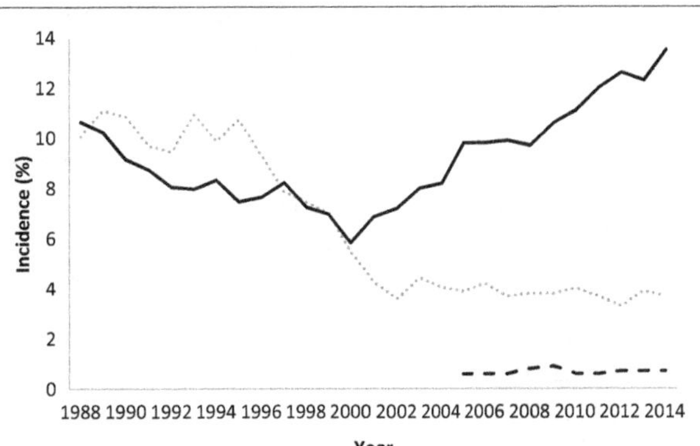

Fig. 1 National incidence of pathological lesions in the respiratory tract of pigs in Sweden at slaughter during a period of 26 years [21]. The *figure* shows the annual incidence of respiratory lesions registered of the entire Swedish pig population. In 1980 around four million pigs were slaughtered. In 2014 around three million pigs were slaughtered. Pneumonia of mycoplasma type *dotted grey line*; Pneumonia of acute *A. pleuropneumoniae* type *dashed black line*; Pleuritis *black line*

The aim of this study was to validate the presence of *A. pleuropneumoniae* and *M. hyopneumoniae*, as well as the secondary invaders *P. multocida* and *Streptococcus suis* in pig herds with a high incidence of pleuritic lesions at slaughter.

Methods

Herds and general health status

Four pig herds (A, B, C and D) with continuously high incidences of pleuritis recorded at slaughter (Table 1) were included in the study. All these herds used age segregated rearing with emptying and cleaning of each unit between consecutive batches of growers. The pigs were weaned at a median age of 31 days (range 28–34) and the growers weighted approximately 28 kg when transferred to the fattening unit and around 120 kg at slaughter. Details of herd sizes are included in Table 2.

Pigs in Sweden are certified free from African swine fever, Aujeszky's disease, hog cholera, porcine epidemic diarrhoea, porcine reproductive and respiratory syndrome, transmissible gastroenteritis, and salmonellosis [24].

Table 1 Incidence of pleuritis and pneumonia registered at slaughter in four fattening herds with high prevalence of pleuritic lesions recorded at slaughter during 1 year (mean percentage ± standard deviation)

	Pleuritis		Pneumonia			
			Mycoplasma-like		Resembling acute *A. pleuropneumoniae*	
	Preceding 4 quarters (%)	Study quarter (%)	Preceding 4 quarters (%)	Study quarter (%)	Preceding 4 quarters (%)	Study quarter (%)
Herd A	32.9 ± 1.0	33.1	0.8 ± 0.8	1.2	0.2 ± 0.1	0.3
Herd B	26.7 ± 5.9	21.5	10.0 ± 2.7	7.5	1.4 ± 1.7	0.8
Herd C	19.3 ± 2.6	20.5	1.1 ± 1.1	0.8	1.5 ± 0.8	0.4
Herd D	26.9 ± 11.5	26.1	3.2 ± 4.4	3.8	0.2 ± 0.2	0.3

The table also shows the prevalence of pleuritis and pneumonia during the quarter of a year when serological profiles were established for individual pigs regarding antibodies to selected bacterial infections. For details, see "Methods" section

Table 2 Information about the four herds that participated in the study

	Herd A	Herd B	Herd C	Herd D
Category	Fattening herd	Farrow to finish	Farrow to finish	Farrow to finish
Pigs slaughtered per year	21,000	15,800	6400	22,000
Merchandise of pigs from	1 herd	None	None	None
Vaccination of growers	None	None	None	None
Season studied	Winter	Winter	Winter	Winter
Pigs in unit studied	400	400	400	400

Endemic viral diseases associated to the respiratory tract include swine influenza that was introduced in 1982. At that time, it caused severe disease outbreaks but today influenza is rarely associated with severe respiratory disease [24]. Porcine respiratory coronavirus (PRCV) entered Sweden in 1987, but has never been associated with severe respiratory disease [24], nor has porcine circovirus type 2 (PCV2). PCV2 was diagnosed for the first time in 1993 in a specific pathogen free (SPF) herd when exudative epidermitis was diagnosed in one batch of piglets [25], which indicated that PCV2 probably had existed earlier in the country.

Animals and collection of blood samplings

The study was carried out during the winter season in four pig herds with fattening units sized for 400 pigs. All herds applied the "all in–all out" system, and clinical signs of respiratory disease were monitored. On arrival to an empty fattening unit, 10 pens in herd B and 12 pens in herd A, C and D were selected. The pens were evenly distributed within the unit. One pig in each pen was randomly selected and tagged. Blood samples were collected, into tubes without additive, from the tagged pig by jugular venipuncture within the first week after arrival and thereafter every 4th week (week 0, 4 and 8 in all herds, and also week 12 in herd A, C and D). The serum was removed and stored at −20 °C until analysis.

Registration of pathological lesions in the respiratory tract at slaughter

At slaughter, every pig was inspected by the Swedish Food Administration, a governmental veterinary authority. Lesions in the respiratory tract were registered according to rules set by The Swedish Food Administration (SLVFS 1996:32 and SLVFS 2002:27). Adhesions between lungs and *pleura intercostalis* larger than 10 cm^2 (a diameter of 3.5 cm) were recorded as pleuritis. Ongoing pneumonic lesions in the cranio-ventral parts of the lungs were recorded as *Mycoplasma*-like pneumonia. Acute pneumonic lesions in other parts of the lung were registered as *A. pleuropneumoniae*-like pneumonia.

Detection of antibodies to *Actinobacillus pleuropneumoniae*

Antibodies to *A. pleuropneumoniae* serotypes 2 and 3 (cross reacting with serotypes 6 and 8) in serum diluted 1/1000 were detected by previously described indirect ELISA systems based on phenol water extracts of the antigens [26]. The absorbance value in serum diluted 1/1000 ($A_{450} = 0.5$) was used as the limit for defining a positive reaction in both tests.

Detection of antibodies to *M. hyopneumoniae*

Antibodies to *M. hyopneumoniae* in serum diluted 1/40 were detected by a commercial ELISA kit (IDEXX *M.*

hyo. Ab test, IDEXX, Westbrook, USA) according the instructions of the manufacturer. The absorbance value in serum diluted 1/40 ($A_{450} = 0.4$) was used as the limit for defining a positive reaction.

Detection of antibodies to *P. multocida*

Antibodies to *P. multocida* in serum diluted 1/1000 was detected by a previously described indirect ELISA system based on a sonicated whole cell antigen [27]. The absorbance value in serum diluted 1/1000 ($A_{450} = 0.5$) was used as the limit for defining a positive reaction.

Detection of antibodies to *S. suis*

Detection of antibodies to *S. suis* was made by an indirect ELISA designed for that purpose. The antigen was produced by cultivating *S. suis* (strain CCUG 4255) for 18 h at 37 °C on horse blood agar plates. From each plate, the whole growth was harvested in 2 ml PBS without Ca and Mg (pH 7.4; SVA art no 302800) and ultrasonicated (MSE, 60 W ultrasonic disintegrator, Measuring Scientific Equipment Ltd, London, UK) for 5 min per 8 ml solution at 1.3 Ampere with an amplitude of 10 μm. The ultrasonicated solution was centrifuged at 12,000*g* for 20 min at 4 °C (RC2B, Sorvall, Newton, USA). Thereafter, the liquid phase was collected and stored at −20 °C.

Each well in a microtiter plate (Greiner Bio-one, Sigma-Aldrich) was coated with 100 μL of the sonicated antigen diluted 1/10,000 in PBS-T in room temperature for 18 h. Thereafter the microtiter plate was washed three times with PBS-T, and 100 μL serum diluted 1/100 in PBS was added to duplicate wells and the plates were incubated at 37 °C for 1 h. The plates were again washed three times with PBS-T and 100 μL of the conjugate (Protein A-horseradish peroxidase conjugate, Bio-Rad, Richmond, USA) diluted 1/5000 with PBS-T was added to each well and the microtiter plates were stored for 1 h in 37 °C. Then the plates were again washed three times with PBS-T and 100 μL of the substrate with tetra methylbenzidine (TMB, SVANOVA Biotech, Uppsala, Sweden) was added to each well. The reaction was stopped with 100 μL H_2SO_4 after 10 min and the absorbance was read at 450 nm by a spectrophotometer (Multiscan MCC/340® MK type II, Labsystem OY, Helsinki, Finland). The results obtained were adjusted to $A_{450} = 1.0$ for a positive standard serum and absorbance values exceeding 0.5 were regarded as positive reactions, based on the mean absorbance value +2 standard deviations of samples from 72 pigs without clinical signs of *S. suis* infection ($A_{450} = 0.26 \pm 0.12$).

Presentation of serum antibody levels and statistical calculations

The levels of serum antibodies are shown as mean absorbance values with standard deviations in Figs. 2, 3, 4, 5. These figures also show statistical differences in antibody levels between consecutive sampling occasions within herds calculated with the Wilcoxon signed-rank test for matched

Bacteria/comparison	4 vs 0	8 vs 4	12 vs 8
A. pleuropneumoniae, 2	*	**	NS
A. pleuropneumoniae, 3	*	**	NS
P. multocida	NS	*	NS
S. suis	*	**	NS
M. hyopneumoniae	NS	NS	NS

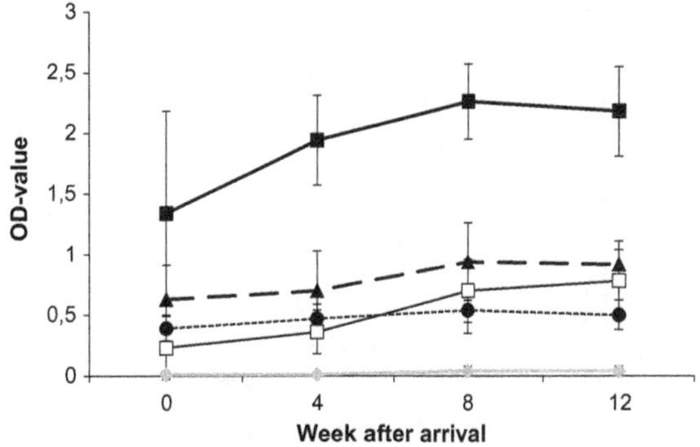

Fig. 2 Herd A. Serological profile (mean absorbance ± standard deviation) of 12 pigs repeatedly analyzed during the fattening period at a time when pleuritis was registered in 33.1 % of the pigs at slaughter. The *figure* shows serum levels of antibodies to *A. pleuropneumoniae* serotype 2 (*filled square*), serotype 3 (*square*), *P. multocida* (*filled triangle*), *S. suis* (*filled circle*) and *M. hyopneumoniae* (*filled diamond*). Statistical differences to the previous sampling occasion are visualized at the *top* of the figure (NS, P > 0.05; *P < 0.05; **P < 0.01; ***P < 0.001)

Bacteria/comparison	4 vs 0	8 vs 4
A. pleuropneumoniae, 2	**	*
A. pleuropneumoniae, 3	***	NS
P.multocida	*	NS
S. suis	*	NS
M. hyopneumoniae	NS	**

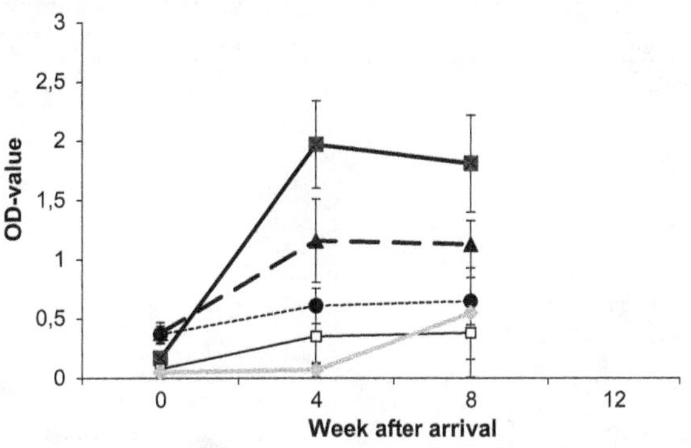

Fig. 3 Herd B. Serological profile (mean absorbance ± standard deviation) of 10 pigs repeatedly analyzed during the fattening period at a time when pleuritis was registered in 21.5 % of the pigs at slaughter. The *figure* shows serum levels of antibodies to *A. pleuropneumoniae* serotype 2 (*filled square*), serotype 3 (*square*), *P. multocida* (*filled triangle*), *S. suis* (*filled circle*) and *M. hyopneumoniae* (*filled diamond*). Statistical differences to the previous sampling occasion are visualized at the *top* of the figure (NS, P > 0.05; *P < 0.05; **P < 0.01; ***P < 0.001)

Bacteria/comparison	4 vs 0	8 vs 4	12 vs 8
A. pleuropneumoniae, 2	NS	**	NS
A. pleuropneumoniae, 3	*	**	**
P.multocida	**	***	*
S. suis	*	*	**
M. hyopneumoniae	NS	*	**

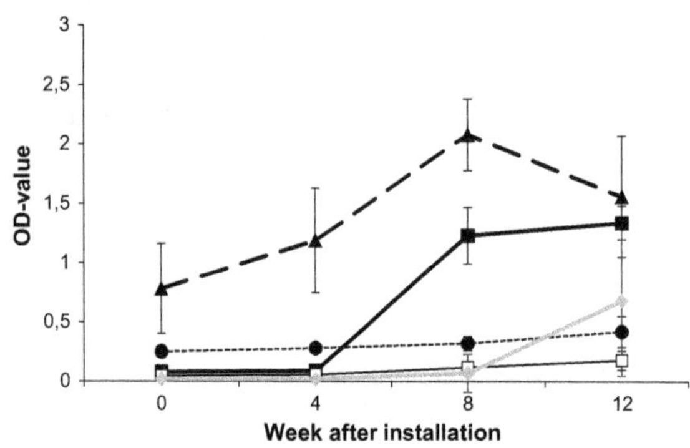

Fig. 4 Herd C. Serological profile (mean absorbance ± standard deviation) of 12 pigs repeatedly analyzed during the fattening period at a time when pleuritis was registered in 20.5 % of the pigs at slaughter. The *figure* shows serum levels of antibodies to *A. pleuropneumoniae* serotype 2 (*filled square*), serotype 3 (*square*), *P. multocida* (*filled triangle*), *S. suis* (*filled circle*) and *M. hyopneumoniae* (*filled diamond*). Statistical differences to the previous sampling occasion are visualized at the *top* of the figure (NS, $P > 0.05$; $^*P < 0.05$; $^{**}P < 0.01$; $^{***}P < 0.001$)

Bacteria/comparison	4 vs 0	8 vs 4	12 vs 8
A. pleuropneumoniae, 2	NS	**	NS
A. pleuropneumoniae, 3	NS	**	*
P.multocida	**	**	NS
S. suis	**	NS	NS
M. hyopneumoniae	NS	NS	**

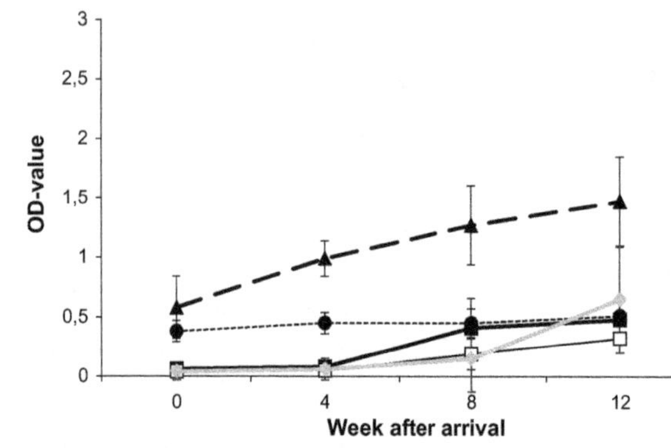

Fig. 5 Herd D. Serological profile (mean absorbance ± standard deviation) of 12 pigs repeatedly analyzed during the fattening period at a time when pleuritis was registered in 26.1 % of the pigs at slaughter. The *figure* shows serum levels of antibodies to *A. pleuropneumoniae* serotype 2 (*filled square*), serotype 3 (*square*), *P. multocida* (*filled triangle*), *S. suis* (*filled circle*) and *M. hyopneumoniae* (*filled diamond*). Statistical differences to the previous sampling occasion are visualized at the *top* of the figure (NS, $P > 0.05$; $^*P < 0.05$; $^{**}P < 0.01$; $^{***}P < 0.001$)

data. Tables 3, 4, 5, 6 show the number of seropositive and the number of pigs tested at each occasion. These tables include no statistical calculations since the number of pigs tested were too few to allow Chi square analysis, and the variance was too low to allow Fisher's exact test.

Results

There were no clinical signs of severe respiratory disease during the rearing of the pigs, but the herd prevalence of pleuritic lesions registered at slaughter at that time ranged from 20.5 to 33.1 % (Table 1).

Table 3 Herd A

	Week after arrival			
	0	4	8	12
A. pleuropneumoniae, type 2	8/12	12/12	12/12	11/11
A. pleuropneumoniae, type 3	0/12	2/12	8/12	8/11
M. hyopneumoniae	0/12	0/12	0/12	0/11
P. multocida	7/12	10/12	12/12	11/11
S. suis	1/12	4/12	5/12	4/11

Number of seropositive pigs in 12 pigs repeatedly analysed during the fattening period at a time when pleuritis was registered in 33.1 % of the pigs at slaughter. At week 12, one of the pigs was slaughtered. For details about serum antibody levels, see the corresponding Fig. 2

Table 4 Herd B

	Week after arrival			
	0	4	8	12
A. pleuropneumoniae, type 2	0/10	10/10	10/10	–
A. pleuropneumoniae, type 3	0/10	3/10	3/10	–
M. hyopneumoniae	0/10	0/10	4/10	–
P. multocida	1/10	10/10	10/10	–
S. suis	0/10	8/10	9/10	–

Number of seropositive pigs in 10 pigs repeatedly analysed during the fattening period at a time when pleuritis was registered in 21.5.1 % of the pigs at slaughter. At week 12, all of the pigs were slaughtered. For details about serum antibody levels, see the corresponding Fig. 3

Table 5 Herd C

	Week after arrival			
	0	4	8	12
A. pleuropneumoniae, type 2	0/12	0/12	12/12	12/12
A. pleuropneumoniae, type 3	0/10	0/12	0/12	0/12
M. hyopneumoniae	0/12	0/12	0/12	5/12
P. multocida	8/12	12/12	12/12	12/12
S. suis	0/12	0/12	0/12	2/12

Number of seropositive pigs in 12 pigs repeatedly analysed during the fattening period at a time when pleuritis was registered in 20.5 % of the pigs at slaughter. For details about serum antibody levels, see the corresponding Fig. 4

Table 6 Herd D

	Week after arrival			
	0	4	8	12
A. pleuropneumoniae, type 2	0/12	0/12	0/12	0/9
A. pleuropneumoniae, type 3	0/12	0/12	0/12	0/9
M. hyopneumoniae	0/12	0/12	1/12	5/9
P. multocida	7/12	12/12	12/12	9/9
S. suis	1/12	4/12	3/12	5/9

Number of seropositive pigs in 12 pigs repeatedly analysed during the fattening period at a time when pleuritis was registered in 26.1 % of the pigs at slaughter. At week 12, three of the pigs were slaughtered. For details about serum antibody levels, see the corresponding Fig. 5

In herd A, the pigs had seroconverted to *A. pleuropneumoniae* serotype 2 already on arrival to the fattening units (Fig. 2; Table 3), and the levels of antibodies increased ($P < 0.05$) during the rearing period. There were also seroreactors to *A. pleuropneumoniae* serotype 3, *P. multocida* and *S. suis* in the herd, but the serum concentrations of antibodies to these microbes remained below $A_{450} = 1.0$. The herd remained seronegative to *M. hyopneumoniae* throughout the rearing period.

In herd B, pigs were seronegative to all microbes tested for on arrival to the fattening unit. After 4 weeks there was a clear seroconversion ($P < 0.001$) to *A. pleuropneumoniae* serotype 2, and also to *P. multocida* ($P < 0.001$) but with a lower concentration of antibodies (Fig. 3; Table 4). There were seroreactors to *S. suis*, *A. pleuropneumoniae* serotype 3 and *M. hyopneumoniae* in the herd, but the serum concentrations of antibodies to these microbes remained below $A_{450} = 1.0$.

In herd C, pigs were seronegative to *A. pleuropneumoniae* serotype 2 and 3, *S suis* and *M. hyopneumoniae* on arrival. At that time they were seropositive to *P. multocida*, and the concentration of antibodies to *P. multocida* increased ($P < 0.05–0.001$) during the two subsequent sampling occasions (Fig. 4; Table 5). Eight weeks after arrival, a clear seroconversion ($P < 0.001$) to *A. pleuropneumoniae* serotype 2 was recorded, whereas antibodies to *M. hyopneumoniae*, *A. pleuropneumoniae* serotype 3 and *S. suis* remained below $A_{450} = 1.0$.

Also in herd D, pigs were seronegative to *A. pleuropneumoniae* serotype 2 and 3, *M. hyopneumoniae* and *S. suis* on arrival. Regarding *P. multocida*, seven out of twelve pigs (58 %) were seropositive on arrival and the antibody concentrations to *P. multocida* increased ($P < 0.05–0.001$) during the two subsequent sampling occasion (Fig. 5; Table 6). In contrast, the antibody concentrations to the other agents remained below $A_{450} = 1.0$ throughout the rearing period.

Discussion

The results obtained confirmed a low pathogen load of *M. hyopneumoniae*, which concurred well with the decreased incidence of pneumonic lesions recorded at slaughter following the implementation of strict age segregated rearing systems (all in–all out) in Sweden during the 1990s [21, 22] as shown in Fig. 1. It could of course, be argued that pulmonary lesions due to *M. hyopneumoniae* heal with time [28, 29], and therefore, infections gained during the early rearing period could escape detection at slaughter. However, the low levels ($A_{450} < 1.0$ in all herds) of antibodies to *M. hyopneumoniae* recorded show that the registrations of pneumonia were correct. Still, the slight increase of serum antibodies to *M. hyopneumoniae* at the end of the rearing period in herds B, C and D indicate the presence of *M. hyopneumoniae* in these herds, and that should not be neglected. The global market weight of pigs varies from around 80–180 kg, and is at present around 120 kg in Sweden, which is reached at an age of 6–7 months. If the market weight increase also the rearing period will be prolonged with more days at risk for each pig, which may pave the way for clinical signs of *M. hyopneumoniae*. Although the pathogen load differs between Sweden and Italy, it is notable that *M. hyopneumoniae*-like lesions were recorded in 2268 out of 4889 pigs (45.4 %) slaughtered at an age of 9–10 months in Italy [30].

Traditionally *A. pleuropneumoniae* has been strongly associated with pleuritis [6], and the capability of *A. pleuropneumoniae* to induce pleuritis was visualized by herd A in this study where the serological profile suggested *A. pleuropneumoniae* serotype 2 to be the sole bacterial cause of the high incidence of pleuritic lesions recorded at slaughter, although a possible influence from viral infections [15, 16] not can be excluded. However, the high levels of serum antibodies to *A. pleuropneumoniae* ($A_{450} > 1.5$) and low levels of antibodies to other bacteria ($A_{450} < 1$) was concluded to illustrate a classic serological pattern (Fig. 2).

Still, the results obtained in herds B, C and D in this study suggest that pleuritis in pigs could be a multifactorial syndrome rather than being linked to a single specific infection as also has been described by others [11–14, 18].

The synergistic influence of a secondary invader was clear in herd B, where high levels ($A_{450} > 1.5$) of antibodies to *A. pleuropneumoniae* serotype 2 were followed by significant levels ($A_{450} > 1.0$) of antibodies to *P. multocida*. This suggested a strong influence from *P. multocida* as also has been suggested earlier [17, 18, 31]. Also the levels of antibodies to *M. hyopneumoniae* and *S. suis* increased to some extent during the end of the rearing period However, as the antibody levels to these microbes remained at low levels ($A_{450} < 1.0$) their influence on the lung score were considered to be less significant. Thus, the serological pattern in herd B suggested *A. pleuropneumoniae* serotype 2 to be the main cause of the pleuritic lesions, but these lesions may have been amplified by subsequent secondary infections—especially with *P. multocida*.

In herd C the serological response to *P. multocida* was strong ($A_{450} > 1.5$) and preceded that to *A. pleuropneumoniae* serotype 2, and the influence of *P. multocida* therefore should be regarded as even more significant in this herd. Still, the increasing levels of antibodies to *A. pleuropneumoniae* serotype 2 at the end of the rearing period suggested an influence of *A. pleuropneumoniae* also in this herd, and it is notable that the levels of antibodies to *M. hyopneumoniae* increased slightly during the end of the rearing period. As *P. multocida* is regarded to be a secondary invader, something else than *A. pleuropneumoniae* or *M. hyopneumoniae* ought to have paved the way for that microbe. Although this remain undiagnosed in the present study, the frequent demonstrations of interferon-α in serum of fattening pigs during the first week after allocation [15, 16] indicate that viral infections may be precursors to *P. multocida* and the frequent findings of different virus in pigs using novel techniques [32] support that hypothesis. The early infections with *P. multocida* may by themselves not necessarily have induced pleuritic lesions, but obviously the infection with *P. multocida* already was established as the pigs became infected with *A. pleuropneumoniae* and colonies of *P. multocida* already on site may have amplified the effect of the subsequent *A. pleuropneumoniae* infection.

The serological pattern in herd D suggested a minor impact of *A. pleuropneumoniae* despite the high frequencies of pleuritic lesions recorded at slaughter. The mean concentration of antibodies to *A. pleuropneumoniae* serotype 2 and 3 remained below the cut off-value during the entire rearing period. Instead, pigs were seropositive to *P. multocida* already on arrival to the fattening unit and the level of serum antibodies to *P. multocida* increased throughout the rearing period in absence of antibodies to the other microbes. This clearly indicated that pleuritic lesions may evolve at high frequencies also in absence of *A. pleuropneumoniae*, as also has been suggested by others [33]. Likewise, no correlation between *A. pleuropneumoniae* and pleuritis at individual level was seen in herds with low incidences of pleuritic lesions recorded at slaughter [34]. Instead seroconversion to *M. hyopneumoniae* during the early fattening period was related to pleuritis at an individual level in such herds, which indicated an influence of secondary infections [34]. Therefore, the common presence of serum antibodies to *P. multocida* is of interest. However, in the present study, *P. multocida* was associated with a high prevalence of pleuritic lesions recorded at slaughter in absence of *M. hyopneumoniae*. Thereby, the true initial cause for these lesions still remains unknown and warrants further investigations. Since viral infections repeatedly has been demonstrated during the early fattening period [15, 16] viral infections may well have preceded the serological response to *P. multocida*.

Conclusion

Pleuritic lesions registered at slaughter ranged from 20.5 to 33.1 % in the four herds. High levels of serum antibodies to *A. pleuropneumoniae* and *P. multocida*, either alone or in combination, were seen. Pigs in this study seroconverted to *M. hyopneumoniae* late during the rearing period (herd B–D), or not at all (herd A), confirming a positive effect of age segregated rearing in preventing or delaying infections with *M. hyopneumoniae*. The results obtained highlight the necessity of diagnostic investigations to define the true disease pattern in herds with a high incidence of pleuritic lesions.

Authors' contributions

PW and CJE designed the study. CJE, EN and BM identified herds and collected blood samples. MP and PW analyzed the samples and designed the *S. suis* ELISA. PW was the main author of the manuscript. All authors read and approved the final manuscript.

Author details

[1] National Veterinary Institute, SVA, 751 89 Uppsala, Sweden. [2] Department of Clinical Sciences, Swedish University of Agricultural Sciences (SLU), Box 7054, 750 07 Uppsala, Sweden. [3] Farm & Animal Health, Kungsängens Gård, 753 23 Uppsala, Sweden.

Acknowledgements

This study was funded by the National Veterinary Institute, SVA (Grant No. DOA 1), and Farm & Animal Health (Grant No. FAH 2).

Competing interests

The authors declare that they have no competing interests.

References

1. Maré CJ, Switzer WP. New species: *Mycoplasma hyopneumoniae*, the causative agent of virus pig pneumonia. Vet Med. 1965;60:841–6.
2. Goodwin RFW, Pomerov AP, Whittlestone P. Production of enzootic pneumoniae in pigs with a mycoplasma. Vet Rec. 1965;77:1247–9.
3. Thacker EL, Minion FC. Mycoplasmosis. In: Zimmermann JJ, Karriker LA, Ramirez A, Schwartz KJ, Stevenson G, editors. Diseases of swine. 10th ed. Wiley-Blackwell: Ames; 2012. p. 779–97.
4. Shope RE, White DC, Leidy G. Porcine contagious pleuropneumoniae II. Studies of the pathogenicity of the etiological agent *Haemophilus pleuropneumoniae*. J Exp Med. 1964;119:369–75.
5. Bieberstein EL, Gunnarsson A, Hurvell B. Cultural and biochemical criteria for the identification of *Haemophilus* culture from swine. Am J Vet Med Assoc. 1976;38:7–11.

6. Gottschalk M. Actinobacillosis. In: Zimmermann JJ, Karriker LA, Ramirez A, Schwartz KJ, Srevenson G, editors. Disieases of swine. 10th ed. Wiley: Ames; 2012. p. 653–69.
7. Betts AO. Respiratory disease of pigs. V. Some clinical and epidemiological aspects of virus pneumonia of pigs. Vet Rec. 1952;64:283–8.
8. Brockmeier SL, Palmer MV, Bolin SR. Effects of intranasal inoculation of porcine reproductive and respiratory syndrome virus, *Bordetella bronchiseptica*, or a combination of both organisms in pigs. Am J Vet Res. 2000;61:892–9.
9. Brockmeier SL, Loving CL, Nicholson TL, Palmer MV. Coinfection of pigs with porcine respiratory coronavirus and *Bordetella bronchiseptica*. Vet Microbiol. 2008;128:36–47.
10. Loving CL, Brockmeier SL, Vincent AL, Palmer MV, Sacco RE, Nicholson TL. Influenza virus coinfection with *Bordetella bronchiseptica* enhances bacterial colonization and host response exacerbating pulmonary lesions. Microb Pathog. 2010;49:237–45.
11. Nicholson TL, Brockmeier SL, Loving CL, Register KB, Kehrly EK, Shore SM. The *Bordetella bronchiseptica* type III secretion system is required for persistence and diseases severity but not transmission in swine. Infect Immun. 2014;82:1092–103.
12. Eze JI, Correia-Gomes C, Borobia-Belsue J, Tucker AW, Sparrow D, Strachan DW, Gunn GJ. Comparison of respiratory disease prevalence among voluntary monitoring systems for pig health and welfare in the UK. PLoS ONE. 2015;10:e0128137.
13. Little TWA. Respiratory disease in pigs: a study. Vet Rec. 1975;96:540–4.
14. Hansen MS, Pors SE, Jensen HE, Bille-Hansen V, Bissgaard M, Flachs EM, Nielsen OL. An investigation of the pathology and pathogens associated with porcine respiratory disease complex in Denmark. J Comp Path. 2010;143:120–31.
15. Artursson K, Wallgren P, Alm GV. Appearance of interferon-α in serum and signs of reduced immune functions in pigs after transport and installation in a fattening farm. Vet Immunol Immunopath. 1989;23:345–53.
16. Wallgren P, Artursson K, Fossum C, Alm GV. Incidence of infections in pigs bred for slaughter revealed by elevated serum levels of interferon and development of antibodies to *Mycoplasma hyopneumoniae* and *Actinobacillus pleuropneumoniae*. J Vet Med B. 1993;40:1–12.
17. Bölske G, Martinsson K, Persson N. The incidence of mycoplasma and bacteria from lungs of swine with enzootic pneumonia in Sweden. In: Nielsen NC, Høgh P, Bille N, editors. International pig veterinary society congress. 6th ed. Copenhagen: Reproset; 1980. p. 213.
18. Ciprian A, Pijoan C, Cruz T, Camacho J, Tortora J, Colmenares G, Lopez-Revilla R, De la Garza M. *Mycoplasma hyopneumoniae* increase the susceptibility of pigs to experimental *Pasteurella multocida* pneumonia. Can J Vet Res. 1988;52:434–8.
19. Wallgren P. First out to ban feed additives in 1986. Veterinary challenges in the Swedish pig production. Part I. Use of antimicrobials and respiratory diseases. Pig J. 2009;62:43–51.
20. Wallgren P. First out to ban feed additives in 1986. Veterinary challenges in the Swedish pig production. Part II. Intestinal and miscellaneous diseases. Pig J. 2009;62:51–60.
21. Holmgren N, Lundeheim N. Rearing systems and health of pigs in Sweden. Svensk VetTidn. 2002;54:469–74.
22. Wallgren P, Lindberg M, Sjölund M, Karlsson Frisch K, Ericsson Unnerstad H. Antimicrobial resistance in *Actinobacillus pleuropneumoniae* and *Pasteurella multocida* isolated from the respiratory tract of pigs in Sweden. Svensk VetTidn. 2015;67(number10):11–7.
23. Wallgren P, Aspán A. *Actinobaccillus pleuropneumoniae*. A comparison of Swedish isolates of serotype 2 and 5 over time. Pig J. 2009;62:88–9.
24. Anonymous. Surveillance of infectious diseases in animals and humans in Sweden 2014. National Veterinary Institute (SVA), Uppsala. SVA:s rapportserie 31. ISSN 1654-7098. http://www.sva.se.
25. Wattrang E, McNelly F, Allan GM, Greko C, Fossum C, Wallgren P. Exudative epidermitis and porcine circovirus-2 infection in a Swedish SPF herd. Vet Microbiol. 2002;86:281–93.
26. Wallgren P, Persson M. Relationship between the amounts of antibodies to *Actinobacillus pleuropneumoniae* serotype 2, detected in blood serum and in fluids collected from muscles of pigs. J Vet Med B. 2000;47:727–38.
27. Sjölund M, Zoric M, Persson M, Karlsson G, Wallgren P. Disease patterns and immune responses in the offspring to sows with high or low antibody levels to *Actinobaccillus pleuropneumoniae* serotype 2. Res Vet Sci. 2011;91:25–31.
28. Noyes EP, Feeny DA, Pijoan C. Comparison of the effect of pneumonia detected during lifetime with pneumonia detected at slaughter on growth in swine. J Am Vet Med Assoc. 1990;197:1025–9.
29. Wallgren P, Beskow B, Fellström C, Renström HML. Porcine lung lesions at slaughter and their correlation to the incidence of infections by *Mycoplasma hyopneumoniae* and *Actinobacillus pleuropneumoniae* during the rearing period. J Vet Med B. 1994;41:441–52.
30. Merialdi G, Dottori M, Bonilauri P, Luppi A, Gozio S, Pozzi P, Spaggiaria B, Martelli P. Survey of pleuritis and pulmonary lesions in pigs at abattoir with focus on the extent of the conditions and herd risk factors. Vet J. 2012;193:234–9.
31. Pijoan C, Fuentes M. Severe pleuritic associated with certain strains of *Pasteurella multocida* in swine. J Am Med Assoc. 1987;191:823–6.
32. Blomström AL, Belák S, Fossum C, McKillen J, Allan G, Wallgren P, Berg M. Detection of a novel porcine boca-like virus in the background of porcine circovirus type 2 induced post weaning multisystemic wasting syndrome. Vir Res. 2009;146:125–9.
33. Fablet C, Marois C, Dorenlor V, Eono F, Eveno E, Jolly JP, Le Devendec L, Kobisch M, Madec F, Rose N. Bacterial pathogens associated with lung lesions in slaughter pigs from 125 herds. Res Vet Sci. 2012;93:627–30.
34. Holmgren N, Lundeheim N, Wallgren P. Infections with *Mycoplasma hyopneumoniae* and *Actinobacillus pleuropneumoniae* in fattening pigs. Influence of piglet production system and influence on production parameters. J Vet Med B. 1999;46:535–44.

5

Survey of otitis externa in American Cocker Spaniels in Finland

Mirja Kaimio*, Leena Saijonmaa-Koulumies and Outi Laitinen-Vapaavuori

Abstract

Background: American Cocker Spaniels are overrepresented among breeds that require surgery as a treatment of end-stage otitis externa. However, the prevalence of otitis externa (OE) in this breed remains unknown. We reviewed the year 2010 medical records of 55 private veterinary clinics in Finland to determine the prevalence of OE in American Cocker Spaniels compared with English Cocker and English and Welsh Springer Spaniels. An American Cocker Spaniel owner questionnaire was designed to identify potential risk factors for end-stage OE.

Results: From the medical records of 98,736 dogs, the prevalence of OE was highest in Welsh Springer Spaniels (149 out of 468, 31.8%, [95% confidence interval 27.6–36.0]), followed by American Cocker (89/329, 27.0%, [22.2–31.7]), English Springer (96/491, 19.6%, [16.1–23.1]) and English Cocker Spaniels (231/1467, 15.7%, [13.8–17.6]). The mean number of OE episodes in ear-diseased dogs and the number of ear surgeries were highest in American Cocker Spaniels. Owner questionnaires were received for 151 American Cocker Spaniels, 85 (56%) of which had suffered from OE. In 47% (40/85) of these dogs, OE occurred without concurrent skin lesions, 46% (33/72) displayed the first signs of OE before 1 year of age. In 24% (20/85) of the dogs, the signs of OE recurred within 1 month or continued despite treatment, 16% (14/85) required surgery ($n = 11$) or were euthanized ($n = 5$; 2 of the operated dogs and 3 others) due to severe OE. The onset of OE before the age of 1 year significantly increased the risk (OR 3.8, 95% CI 1.1–13.6) of end-stage OE.

Conclusions: The prevalence of OE in American Cocker Spaniels in Finland was higher than previously reported in Cocker Spaniels, but the highest prevalence of OE was found in Welsh Springer Spaniels. Compared to the other Spaniels, OE was more often recurrent and more frequently surgically managed in American Cocker Spaniels. Based on the questionnaire, early onset (<1 year) of OE increased the risk of end-stage OE. In American Cocker Spaniels, OE requires an intensive approach from the first treatment, and prevention of recurrence should be emphasised. The causes and treatment of OE in this breed warrant further study.

Keywords: American Cocker Spaniel, Otitis externa, Prevalence, End-stage otitis externa, Owner questionnaire

Background

Otitis externa (OE) is a relatively common disease in dogs [1]. In previous studies, the estimated prevalence of OE in primary-care veterinary practice has varied from 4.5% [2] and 10.2% [3] in the UK and England to 13% in the US. [4] Successful treatment of OE requires recognition and control of all the causative factors of OE, including primary and secondary causes, as well as predisposing and perpetuating factors [1, 5–7]. Cocker Spaniels have a breed predisposition to OE [8–10]. However, in the literature the term "Cocker Spaniel" is used to describe both English and American Cocker Spaniels; consequently the prevalence of OE in American Cocker Spaniels remains unknown. Some reports suggest, however, that American Cocker Spaniels are overrepresented among breeds that require total ear canal ablation and bulla osteotomy (TECABO) surgery as a treatment of end-stage OE [11–15].

This study aimed to evaluate the prevalence of OE in American Cocker Spaniels in Finland in comparison with other Spaniel breeds. We also aimed to evaluate

*Correspondence: mirja.kaimio@evidensia.fi
Department of Equine and Small Animal Medicine, Faculty of Veterinary Medicine, University of Helsinki, P.O. Box 57, 00014 Helsinki, Finland

American Cocker Spaniel owners' assessments of the clinical signs and management of OE, and to identify potential risk factors for end-stage OE.

Methods

Prevalence study

We conducted a retrospective cross-sectional study, reviewing the medical records of all dogs visiting 55 privately owned first opinion small animal veterinary clinics during 2010. The clinics varied in size and geographical location throughout Finland, but shared a database. These clinics covered 17–33% (the percentage varied regionally) of the total companion animal veterinary market in Finland [16]. The total number of dogs in Finland in 2010 is unknown; but according to Statistics Finland, it stood at approximately 630,000 in 2012 [17].

Information retrieved from the database included dog breed, the number of dogs with veterinary consultations (for any reason) and the number of dogs with ear-related consultations (a keyword "ears" as the presenting sign), as well as topical ear-medication prescriptions. Since the keyword "ears" and the use of topical ear medications also included diagnoses other than OE, these figures were only used to determine the relative frequency of ear diseases in different breeds, not the true prevalence. We further classified topical ear medications according to national recommendations from the Finnish Food Safety Authority Evira [18] into first-line (primary) and second-line (secondary) medications. First-line topical ear medications contain miconazole and polymyxin-B or fusidic acid, framycetin and nystatin as antimicrobials. Second-line topical ear medications contain fluoroquinolones or gentamicin and should only be used after bacterial culture and sensitivity testing [18].

In order to determine the prevalence of OE in different Spaniel breeds, we further examined the medical records of American and English Cocker Spaniels as well as Welsh and English Springer Spaniels, and then calculated the number of dogs with at least 1 diagnosed OE episode during 2010. The diagnosis of OE was based on clinical and otoscopic examinations by a veterinarian (this information was extracted from the free text notes), cytology of the aural exudate (when available) and treatment information. The dogs were required to have clinical evidence of OE together with relevant treatment prescription, to be classified as having OE. In most of the cases, the medical record data did not contain sufficient information to rule in or out concurrent otitis media, so we used only one diagnosis term "otitis externa". In addition, for each breed, we recorded the total number of consultations, the total number of OE episodes in each ear-diseased dog and the number of dogs undergoing ear canal surgery during 2010.

Owner questionnaire

An online owner questionnaire on ear and skin diseases in American Cocker Spaniels was developed to evaluate the owners′ assessments of the clinical signs and management of OE among this breed. The questionnaire was in Finnish, and a small pilot survey with a subsample of owners evaluated its ease of completion prior to the full-scale launch. Veterinarians, breeders and the American Cocker Spaniel Kennel Club informed private dog owners about the questionnaire from October 2009 to June 2010. Owners were invited to participate in this voluntary and open study regardless of whether their dog had suffered from otitis. The questionnaire was freely downloadable via the Internet and also available in print format. In addition to questions on ear and skin conditions, the questionnaire consisted of multiple-choice questions on signalment (age, sex, colour and weight), overall health and general dog management.

Questions about ear conditions covered the age of onset, clinical signs and the development of OE as noticed by the owner. The owners were also requested whether they had consulted a veterinarian after noticing the signs of otitis. The treatment of OE included questions on possible medication(s), the recurrence of signs after treatment(s) and whether the ears were re-evaluated by a veterinarian following treatment. Table 1 presents the most relevant questions on ears.

Questions about skin diseases covered the age of onset, continuity, seasonality, appearance, localisation and the development of skin lesions as noticed by the owner. The level of pruritus, explained as scratching, biting, chewing, licking and/or rubbing, at the time of answering the questionnaire was solicited using a 0–10 visual analogue scale (modified from Hill et al. [19]).

Statistical analysis

Prevalence study

The breeds of dogs were divided into "Spaniel breeds" and "other breeds" as well as into "dogs with pendulous ears" and "dogs with erect ears" according to the appearance of the breed. The group "Spaniel breeds" included all Spaniel breeds in the database. The proportion of ear-related consultations between Spaniels and dogs of other breeds and between dogs with pendulous and erect ears was assessed using univariate logistic regression models. The proportion of first-line and second-line topical ear medication prescriptions were analysed in the same way.

Owner questionnaire

We defined one dichotomous (yes or no) endpoint for the owner questionnaire database: incidence of end-stage OE. Dogs that were treated with surgery or dogs that were euthanized due to severe OE were classified

Table 1 The most relevant questions concerning ears in the American Cocker Spaniel owner questionnaire

Question	Responses								Response rate without I don´t know responses (%)
1. Has your dog suffered from ear or skin problems?	No	Only ear problems	Only skin problems	Both ear and skin problems					100
2. At what age did your dog experience the first signs of otitis?	Less than 3 months	3 months to less than 6 months	6 months to less than 12 months	1 year to less than 3 years	More than 3 years	I don't know			85
3. What were the most common signs of ear disease?	Scratching of the ears	Redness of the ears (erythema)	Foul smelling ears	Increased ear secretion	Head shaking	Head tilting	Ear soreness	Rash on pinnae	100
4. How many times has your dog been treated for otitis?	Never	Once	Twice	3 times	4–5 times	At least 6 times			100
5. List the medications which you have used to treat your dog´s otitis									91
6. For how long did the signs of otitis subside following treatment?	Less than 1 week	1 week to less than 2 weeks	2 weeks to less than 4 weeks	1–3 months	Signs continued despite treatment	I don't know			63–75
7. Did you bring your dog for a veterinary re-check after treatment?	Yes, every time	Yes, sometimes after treatment	No						99
8. Has surgery been performed to treat your dog's ears?	No	Yes, Zepp[a]	Yes, TECABO[a]						87

[a] *Zepp* ear surgery where only part of the ear canal is removed, *TECABO* ear surgery where the entire ear canal is removed and the bony bulla is opened

as having end-stage OE. We determined predefined lists of potential explanatory factors for the response: signalment (age, gender and body weight), diet (commercial diet, raw food diet, veterinary prescription diet for skin patients, use of nutritional oils or use of other additional nutritional supplements), owner's management of the ears (ear inspection frequency, ear cleaning frequency, frequency of shaving the dog´s pinnae and cheeks, swimming, rapidness of seeking veterinary consultations and whether a veterinary re-evaluation was performed after treatment) and clinical signs of disease (presence of skin lesions, age of onset of first OE episode, ear scratching, ear erythema, foul smell from the ears, increased ear secretion, head shaking, head tilting, rash on the pinnae or ear soreness). Some of these factors had low frequencies in some categories. Therefore, we created a few combinations in order to analyse the data (Table 2).

Each explanatory factor was first assessed separately using univariate logistic regression models with the explanatory factor in question as the sole fixed term in the model. Second, a penalised least absolute shrinkage and selection operator (LASSO) logistic regression model [20, 21] was fitted for our response variable. LASSO is a regression analysis method that performs both variable selection and regularisation in order to enhance the predictive accuracy and interpretability of the fitted statistical model. We used Akaike Information Criteria (AIC) for the optimal model selection and the Newton–Raphson Optimisation as the optimisation technique.

Least absolute shrinkage and selection operator regression was applied separately for four different groups of explanatory variables: (1) signalment, (2) diet, (3) owner's management of the ears and (4) clinical signs.

We calculated the odds ratios (OR) with a 95% confidence interval (CI) to quantify the results. We considered $P < 0.05$ statistically significant. All statistical analyses were completed at 4Pharma Ltd using SAS® System for Windows, version 9.3 (SAS Institute Inc., Cary, NC, USA).

Results

Prevalence study

The medical record search yielded information on 98,736 dogs, comprising 220 different breeds and mongrels, which represented 15.7% of the estimated total dog population in Finland [17]. Of these dogs, 11,281 (11.4%) had ear-related consultations. Among the 178 most prevalent breeds in the dataset (with a minimum of 50 individuals receiving veterinary consultations in each breed), the relative frequency of ear-related consultations was highest among Welsh Springer Spaniels (34.2%), followed by Shar-Peis (27.6%) and American Cocker Spaniels (27.1%) (Table 3). The OR for the proportion of dogs having ear-related consultations compared to consultations for other reasons was 1.5 (95% CI 1.4–1.6) in both group comparisons: that is, Spaniel breeds compared to dogs of other breeds and dogs with pendulous ears compared to dogs with erect ears.

Of the 98,736 dogs, 8761 (8.9%) were treated with topical ear therapy. First-line topical ear medications were prescribed to 8041 (8.1%) dogs and second-line ear-medications to 1136 (1.2%) dogs, while 416 dogs (0.4%) received both (Table 3). Second-line topical ear medications were prescribed at a higher proportion to Shar-Peis (10.5%) and American Cocker Spaniels (8.8%). When Spaniel breeds were compared to other breeds, the OR of first-line topical ear medications was 1.4 (95% CI 1.3–1.6), while second-line topical ear medications resulted in an OR of 2.6 (95% CI 2.2–3.0). Comparing dogs with pendulous and erect ears, the ORs of first and second-line topical ear medications were 1.7 (95% CI 1.6–1.8) and 1.6 (95% CI 1.4–1.9), respectively.

In Cocker and Springer Spaniel breeds, the prevalence of OE was highest in Welsh Springer Spaniels, but the mean number of OE episodes was 1.5-fold higher in

Table 2 Variable modifications for the statistical analysis

Variable	Categories	Action
Age of onset of signs	"Less than 3 months", "3 months to less than 6 months", "6 months to less than 12 months"	Combined to "less than 1 year"
Recurrence of signs of otitis	"Less than 1 week", "1 week to less than 2 weeks", "2 weeks to less than 4 weeks"	Combined to "less than 4 weeks"
Ear inspection frequency	"Once a week", "once every 2 weeks", "more seldom"	Combined to "once a week or more seldom"
Frequency of shaving the dog´s pinnae and cheeks	"Once every fortnight", "biannually", "once a year"", "never"	Combined
Rapidness of seeking veterinary advice	"1–3 days after noticing signs of otitis", "4–7 days after noticing signs of otitis"	Combined
Rapidness of seeking veterinary advice	"8–14 days after noticing signs of otitis", "I did not seek veterinary advice"	Combined

The data were collected from the American cocker spaniel owner questionnaire

Table 3 Relative frequency of ear-related consultations and topical ear medication prescriptions in different dog breeds

Breed	Dogs with veterinary consultations	Ear-related consultations n	% (95% CI)	Topical ear medication prescriptions n	% (95% CI)	Second-line[a] topical ear medication prescriptions n	% (95% CI)
Welsh Springer Spaniel	468	160	34.2 (29.9–38.5)	136	29.1 (25.0–33.2)	29	6.2 (4.0–8.4)
Shar-Pei	76	21	27.6 (17.6–37.7)	21	27.6 (17.6–37.7)	8	10.5 (3.6–17.4)
American Cocker Spaniel	329	89	27.1 (22.3–31.9)	75	22.8 (18.3–27.3)	29	8.8 (5.7–11.9)
West Highland White Terrier	1341	361	26.9 (24.5–29.3)	314	23.4 (21.1–25.7)	63	4.7 (3.6–4.8)
Bullmastiff	243	60	24.7 (19.3–30.1)	46	18.9 (14.0–23.8)	14	5.8 (2.9–8.7)
Pug	763	187	24.5 (21.4–27.6)	156	20.4 (17.5–23.3)	30	3.9 (2.5–5.3)
Dogue de Bordeaux	98	24	24.5 (16.0–33.0)	18	18.4 (10.7–26.1)	2	2.0 (−0.8 to 4.8)
Basset Hound	147	34	23.1 (16.3–29.9)	29	19.7 (13.3–26.1)	8	5.4 (1.7–9.1)
Grand Basset Griffon Vendeen	59	13	22.0 (11.4–32.6)	13	22.0 (11.4–32.5)	2	3.4 (−1.2 to 8.0)
Dogo Argentino	97	21	21.6 (13.4–29.8)	23	23.7 (15.2–32.2)	2	2.1 (−0.8 to 5.0)
Bull Terrier	188	40	21.3 (15.4–27.2)	33	17.6 (12.2–23.0)	11	5.9 (2.5–9.3)
Bulldog	596	122	20.5 (17.3–23.7)	105	17.6 (14.5–20.7)	27	4.5 (2.8–6.2)
Labrador Retriever	3708	737	19.9 (18.6–21.2)	644	17.4 (16.2–18.6)	75	2.0 (1.5–2.5)
Lagotto Romagnolo	426	84	19.7 (15.9–23.5)	70	16.4 (12.9–19.9)	3	0.7 (−0.1 to 1.5)
English Springer Spaniel	491	97	19.8 (16.3–23.3)	89	18.1 (14.7–21.5)	28	5.7 (3.6–7.5)
English Cocker Spaniel	1467	274	18.7 (16.7–20.7)	165	15.1 (13.3–16.9)	56	3.8 (2.8–4.8)
Swedish Elkhound	289	8	2.8 (0.9–4.7)	5	1.7 (0.2–3.2)	0	0
Japanese Spitz	344	9	2.6 (0.9–4.3)	12	3.5 (1.6–5.4)	2	0.6 (−0.2 to 1.4)
Greyhound	187	4	2.1 (0.0–4.2)	2	1.1 (−0.4 to 2.6)	0	0
German Spitz (klein)	171	3	1.8 (−0.2 to 3.8)	3	1.8 (−0.2 to 3.8)	0	0
Norrbottenspets	140	2	1.4 (−0.5 to 3.3)	3	2.1 (−0.3 to 4.5)	1	0.7 (−0.7 to 2.1)
All dogs (220 breeds)	98,736	11,281	11.4 (11.2–11.6)	8761	8.9 (8.7–9.1)	1136	1.2 (1.1–1.3)

This table presents the relative frequencies for all dogs and for the 16 most prevalent and 5 least prevalent breeds with ear-related consultations for the year 2010, from the medical records of 55 private veterinary clinics in Finland. n = the number of dogs

[a] A topical product containing marbofloxacin, clotrimazole and dexamethasone (Aurizon®, Vetoquinol S.A., Cedex, France); gentamicin, betamethasone and clotrimazole (Otomax®, Intervet International B.V., Boxmeer, the Netherlands); or hydrocortisone aceponate, gentamicin and miconazole (Easotic®, Virbac, Carros, France)

ear-diseased American Cocker Spaniels compared with Welsh Springer Spaniels (Table 4). Ear surgery was performed on eight of 89 (9.0%) American Cocker Spaniels, consisting of a Zepp operation (n = 2), a vertical ear canal ablation (n = 1) or TECABO (n = 5). TECABO (n = 1) or Zepp (n = 1) was also performed on two of 231 (0.9%) English Cocker Spaniels, while one of 96 (1.0%) English Springer Spaniels underwent the Zepp operation. None of the Welsh Springer Spaniels underwent surgery.

Owner questionnaire

Questionnaires were received from 117 owners, providing information on 151 dogs. This comprises approximately 10% of the American Cocker Spaniel population in Finland (American Cocker Spaniel Kennel Club, personal communication). Among these, 67 (44%) dogs were male and 84 (56%) were female. Their ages ranged from 0.3 to 14.4 years (mean 4.9 years, SD ± 3.15). In total, 25 of the dogs had already been euthanized, five due to serious ear disease. Of the 151 dogs, 85 (56%) had suffered from OE and 51 (34%) from skin disease. Only 6 dogs (4%) had experienced skin lesions without OE.

Clinical signs of ear and skin disease

Approximately half of the dogs with OE (47%, 40 out of 85) had no concurrent reported skin lesions. Most dogs (88%, 75 out of 85) had bilateral ear disease. The first episode of OE appeared before the age of 1 year in 46% (33 out of 72) of the dogs, 39% (13 out of 33) of these dogs also showed skin lesions before the age of 1 year and 12% (4 out of 33) after the age of 1 year. Only 22% (16 out of 72) of the dogs displayed the first signs of OE after the age of 3 years.

Half of the ear-diseased dogs' owners (54%, 46 out of 85) examined their dog's ears 1–2 times per week and 37% (31 out of 85) every day. The most common reported sign of OE was scratching of the ears (85%, 72 out of 85) followed by a foul smell (62%, 53 out of 75). Of the symptoms related to the skin, scratching (63%, 32 out of 51) and scaling (33%, 17 out of 51) were most commonly

Table 4 The prevalence of otitis externa (OE) in Cocker and Springer Spaniels in Finland

Breed	Number of dogs with veterinary consultations	Number of dogs with diagnosed OE	Prevalence of OE (95% CI)	Total number of veterinary consultations	Total number of OE episodes	Mean number of OE episodes in ear-diseased dogs	Median number of OE episodes in ear-diseased dogs
American Cocker Spaniel	329	89	27.0 (22.2–31.7)	847	231	2.6	2.0
Welsh Springer Spaniel	468	149	31.8 (27.6–36.0)	1286	257	1.7	1.0
English Springer Spaniel	491	96	19.6 (16.1–23.1)	1176	196	2.0	1.0
English Cocker Spaniel	1467	231	15.7 (13.8–17.6)	3609	449	1.9	1.0

The data were collected from the medical records of 55 private veterinary clinics in Finland during 2010

reported. The most frequent locations of the skin lesions were the axillae (29%, 15 out of 51), the back (25%, 13 out of 51), the interdigital skin (22%, 11 out of 51) and the paws (20%, 10 out of 51). The pruritus score ranged from 1 to 10, but pruritus was mild or moderate in most of the dogs (mean 4.8, SD $\pm$ 2.59).

Treatment of the ears

After noticing signs of otitis, 94% of the owners (80 out of 85) consulted a veterinarian. Altogether, topical ear medications were used in 79 (93%) dogs with OE, of these 27 (32%) received second-line medications. Half of the ear-diseased dogs (49%, 42 out of 85) received systemic antibiotics, most often amoxicillin and clavulanic acid or cephalexin. Systemic glucocorticoids were used on 19 (22%) and cyclosporine on three (4%) of 85 dogs. Ear cleaning under sedation or anaesthesia was performed on 22 (26%) of 85 dogs.

Most ear-diseased dogs′ owners (81%, 65 out of 80) received instructions from their veterinarian regarding how to clean their dog's ears at home. Almost all owners (84%, 71 out of 85) used commercially available cleaning products to clean their dog's ears. The most common product mentioned (81%, 57 out of 70) contained salicylic acid and EDTA (Epi-Otic®, Virbac, Carros, France).

Recurrence of signs

A veterinarian re-evaluated the ears each time after treatment for 32% (25 out of 79) and occasionally among 39% (31 out of 79) of the dogs; but, 29% (23 out of 79) of the owners never brought their dog for a re-evaluation. Approximately half of dog owners (48%, 41 out of 85) reported that the signs of OE resolved for a period of at least 1–3 months after treatment. Signs of OE recurred rapidly within less than 4 weeks or continued despite any medical therapy in 20 of 85 dogs (24%). The incidence of medically unmanageable end-stage OE was 16% (14 out of 85). Surgery was performed on 11 (13%) dogs consisting of either Zepp (n = 5) or TECABO (n = 6). Two dogs undergoing Zepp and three other dogs were euthanized due to severe OE.

Diet and general health

A commercial pet diet was fed to 90% (136 out of 151) of the dogs, either exclusively or in conjunction with home-cooked food. In addition, 8% of the dogs (12 out of 151) received only home-cooked or raw food. Among those who were on a commercial diet, a veterinary prescription diet formulated for skin patients was fed to 13 dogs–nine dogs with both ear and skin symptoms, three dogs with only skin symptoms and one dog with only OE. Nearly one-quarter of the dogs (23%, 35 out of 151) received nutritional oils and 11% (16 out of 151) received other nutritional supplements. One-third of the dogs (31%, 46 out of 151) had other illnesses such as hypothyroidism, cardiac failure, epilepsy, orthopaedic conditions and ophthalmic disease. Furthermore, eight of 151 (5%) dogs suffered from hypothyroidism, seven of which had both ear and skin symptoms, although none of these had end-stage OE.

Factors associated with end-stage OE

Based on the univariate logistic regression analyses, the onset OE before the age of 1 year (P = 0.040, OR = 3.804) and head tilting (P = 0.011, OR = 5.167) were risk factors for end-stage OE (Fig. 1). In the multivariate logistic regression model, in addition to head tilting (OR = 7.111) and onset of OE before the age of 1 year (OR = 2.326), erythema of the ears (OR = 1.460) and ear soreness (OR = 1.226) increased the risk, but the presence of symptoms related to the skin decreased (OR = 0.641) the risk of end-stage OE. None of the variables in the signalment, diet and owner's management of the ears groups were identified as risk factors for end-stage OE in the logistic regression analyses.

Discussion

In this study, the prevalence of otitis externa among American Cocker Spaniels visiting 55 private veterinary clinics in Finland during 2010 was high, reaching 27%. This is 1.4- to 5.9-fold higher than the figures reported in other studies for Cocker Spaniels [3, 22], for dogs with pendulous hairy ears [23] or for dogs in general

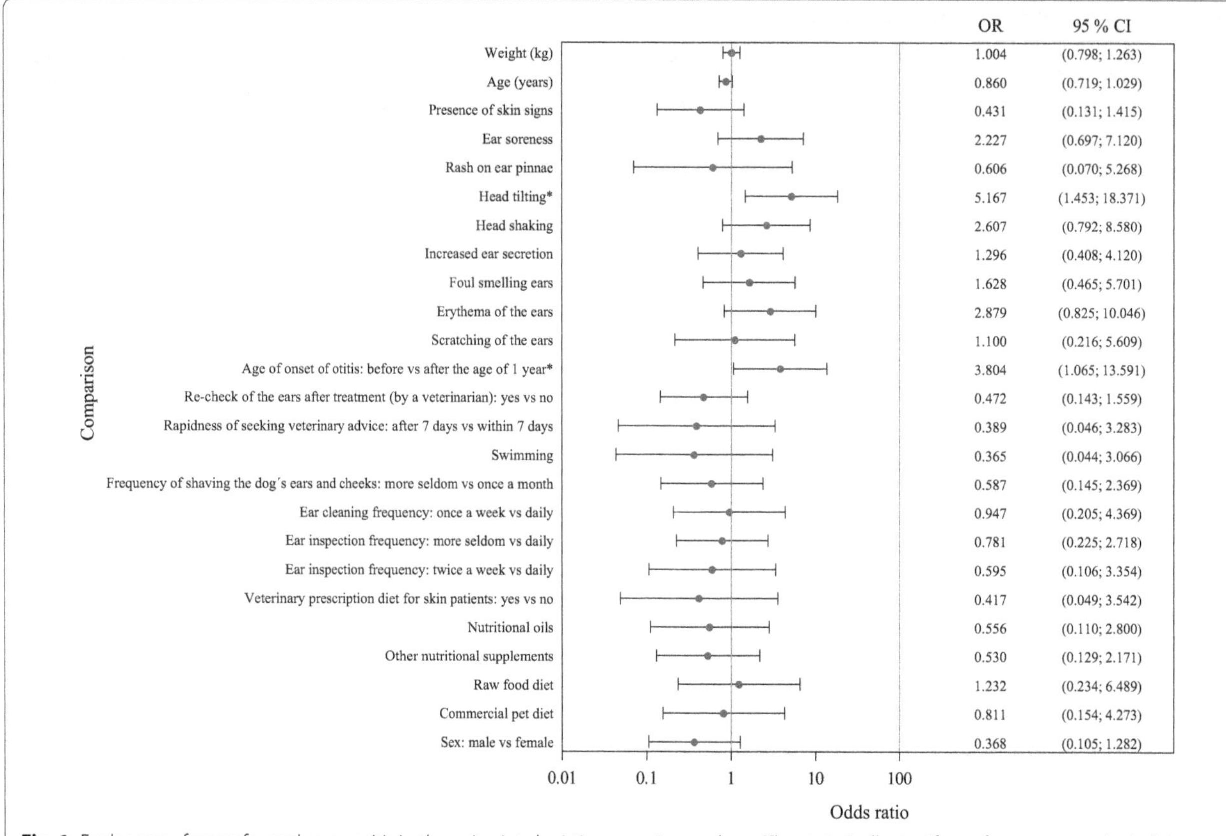

Fig. 1 Explanatory factors for end-stage otitis in the univariate logistic regression analyses. The statistically significant factors are marked with *asterisk*

[2–4]. Furthermore, among all breeds of dogs, ear-related consultations were most frequent in Welsh Springer Spaniels, followed by Shar-Peis and American Cocker Spaniels. Our finding that Spaniel breeds, compared to other dog breeds, had an increased risk for ear-related consultations and for the use of topical ear medications is in line with previous studies showing a predisposition to OE among these breeds [8–10].

When the four Spaniel breeds were studied more closely, American Cocker Spaniels and Welsh Springer Spaniels suffered more often from OE than English Cocker and Springer Spaniels. Interestingly, the highest prevalence of OE occurred among Welsh Springer Spaniels. To our knowledge, the high prevalence of OE in this breed has not been documented previously, a finding that warrants further study. However, our study reflected the situation during 1 year only and the 95% confidence intervals of the prevalence estimates of American Cocker Spaniels overlapped with those of English and Welsh Springer Spaniels. Thus, the role of chance in sampling should be remembered within these results. The mean and median number of OE episodes in ear-diseased dogs were highest among American Cocker Spaniels, which may indicate that OE recurs more often in this breed. Moreover, the number of ear surgeries on American Cocker Spaniels was high in comparison to other Spaniels, indicating that OE was also more difficult to manage medically in this breed. Difficulties in treatment were also reported by owners, whereby 24% of the owners of the ear-diseased dogs reported that the signs of OE recurred within one month or continued despite treatment. Furthermore, in 16% of the dogs, medical treatment failed, and 5.6% of dogs were euthanized due to severe OE.

According to the owner questionnaire, half of the dogs with OE displayed initial signs of OE before reaching 1 year of age. This could be explained in part by predisposing anatomical factors. Cocker Spaniels have long, hairy pendulous pinnae and, compared to Greyhounds and mongrels, a greater density of compound hair follicles and ceruminous glands in the ear canal [24]. Pendulous conformation is considered a predisposing factor for OE [25, 26], as also found in our study. In addition, the accumulation of cerumen in the external ear canal is thought to predispose dogs to OE [5], and sometimes the only underlying cause for chronic OE appears to be excessive cerumen production [1].

The early onset of first OE before the age of 1 year was a significant risk factor for end-stage OE. This is an interesting finding and, to our knowledge, not previously reported. It is possible that genetic predisposing factors play a larger role in the development of end-stage OE in this breed than previously understood. Other risk factors identified for end-stage OE such as ear soreness and head tilting appear to be clinical signs rather than risk factors for chronic otitis. These signs merely indicate that such dogs most probably suffered from severe otitis externa and otitis media. It is known that on-going inflammation can lead to permanent changes in the physiology and microanatomy of the ear canal [6]. American Cocker Spaniels in particular have a strong breed predisposition to proliferative ceruminous gland hyperplasia and ectasia, resulting in end-stage OE without proper care [13]. These facts and the results of this study imply that, in order to reduce the likelihood of chronic changes, the treatment of OE in a young American Cocker Spaniel should be intensive from the very first treatment, with greater emphasis placed on preventing recurrence. Unfortunately, after ear treatment many dogs did not undergo a re-evaluation. It is uncertain, however, whether a re-evaluation was requested. The re-check of the ears is of utmost importance in recognising and controlling perpetuating factors [27]. Increasing the frequency of veterinary re-checks through client and veterinary education might lead to better outcomes.

Skin symptoms were reported in only half of the dogs with OE; 29% of these dogs showed initial signs of OE before the age of 1 year. Interestingly, the presence of symptoms related to the skin decreased the risk of end-stage OE. Possible explanations for this surprising finding are that veterinarians may have neglected determining the primary cause of OE in dogs without concurrent skin disease, or that the primary cause of OE may have been more difficult to identify or control in these dogs. Thus, it would be useful to identify the primary cause of OE, particularly in these cases, through a more detailed study. In 1994, Rosychuck described "idiopathic inflammatory or hyperplastic otitis" in American Cocker Spaniels with chronic OE without other significant skin disease, but the cause of this ear disease remains unknown [28]. In our study, veterinary prescription diets for skin patients were fed more often to dogs with concurrent skin disease, suggesting that hypersensitivities were not considered a likely primary cause in dogs with OE only. However, allergies have been noted as the most common primary cause of OE [9, 10] and Cocker Spaniels are predisposed to atopic dermatitis [29]. Furthermore, food allergies [30] and canine atopic dermatitis [31] may be manifested solely by OE or otitis may precede other signs in allergic dermatitis [32]. An undiagnosed allergic disease may have been the primary cause of recurrent OE in some of the dogs in our study. Our results underline the need for a thorough investigation to identify the primary cause of otitis in all cases of recurrent OE.

We should consider the results in relation to limitations of our study. In the prevalence study, the diagnosis of OE was based on medical record data. Thus, it was not possible to verify the accuracy of the diagnosis. Because we distributed the owner questionnaire through veterinarians, breeders and the American Cocker Spaniel Kennel Club, we may not have reached all owners. The differences in the prevalence estimates of OE among American Cocker Spaniels between the questionnaire and the prevalence study indicate that the owners of dogs with ear-disease may have been more willing to participate in the questionnaire study, resulting in a nonresponse error. In addition, responses may have been influenced by the owners' perceptions or memory of various facts. However, the prevalence estimates of ear-diseased dogs receiving second-line topical ear medications and undergoing surgery were similar in both studies. The temporal sequence of events can be difficult to establish in cross sectional studies. Also in our study, there was potential reverse causality for some of the factors, such as ear-cleaning, because it was not known, whether ear-cleaning preceded OE or was introduced as a treatment of OE. In addition, certain factors, such as owner's management of the ears, may have changed over time, but data were only captured for one point of time. Some questions appeared to be more difficult to answer, resulting in a lower response rate and a higher number of "I don't know" responses, thus increasing measurement error. The problem regarding missing data was greater in the multivariate analyses, since the analysis can only be conducted using complete data for all of the explanatory variables included in our model. Reducing the number of observations rendered the results less reliable and, similarly, the results between the univariate and multivariate analyses were not completely comparable since they relied on somewhat different data. Because our questionnaire was freely downloadable from the internet, the total survey error is impossible to calculate. These limitations, many of which are inherent for cross sectional studies, should be kept in mind when interpreting our results.

Conclusions

We conclude that the prevalence of OE in American Cocker Spaniels in Finland was higher than previously reported among Cocker Spaniels. Interestingly, the highest prevalence of OE was found in Welsh Springer Spaniels. The recurrence of OE and the number of ear surgeries were highest among American Cocker Spaniels in comparison with other spaniels. Based on an owner questionnaire, half of the American Cocker Spaniels displayed the initial signs of OE before the age of 1 year and half of the dogs with OE showed no concurrent skin lesions. Furthermore, the onset of OE before the age of 1 year significantly increased the risk of end-stage OE. In this breed, OE requires an intensive approach from the first treatment, and emphasis should be placed on preventing recurrence. Further studies should focus on the causes and treatment of OE in this breed.

Authors' contributions

MK collected the prevalence study data, analysed all data and drafted the manuscript. LS-K and OL-V formulated the questionnaire and helped to draft the manuscript. All authors read and approved the final manuscript.

Acknowledgements

We thank Evidensia Finland for sharing their electronic patient record data, Hannele Ylitalo, DVM, for collecting the questionnaire data and Jouni Junnila, MSc, for the statistical analysis.

Competing interests

The authors declare that they have no competing interests.

Funding

This study was funded by the Finnish Veterinary Foundation.

References

1. Miller WH, Griffin CE, Campbell KL. Diseases of eyelids, claws, anal sacs, and ears. In: Muller & Kirk's Small Animal Dermatology. 7th edn. St. Louis: Elsevier Inc.; 2013. p. 724–73.
2. Hill PB, Lo A, Eden CAN, Huntley S, Morey V, Ramsey S, et al. Survey of the prevalence, diagnosis and treatment of dermatological conditions in small animals in general practice. Vet Rec. 2006;158:533–9.
3. O'Neill DG, Church DB, McGreevy PD, Thomson PC, Brodbelt DC. Prevalence of disorders recorded in dogs attending primary-care veterinary practices in England. PLoS ONE. 2014. doi:10.1371/journal.pone.0090501.
4. Lund EM, Armstrong PJ, Kirk CA, Kolar LM, Klausner JS. Health status and population characteristics of dogs and cats examined at private veterinary practices in the United States. J Am Vet Med Assoc. 1992;214:1336–41.
5. August JC. Otitis externa. A disease of multifactorial etiology. Vet Clin North Am Small Anim Pract. 1988;18:731–42.
6. Logas DB. Diseases of the ear canal. Vet Clin North Am Small Anim Pract. 1994;24:905–18.
7. Rosser EJ Jr. Causes of otitis externa. Vet Clin North Am Small Anim Pract. 2004;34:459–68.
8. Carlotti D. Diagnosis and medical treatment of otitis externa in dogs and cats. J Small Anim Pract. 1991;32:394–400.
9. Saridomichelakis MN, Farmari R, Leontides LS, Koutinas AF. Aetiology of canine otitis externa: a retrospective study of 100 cases. Vet Dermatol. 2007;18:341–7.
10. Zur G, Lifshitz B, Bdolah-Abram T. The association between the signalment, common causes of canine otitis externa and pathogens. J Small Anim Pract. 2011;52:254–8.
11. Matthiesen DT, Scavelli T. Total ear canal ablation and lateral bulla osteotomy in 38 dogs. J Am Anim Hosp Assoc. 1990;26:257–67.
12. White RAS, Pomeroy CJ. Total ear canal ablation and lateral bulla osteotomy in the dog. J Small Anim Pract. 1990;31:547–53.
13. Angus JC, Lichtensteiner C, Campbell KL, Schaeffer DJ. Breed variations in histologic features of chronic severe otitis externa in dogs: 80 cases (1995–2001). J Am Vet Med Assoc. 2002;221:1000–6.
14. Mason LK, Harvey CE, Orsher RJ. Total ear canal ablation combined with lateral bulla osteotomy for end-stage otitis in dogs. Vet Surg. 1988;17:263–8.
15. Coleman KA, Smeak DD. Complication rates after bilateral versus unilateral total ear canal ablation with lateral bulla osteotomy for end-stage inflammatory ear disease in dogs: 79 ears. Vet Surg. 2016;45:659–63.
16. Finnish Competition and Consumer Authority, Dnro 6/KKV14.00.10/2015. http://www.kkv.fi/globalassets/kkv-suomi/ratkaisut-aloitteet-lausunnot/ratkaisut/kilpailuasiat/2015/yk—hyvaksytyt/paatos_ii_vaihe_eqv.pdf. Accessed 15 March 2016.
17. http://tietotrendit.stat.fi/mag/article/60/. Accessed 3 Dec 2016.
18. Permanent work group on antimicrobials of the Ministry of Agriculture and Forestry. Recommendations for the use of antimicrobials against the most common infectious diseases on animals. Finnish Food Safety Authority Evira, Evira publications. 2009; 3: 44.
19. Hill PB, Lau P, Rybnijek J. Development of an owner-assessed scale to measure the severity of pruritus in dogs. Vet Dermatol. 2007;18:301–8.
20. Tibshirani R. Regression shrinkage and selection via the lasso. J R Stat Soc Ser B. 1996;58:267–88.
21. Yuan M, Lin L. Model selection and estimation in regression with grouped variables. J R Stat Soc Ser B. 1996;68:49–67.
22. Baba E, Fukata T. Incidence of otitis externa in dogs and cats in Japan. Vet Rec. 1981;108:393–5.
23. Sharma VD, Rhoades HE. The occurrence and microbiology of otitis externa in the dog. J Small Anim Pract. 1975;16:241–7.
24. Stout-Graham M, Kainer RA, Whalen LR, Macy DW. Morphometric measurements of the external ear horizontal ear canal of dogs. Am J Vet Res. 1990;51:990–4.
25. Cafarchia C, Gallo S, Capelli G, Otranto D. Occurrence and population size of Malassezia spp. in the external ear canal of dogs and cats both healthy and with otitis. Mycopathologia. 2005;160:143–9.
26. Lehner G, Sauter Louis C, Mueller RS. Reproducibility of ear canal cytology in dogs with otitis externa. Vet Rec. 2010;167:23–6.
27. Morris DO. Medical therapy of otitis externa and otitis media. Vet Clin North Am Small Anim Pract. 2004;34:541–55.
28. Rosychuck R. Management of otitis externa. Vet Clin North Am Small Anim Pract. 1994;24:921–52.
29. Jaeger K, Linek M, Power HT, Bettanay SV, Zabel S, Rosychuck RAW, et al. Breed and site predispositions of dogs with atopic dermatitis: a comparison of five locations in three continents. Vet Dermatol. 2010;21:119–23.
30. Harvey RG, Harari J, Delauche AJ. Ear diseases of the dog and cat. London: Manson Publishing Ltd; 2001.
31. Hillier A, Griffin CE. The ACVD task force on canine atopic dermatitis (I): incidence and prevalence. Vet Immunol Immunopathol. 2001;81:147–51.
32. Picco F, Zinit E, Nett C, Naegeli C, Bigler B, Rüfenacht S, et al. A prospective study on canine atopic dermatitis and food-induced allergic dermatitis in Switzerland. Vet Dermatol. 2008;19:150–5.

6

Comparison of the porcine uterine smooth muscle contractility on days 12–14 of the estrous cycle and pregnancy

Włodzimierz Markiewicz[1*], Marek Bogacki[2], Michał Blitek[2] and Jerzy Jan Jaroszewski[1]

Abstract

Background: Uterine contractile activity is very important for many reproductive functions including embryo transport, implantation, gestation and parturition. Abnormal contractility leads to implantation failure, spontaneous miscarriage, preterm birth and many other disorders. The objective of the present study was to assess the effects of acetylcholine (ACh), noradrenaline (NA), oxytocin (OT) and prostaglandins $F_{2α}$ ($PGF_{2α}$) and E_2 (PGE_2) on the contraction of uterine strips collected from the horns of cyclic gilts (12–14 days of the estrous cycle—group I) and from pregnant (12–14 days after first insemination gilts in which one of the uterine horn was gravid (group IIa) and the second one was non-gravid (group IIb). Uterine strips consisting of the endometrium with the myometrium and myometrium alone were examined.

Results: ACh increased the tension in all groups as compared to the pretreatment period, and the increase was the highest in group IIb; the amplitude decreased in all groups, and the frequency increased mainly in groups I and IIa. NA did not affect the tension in any group, but decreased the amplitude and frequency in group IIb as compared to groups I and IIa. OT caused the highest increase in the tension in group IIb, a decrease in the amplitude and an increase in the frequency of contractions as compared to the pretreatment period. $PGF_{2α}$ induced the highest increase in the tension and amplitude in group IIb, with a decline in the frequency in this group. PGE_2 increased the tension and frequency only in group IIb, and caused the greatest eduction in the amplitude in this group.

Conclusions: These results indicate that contractility of the porcine smooth muscle collected from uterine horns with embryos was different from those obtained from the uterine horns without embryos and the horns of cyclic gilts.

Keywords: Early pregnancy, Embryos, Gilts, Uterine contractility

Background

It is generally acknowledged that uterine contractility is regulated by complex interactions between many factors. Contractions determine the motor activity of the uterus which is particularly important during the migration of embryos and its implantation in the uterus. Contractions and relaxations of the porcine myometrium are controlled by the autonomic nerve system [1]. Moreover many endocrine and auto/paracrine/factors are also involved in this regulation [2–4]. Uterine contractions in pigs can be stimulated by compounds such as acetylcholine (ACh) [5], oxytocin (OT) [6–8], prostaglandins $F_{2α}$ ($PGF_{2α}$) [7–9] and E_2 (PGE_2) [7, 8, 10], histamine [11], neuropeptide Y (NPY) [12], and endothelin [13]. On the other hand, the relaxation of the porcine myometrium may be caused by noradrenaline (NA), serotonin (5-HT) [14], and nitric oxide [15]. These factors influence smooth muscle contractility directly or indirectly by affecting the synthesis and release of other substances. It has been shown that both exogenous and endogenous ACh cause contraction of the myometrium through the activation of the muscarinic M_3 receptor [5]. Other data have shown that NA causes an excitatory response, pre-

*Correspondence: mark@uwm.edu.pl
[1] Department of Pharmacology and Toxicology, Faculty of Veterinary Medicine, University of Warmia and Mazury, Oczapowskiego Street 13, 10-718 Olsztyn, Poland

dominantly via α_2-adrenergic receptors, and stimulation of β_2-adrenergic receptors inhibits contractile activity of the porcine myometrium [1]. It is also generally accepted that OT stimulates uterine contractile activity via its receptors [6], which are present in the porcine uterus [16]. Oxytocin, acting through its receptors in the endometrium and myometrium, is involved in the control of $PGF_{2\alpha}$ and PGE_2 secretion in pigs [17, 18]. Prostaglandin $F_{2\alpha}$ contracts the uterine muscle indirectly by enhancing the responsiveness to OT followed by the prostaglandin PGF_2 receptor (FP) mediated regression of the corpora lutea (decrease in plasma progesterone levels) [2]. However, the direct action of $PGF_{2\alpha}$ on contractile (FP, EP_1, EP_3) and relaxatory (DP, IP, EP_2) receptors in porcine uterine smooth muscle has also been described [2]. Similarly, PGE_2 may cause contraction or relaxation through its impact on particular EP receptor subtypes [10].

In gilts, myometrial activity undergoes changes during the oestrous cycle [2, 9, 10, 14, 19], at the time of mating and insemination [20, 21], and during the course of pregnancy [3, 22]. The early pregnancy in the pig is divided into three periods: post-conception (days 1–10 of pregnancy), the maternal recognition of pregnancy (days 11–13) and implantation (days 14–19) [23]. Thus, the period between the 12th and 14th days of the pregnancy is crucial for the successful implantation. The effects of various substances on motor activity of non-pregnant and pregnant porcine uteri have been studied, however, a comparison of the contractile activity between 12–14 days of the estrous cycle and pregnancy has not yet been made, especially in regard to the presence or not of embryos in the uterine horns. Therefore, the aim of our study was to examine the effects of ACh, OT, $PGF_{2\alpha}$, and PGE_2 on the contraction of uterine strips collected from the horns of cyclic gilts and from the horns with and without embryos of early pregnant pigs. Selection of the substances was made on their importance in the regulation of reproductive processes and the endogenous activity in the reproductive tract. The receptor mechanisms of these substances are also used in the case of drugs that interfere with the processes of uterine contractility. Until now, the differences in the impact of tested substances within the a period that is a crucial for a successful implantation compared to the analogous period of the estrous cycle are unknown. Therefore, we hypothesize that the uterine contractile response to stimuli will be affected by the presence of embryos within the uterus.

Methods

Animals

Prepubertal crossbred gilts (n = 10) with a body weight of 106 ± 4.8 kg and approximately 7 months of age were used. The gilts were subjected to surgical procedure under general anaesthesia. The animals were premedicated with azaperone (2 mg/kg bw i.m.; Stresnil, Janssen Animal Health, Belgium) and ketamine (12 mg/kg bw i.m.; VetaKetam, Vet-Agro, Poland), and anaesthetized with thiopental (20–30 mg/kg bw i.v.; Thiopental, Sandoz, GMBH, Austria). In five gilts one of the uterine horns was separated according to a surgically-generated model described previously by [24]. Briefly, the uterus was presented by a midventral opening of the caudal part of the abdomen. Thereafter, one horn was cut transversely and the ends were closed by a suture. This way the uterus consisted of one whole uterine horn and a part of the second horn, both connected with the uterine corpus. The remaining part of the second horn, connected with the contiguous ovary, was surgically detached from the uterine corpus. Ten days after surgery gilts were treated hormonally by an intramuscular injection of 750 I.U. of eCG (Folligon, Intervet, Poland) and 500 I.U. of hCG (Chorulon, Intervet) given 72 h later. Subsequently, 24 h after the hCG treatment the gilts were inseminated twice at 12 h intervals. Only gilts with the symptoms of heat were used for the next stages of procedures. Heat were checked by observation of symptoms: sticky discharge from vulva, clitoris red and protruding and the standing behaviour after applying pressure on the back and flanks of the gilt. The remaining five gilts were treated hormonally in the same way but they were not inseminated. On days 12–14 after insemination or for non-bred animals the gilts were slaughtered. To confirm pregnancy, the uterine horns were flushed with 10 ml PBS to determine the presence of embryos in uterine flushings [24]. The exact number of embryos was not possible to count because of their defragmentation caused by flushing. All procedures involving animals were conducted in accordance with the rules approved by the Local Ethics Commission of the University of Warmia and Mazury in Olsztyn.

Preparation of the uterine strips and measurements of their contraction

Fragments of the uterine horns, collected from the middle part of the horns, were transferred to ice, moved to the laboratory and immediately processed for examination of contractile activity. Uterine tissue was collected from the horns of cyclic gilts (group I) and the horns of pregnant gilts without (group IIa) and with embryos (group IIb). The contractile activity was examined according to the method described previously [4, 19]. Briefly, two kinds of the uterine strips (3 × 5 mm) consisting of the endometrium with myometrium (ENDO/MYO) and myometrium (MYO) alone were resected. The study involved these two types of strips because in previous studies we found that the presence of endometrium affected the contractile activity of myometrium [20]. From each examined horn of the uterus two ENDO/MYO and two MYO strips were selected. After resection the strips were washed in saline and mounted between two stainless steel hooks in 5 ml of an organ bath (Schuler Organ bath type 809; Hugo Sachs Electronic, Germany) under conditions of resting tension of 5 mN. The strips were kept in the Krebs-Ringer solution of the following composition (mM/l): NaCl, 120.3; KCl, 5.9; $CaCl_2$, 2.5; MCl_2 1.2; $NaHCO_3$ 15.5; glucose, 11.5; 37 °C, pH 7.4. The solution was maintained at 37 °C and continuously saturated with a mixture of 95 O_2 and 5 % CO_2. Measurements of smooth muscle contraction were conducted using a force transducer (HSE F-30 type 372), and a bridge coupler type 570, while the graphic recording was made on a recorder (Hugo Sachs Elektronik) with HSE-ACAD W software.

Schedule of contractile activity examination

The recording was started after prior equilibration for at least 60 min. Thereafter, the strips were incubated with ACh (10^{-5}–10^{-4} M; Sigma, St. Louis, MO, USA), NA (10^{-7}–10^{-6} M; Levonor Polfa, Poland), OT (10^{-7}–10^{-6} M, Vet-Agro, Poland), $PGF_{2\alpha}$ (10^{-8}–10^{-7} M; Sigma), and PGE_2 (10^{-8}–10^{-7} M; Sigma). The doses of the substances tested were based on previous studies [9, 10, 19, 22]. Contractile activity was measured for 10 min after the administration of each concentration of the examined substance. At the end of the examination of each substance tissue chambers were washed three times with 15 ml of Krebs-Ringer solution at 10 min intervals. Finally, at the end of treatment with examined substances to determine the viability of tissues, ACh was repeatedly administered in the same doses as given before. Only those results for which the difference in response to the stimulation by ACh at the beginning and the end of the treatment were less than 20 % were included into the statistical analysis.

Statistical analysis

Numerical values of the contractile activity (intensity, amplitude and frequency) of the strips before the application of the examined substances were calculated for 10 min and accepted as 100 %. The results calculated for 10-min periods after treatments were expressed as a percentage (mean ± SD) of the contraction intensity, amplitude and frequency before drug administration. The statistical significance of the differences was assessed by one-way analysis of variance ANOVA (Graphpad PRISM 3.1; Graphpad Software, San Diego, CA, USA), followed by Bonferroni's multiple comparison test. Differences at $P < 0.05$ were considered statistically significant.

Results

The spontaneous contractile activity before ACh administration in all examined tissues is shown in Fig. 1. Analysis of this activity did not demonstrate statistically significant differences between groups. Therefore, in the further statistical analysis the changes in the contractile activity after administration of the tested substances were compared to the pretreatment period.

Influence of ACh on uterine contractile activity

The administration of ACh in both doses caused a significant ($P < 0.001$) increase in the tension in all groups as compared to the pretreatment period (Fig. 2A). The magnitude of the increase was greater ($P < 0.01$–$P < 0.001$)

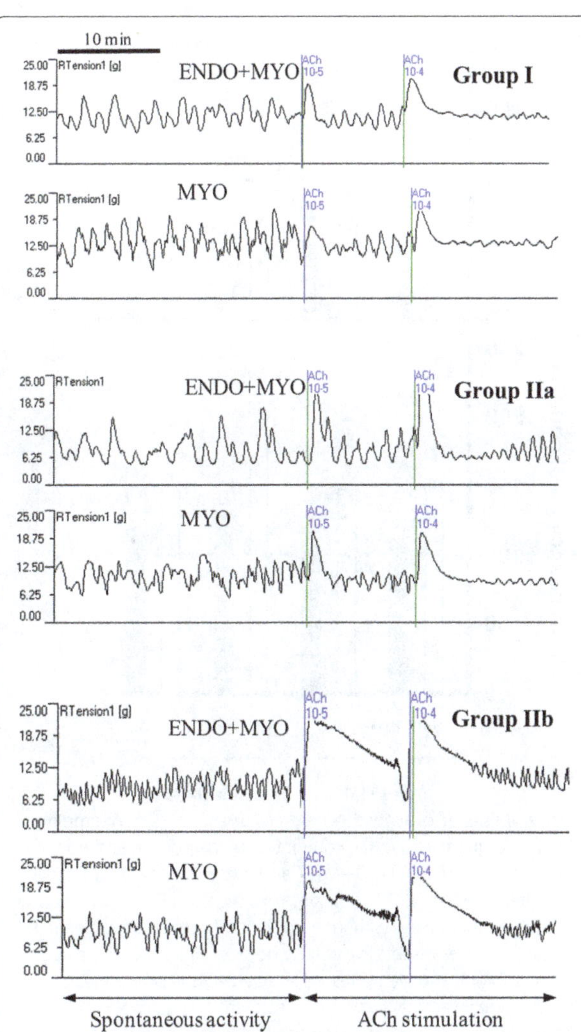

Fig. 1 A representative diagram showing spontaneous contractile activity and motor activity after acetylcholine (ACh) administration at doses 10^{-5} and 10^{-4} M in the endometrium/myometrium (ENDO+MYO) and myometrium (MYO) strips collected on days 12–14 of the oestrous cycle (Group I) or after first insemination (groups without embryos—Group IIa and with embryos—Group IIb)

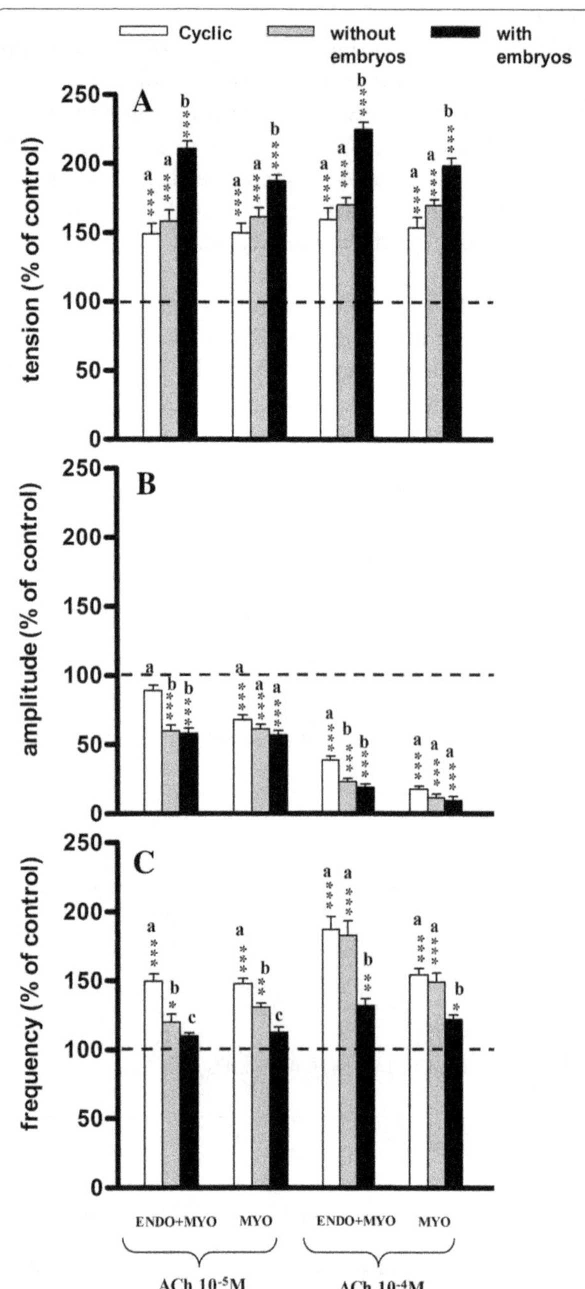

Fig. 2 Influence of acetylcholine (ACh) on the tension (**A**) amplitude (**B**) and frequency (**C**) of the contraction of the porcine endometrium/myometrium (ENDO+MYO) and myometrium (MYO) strips collected on days 12–14 of the oestrous cycle (cyclic) or after first insemination) (groups without embryos and with embryos). Values (mean ± SD) represents five uterine horns examined in two strips from each one and are expressed as a percentage of changes in the contractile activity before the treatment. *$P < 0.05$, **$P < 0.01$, ***$P < 0.001$ as compared to the contractile activity before the treatment; *a*, *b*, *c* indicates differences between groups (cyclic, without embryos and with embryos)

for strips from gravid horns than from non-gravid horns or cyclic gilt strips.

Administration of ACh caused a significant ($P < 0.001$) decrease in the amplitude in all groups (except ENDO/MYO in group I at a concentration of 10^{-5} M) as compared to the pretreatment period (Fig. 2B). Moreover, significantly smaller changes in the amplitude of the ENDO/MYO strips were determined in group I as compared to groups IIa and IIb ($P < 0.001$ after a dose of 10^{-5} M and $P < 0.05$ after a higher dose); such differences were not observed in the MYO strips.

The frequency of contractions in ENDO/MYO and MYO increased significantly ($P < 0.05$–$P < 0.001$) after the application of ACh at both doses in groups I and IIa as compared to the pretreatment period (Fig. 2C). In group IIb a significant increase ($P < 0.05$–$P < 0.01$) was observed only after the higher dose of ACh. After the lower dose of ACh the increase in frequency of contractions was significantly higher in the ENDO/MYO of group I as compared to groups IIa and IIb ($P < 0.001$), and in group IIa as compared to group IIb ($P < 0.05$); also in MYO strips a significantly greater increase was observed in group I as compared to groups IIa ($P < 0.01$) and IIb ($P < 0.001$), and in group IIa as compared to group IIb ($P < 0.05$). After the higher dose of ACh there were no differences between groups I and IIa, while a significantly ($P < 0.05$–$P < 0.001$) lower increase in group IIb was observed in both kind of strips as compared to groups I and IIa.

Influence of NA on uterine contractile activity

Administration of NA at both doses insignificantly influenced tension as compared to the pretreatment period (Fig. 3A); such differences were also not observed between the experimental groups.

The amplitude of contractions was significantly ($P < 0.001$) decreased after both doses in the ENDO/MYO and MYO in group IIb, and only after the smaller dose in groups I and IIa as compared to the pretreatment period (Fig. 3B). After NA administration in a dose of 10^{-7}M significantly lower amplitude was observed in group IIb as compared to group I ($P < 0.001$), but this change was less evident as compared to group IIa ($P < 0.05$); significantly lower ($P < 0.05$–$P < 0.01$) amplitude was also observed in group IIa as compared to group I in both kinds of the strips.

The frequency of contractions decreased significantly ($P < 0.01$–$P < 0.001$) only in group IIb as compared to the pretreatment period (Fig. 3C), as well as compared to groups I and IIa.

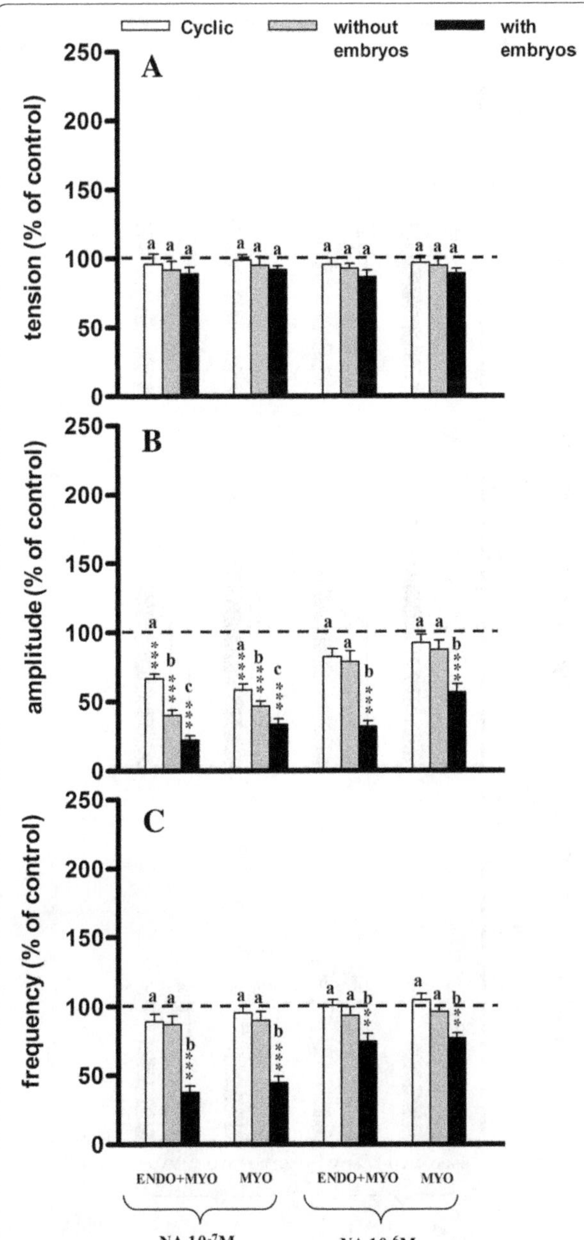

Fig. 3 Influence of acetylcholine (NA) on the tension (**A**) amplitude (**B**) and frequency (**C**) of the contraction of the porcine endometrium/myometrium (ENDO+MYO) and myometrium (MYO) strips collected on days 12–14 of the oestrous cycle (cyclic) or after first insemination) (groups without embryos and with embryos). Values (mean ± SD) represents five uterine horns examined in two strips from each one and are expressed as a percentage of changes in the contractile activity before the treatment. $^{**}P < 0.01$, $^{***}P < 0.001$ as compared to the contractile activity before the treatment; *a*, *b*, *c* indicates differences between groups (cyclic, without embryos and with embryos)

Influence of OT on uterine contractile activity

In the ENDO/MYO strips OT at both doses and in all groups caused a significant ($P < 0.01$–$P < 0.001$) increase in tension as compared to the pretreatment period (Fig. 4A); a significant increase was also observed in the MYO strips in groups IIa and IIb. Insignificant differences ($P > 0.05$) were noticed in tension in both ENDO/MYO and MYO strips between groups I and IIa, while significantly higher ($P < 0.001$) tension was found in group IIb as compared to groups I and IIa.

A significant ($P < 0.05$) increase in amplitude was observed after OT application at both doses in the ENDO/MYO and MYO strips in groups I and IIa, with a significant ($P < 0.05$) decrease in group IIb as compared to the pretreatment period (Fig. 4B). Significantly ($P < 0.001$) lower amplitude was also determined between group IIb as compared to groups I and IIa in both kinds of strip.

In ENDO/MYO and MYO strips the frequency of contractions decreased significantly in group I ($P < 0.01$–$P < 0.001$) but increased in group IIb ($P < 0.001$), and was not changed in group IIa as compared to the pretreatment period (Fig. 4C). The frequency of contractions was significantly lower in group I as compared to groups IIa ($P < 0.01$) and IIb ($P < 0.001$), and in group IIa as compared to group IIb ($P < 0.01$–$P < 0.001$).

Influence of $PGF_{2\alpha}$ on uterine contractile activity

In both kinds of strip a significant increase ($P < 0.01$–$P < 0.001$) in tension after $PGF_{2\alpha}$ administration was observed only in group IIb as compared to the pretreatment period (Fig. 5A). There were no significant changes in tension between groups I and IIa, while significantly higher tension ($P < 0.05$–$P < 0.01$) was observed in group IIb as compared to groups I and IIa.

$PGF_{2\alpha}$ significantly increased the amplitude in the ENDO/MYO strips in groups I ($P < 0.05$) and IIb ($P < 0.001$), and in the MYO strips in group IIb ($P < 0.01$) as compared to the pretreatment period (Fig. 5B). There were no significant changes in amplitude between groups I and IIa, while significantly higher ($P < 0.01$–$P < 0.001$) amplitude was observed in group IIb as compared to groups I and IIa.

In the ENDO/MYO and MYO strips the frequency of contractions after $PGF_{2\alpha}$ administration decreased significantly ($P < 0.001$) in group IIb as compared to the pretreatment period (Fig. 5C). There were no significant changes in the frequency of contractions between groups I and IIa, while significantly ($P < 0.01$–$P < 0.001$) lower

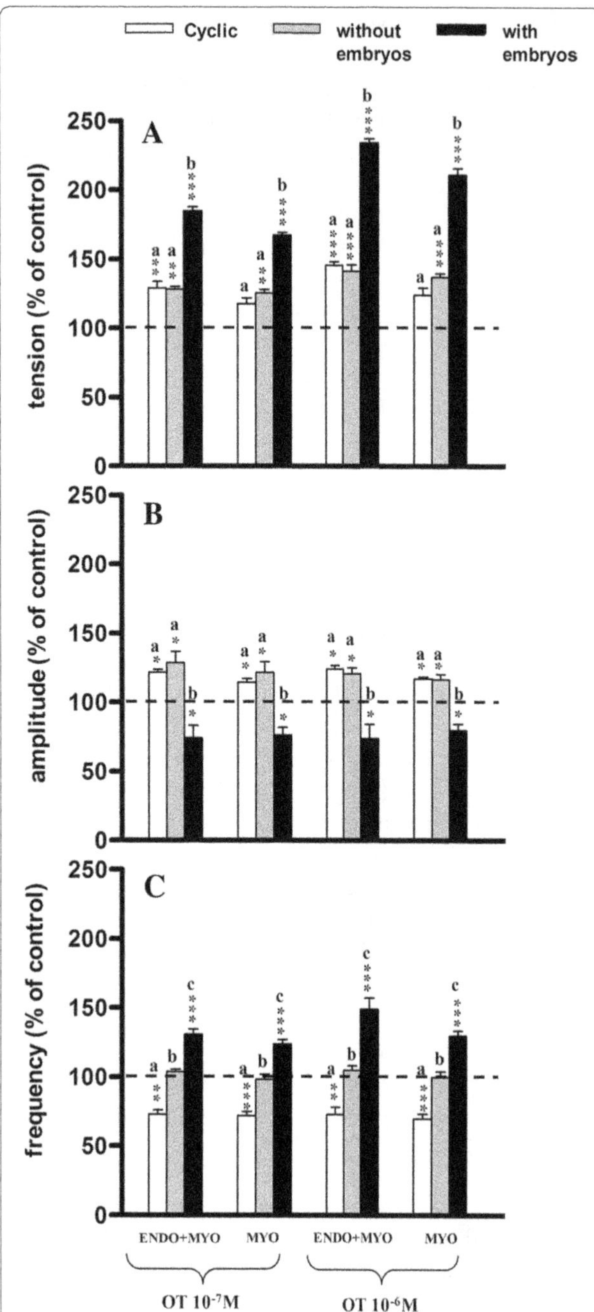

Fig. 4 Influence of oxytocin (OT) on the tension (**A**) amplitude (**B**) and frequency (**C**) of the contraction of the porcine endometrium/myometrium (ENDO+MYO) and myometrium (MYO) strips collected on days 12–14 of the oestrous cycle (cyclic) or after first insemination) (groups without embryos and with embryos). Values (mean ± SD) represents five uterine horns examined in two strips from each one) and are expressed as a percentage of changes in the contractile activity before the treatment. $*P < 0.05$, $**P < 0.01$, $***P < 0.001$ as compared to the contractile activity before the treatment; *a*, *b*, *c* indicates differences between groups (cyclic, without embryos and with embryos)

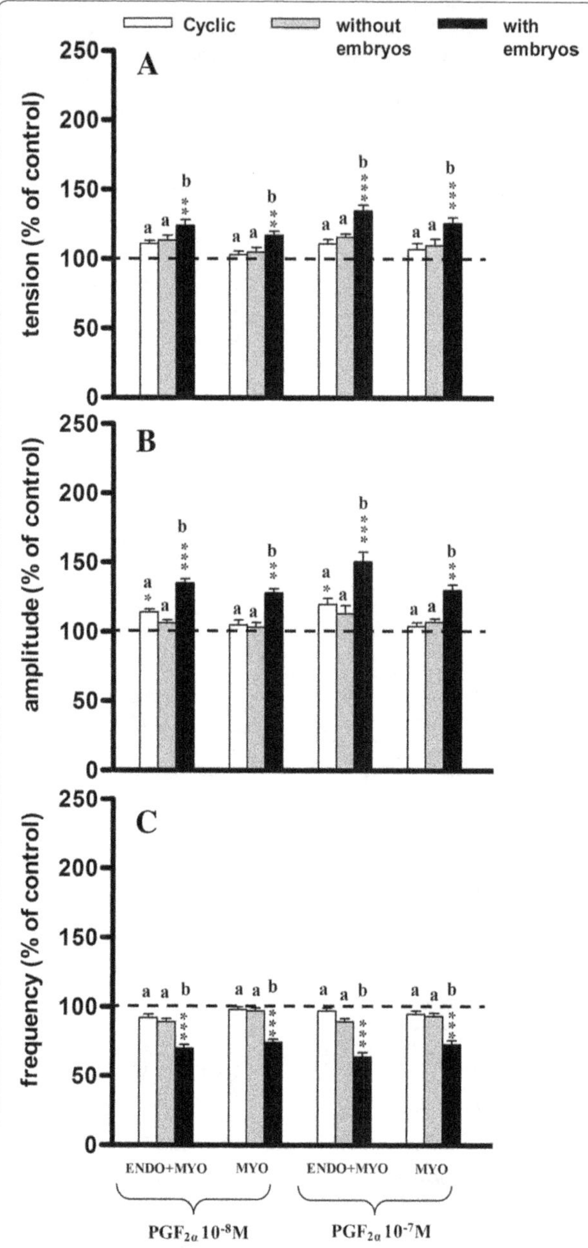

Fig. 5 Influence of prostaglandin $F_{2\alpha}$ ($PGF_{2\alpha}$) on the tension (**A**) amplitude (**B**) and frequency (**C**) of the contraction of the porcine endometrium/myometrium (ENDO+MYO) and myometrium (MYO) strips collected on days 12–14 of the oestrous cycle (cyclic) or after first insemination) (groups without embryos and with embryos). Values (mean ± SD) represents five uterine horns examined in two strips from each one and are expressed as a percentage of changes in the contractile activity before the treatment. $*P < 0.05$, $**P < 0.01$, $***P < 0.001$ as compared to the contractile activity before the treatment; *a*, *b*, *c* indicates differences between groups (cyclic, without embryos and with embryos)

frequency was observed in group IIb as compared to groups I and IIa.

Influence of PGE_2 on uterine contractile activity

At both doses PGE_2 caused a significant increase ($P < 0.001$) in tension only in the ENDO/MYO strips from group IIb as compared to the pretreatment period (Fig. 6A), as well as compared to groups I and IIa ($P < 0.01$–$P < 0.001$).

In the ENDO/MYO strips PGE_2 at the smaller dose decreased the amplitude in group IIb ($P < 0.001$), whereas it decreased the amplitude at the higher dose in all groups ($P < 0.01$–$P < 0.001$) as compared to the pretreatment period (Fig. 6B). Significantly lower amplitude was observed in the ENDO/MYO in group IIb as compared to group I ($P < 0.01$) and group IIa ($P < 0.05$).

The frequency of contractions did not change significantly in any of the analysed groups as compared to the pretreatment period (Fig. 6C). The frequency of contractions significantly ($P < 0.05$) increased in the ENDO/MYO strips of group IIb as compared to groups I and IIa.

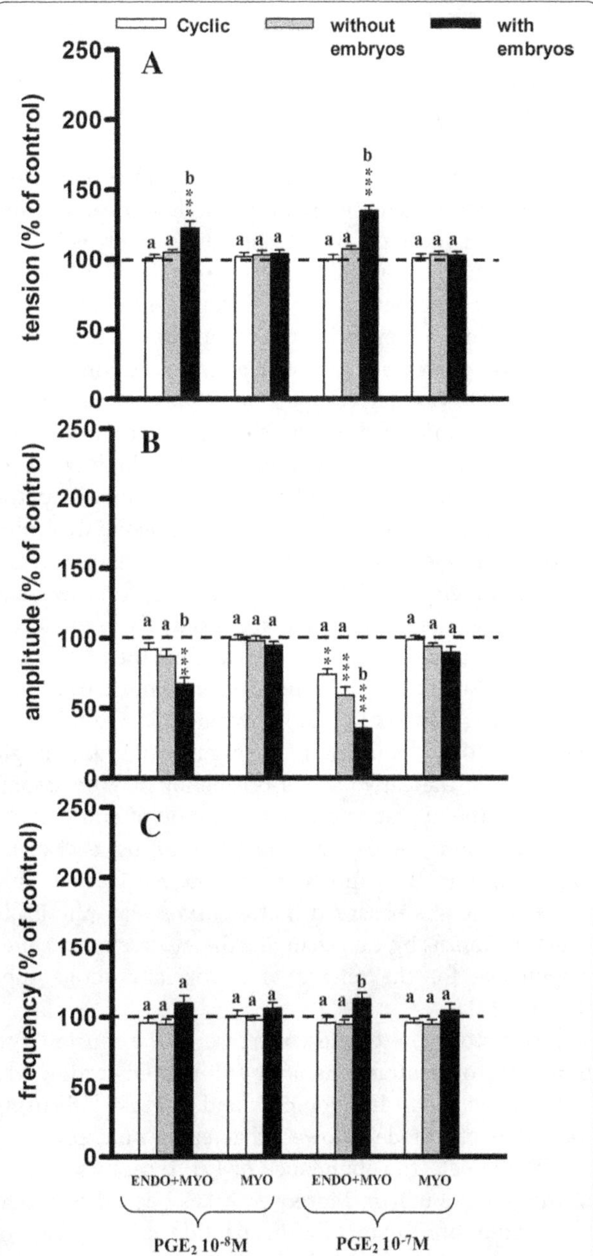

Fig. 6 Influence of prostaglandin E_2 (PGE_2) on the tension (**A**) amplitude (**B**) and frequency (**C**) of the contraction of the porcine endometrium/myometrium (ENDO+MYO) and myometrium (MYO) strips collected on days 12–14 of the oestrous cycle (cyclic) or after first insemination) (groups without embryos and with embryos). Values (mean ± SD) represents five uterine horns examined in two strips from each one and are expressed as a percentage of changes in the contractile activity before the treatment. $^{**}P < 0.01$, $^{***}P < 0.001$ as compared to the contractile activity before the treatment; *a*, *b*, *c* indicates differences between groups (cyclic, without embryos and with embryos)

Discussion

The presented results demonstrate the influence of biologically active substances on smooth muscle contractility collected from cyclic gilts and uterine horns with or without embryos. The results indicate that in the uterus with embryos contractile activity is increased in comparison to the uterus with not embryos. These differences were clearer when compared to contractility in the uterus of cyclic gilts. The experiments in vitro of Pope et al. [25] showed that myometrial contractility increased concomitantly with embryo migration.

In our studies the ACh increased tension in the smooth muscle of the uterus, which was the highest in the strips of pregnant uterus, with a simultaneous decrease in amplitude. Moreover, the frequency of contractions in the strips of the uterus without embryos was higher as compared to the uterine horn with embryos. Our results are consistent with the results of other authors. Kim et al. [26] observed that after administration of carbachol, a muscarinic receptor agonist, the force of contraction of the uterus in pregnant rats was several times higher than in the non-pregnant uterus. Kitazawa et al. [5] found that both exogenous and endogenous ACh cause contraction of the uterine muscle in the pig by the activation of the muscarinic M_3 receptor. Our results also indicated that in the uterine strips with embryos the highest increase in tension is combined with a higher decrease of amplitude and a lower increase in the frequency of contractions as compared to the other groups examined. This data indicate that the high motor activity in the gravid horn can promote uniform distribution of the multiple embryos in the lumen of the pig uterus.

One of the regulatory mechanisms affecting uterine contractile activity is the stimulation of α- and β-adrenergic receptors by catecholamines such as NA. In our study, we observed that NA had no significant effect on muscle tension in any group during the 10-min observation period, although in some strips (in each group) a short-term increase in tension after its administration was seen. However, in comparison to the group I NA had a significant influence on the changes of amplitude and frequency of contractions in group IIb, which suggests that the presence of the embryo in the uterus affects the regulation of contractile activity. It is suggested that inhibition of uterine contractile activity is due to a prevalence of β-adrenergic over the α-adrenergic receptors, and may be related to hormonal changes, particularly in the levels of ovarian steroid hormones, which affect the concentration and distribution of the population of muscarinic and adrenergic receptors [27–30]. Rexroad and Guthrie [31] suggested that a reduction in the number of α-adrenergic receptors in the early days of pregnancy may be associated with the migration and implantation of embryos. In this way, the embryos may affect the uterus, e.g., causing changes in the expression of maternal factors. Furthermore, it was observed that embryos may physically affect the uterus by, e.g., changing the expression of genes responsible for the release of biologically active substances [32].

In our study the greatest increase in the tension and frequency of contractions after OT administration was observed in group IIb. Franczak and Bogacki [18] using the same pig model showed that embryonic products locally regulate the abundance of OT receptors mRNA in the porcine uterus. Moreover, it has been shown that the number of receptors for this peptide at 14–16 days of gestation, compared with days 14–16 of the cycle, is similar in MYO but much higher in ENDO [16]. The role of OT receptors in early pregnancy is not fully understood. It is assumed that the peptide, by interaction with its receptors, affects the secretion of prostaglandins, including $PGF_{2\alpha}$ and PGE_2.

In our study, $PGF_{2\alpha}$ caused the largest increase in tension and amplitude in group IIb, with a decline in frequency in all groups. The weakest effect among all the tested substances was observed after PGE_2 treatment. However, in the ENDO/MYO strips of group IIb it increased the tension and frequency and decreased the amplitude of contractions. In the reproductive system prostaglandin $F_{2\alpha}$ and E_2 participates in the control of many process, including implantation of embryos and causing contractions of the uterus [33]. Dittrich et al. [34] demonstrated that human seminal plasma (consisting among others prostaglandins) has a direct effect on enhancing uterine contractility, which could facilitate sperm transport. It is suggested that prostaglandin secretion disorders during pregnancy are one of the causes of miscarriages and premature births. Currently, it is known that the myometrium secretes more PGE_2 than $PGF_2\alpha$ regardless of pregnancy status, and that the myometrium may be an additional important source of luteotrophic PGE_2 action during early pregnancy [17]. It was also found that PGs may play a significant role in embryo implantation and decidualization of the endometrium [23].

Kitazawa et al. [3], studying the activity of smooth muscle of the uterus of pregnant pig, stated, similarly to our study, that ACh, OT and $PGF_{2\alpha}$ increased contractility in muscle. However, in our study the tension and frequency of contractions were increased, while Kitazawa et al. [3] observed a reduction in the frequency of contractions. This difference may be due to the fact that in our study strips were taken at 12–14 days after first insemination, whereas Kitazawa et al. [3] used tissue from 25–60 days of pregnancy. It is accepted that pregnancy changes the expression of receptors, such as oxytocin receptor [35, 36] α_2-adrenoceptor [37] and prostanoids receptors [38]. Therefore, the increase in the expression of contractile receptors in the uteri of pregnant pigs was suggested to be another mechanism for the pregnancy-associated increase in the contractile responses.

Conclusions

Summarizing, ACh, OT, $PGF_{2\alpha}$ and PGE_2 significantly increased the tension and decreased the amplitude of contraction (except $PGF_{2\alpha}$ whose administration increased the amplitude) in gravid horns compared to non-gravid horns and cyclic gilts. The frequency of contractions was increased in the uterine horn with embryos after the administration of ACh and OT, but this parameter decreased after NA and $PGF_{2\alpha}$, and remained practically unchanged after the administration of PGE_2. Surprisingly, the contractility of the uterine smooth muscle collected from gravid horns exhibited higher activity than that obtained from non-gravid horns and cyclic gilts. Perhaps this is connected with the time of implantation and uniform distribution of embryos. From the data of this study it seem possible to speculate that the presence of embryos may increase the release of some substances which, by auto and paracrine regulation, affect uterine contractile activity.

Authors' contributions

MW conceived the study, and participated in its design, coordination and carried, and drafted the manuscript. MB took part in planning the experimental in vivo study and contributed to the set-up of the materials and methods. MB performed surgical procedures and collected materials for in vitro examinations. JJJ have been involved in revising it critically for important intellectual content and approval of the version to be published. All authors read and approved the final manuscript.

Author details

[1] Department of Pharmacology and Toxicology, Faculty of Veterinary Medicine, University of Warmia and Mazury, Oczapowskiego Street 13, 10-718 Olsztyn, Poland. [2] Institute of Animal Reproduction and Food Research, Polish Academy of Sciences, Bydgoska Street 7, 10-243 Olsztyn, Poland.

Acknowledgements

The study was supported by the Grant No. 15.610.008-300 from the University of Warmia and Mazury in Olsztyn. Publication costs were covered by KNOW (Leading National Research Centre) Scientific Consortium "Healthy Animal-Safe Food", decision of Ministry of Science and Higher Education No. 05-1/KNOW2/2015.

Competing interests

The authors declare that they have no competing interests.

References

1. Taneike T, Narita T, Kitazawa T, Bando S, Teraoka H, Ohga A. Binding and functional characterization of alpha-2 adrenoceptors in isolated swine myometrium. J Auton Pharmacol. 1995;15:93–105.
2. Cao J, Shayibuzhati M, Tajima T, Kitazawa T, Taneike T. In vitro pharmacological characterization of the prostanoid receptor population in the non-pregnant porcine myometrium. Eur J Pharmacol. 2002;442:115–23.
3. Kitazawa T, Hatakeyama H, Cao J, Taneike T. Pregnancy-associated changes in responsiveness of the porcine myometrium to bioactive substances. Eur J Pharmacol. 2003;469:135–44.
4. Markiewicz W, Kamińska K, Bogacki M, Maślanka T, Jaroszewski JJ. Participation of analogues of lysophosphatidic acid (LPA): oleoyl-sn-glycero-3-phosphate (L-alpha-LPA) and 1-oleoyl-2-O-methyl-rac-glycerophosphothionate (OMPT) in uterine smooth muscle contractility of the pregnant pigs. Pol J Vet Sci. 2012;15:635–43.
5. Kitazawa T, Uchiyama F, Hirose K, Taneike T. Characterization of the muscarinic receptor subtype that mediates the contractile response of acetylcholine in the swine myometrium. Eur J Pharmacol. 1999;367:325–34.
6. Kitazawa T, Kajiwara T, Kiuchi A, Hatakeyama H, Taneike T. Muscle layer- and region-dependent distributions of oxytocin receptors in the porcine myometrium. Peptides. 2001;22:963–74.
7. Mueller A, Maltaris T, Siemer J, Binder H, Hoffmann I, Beckmann MW, et al. Uterine contractility in response to different prostaglandins: results from extracorporeally perfused non-pregnantswine uteri. Hum Reprod. 2006;21:2000–5.
8. Dittrich R, Mueller A, Oppelt PG, Hoffmann I, Beckmann MW, Maltaris T. Differences in muscarinic-receptor agonist-, oxytocin-, and prostaglandin induced uterine contractions. Fertil Steril. 2009;92:1694–700.
9. Kucharski J, Jaroszewski JJ, Jana B, Górska J, Kozłowska A, Markiewicz W. The influence of inflammatory process on prostaglandin F2alpha contractile activity in porcine uterus. J Anim Feed Sci. 2007;16:654–67.
10. Jana B, Jaroszewski JJ, Kucharski J, Koszykowska M, Górska J, Markiewicz W. Participation of prostaglandin E2 in contractile activity of inflamed porcine uterus. Acta Vet Brno. 2010;79:249–59.
11. Kitazawa T, Shishido H, Sato T, Taneike T. Histamine mediates the muscle layer-specific responses in the isolated swine myometrium. J Vet Pharmacol Ther. 1997;20:187–97.
12. Markiewicz W, Jaroszewski JJ, Bossowska A, Majewski M. NPY: its occurrence and relevance in the female reproductive system. Folia Histochem Cytobiol. 2003;41:183–92.
13. Isaka M, Takaoka K, Yamada Y, Abe Y, Kitazawa T, Taneike T. Characterization of functional endothelin receptors in the porcine myometrium. Peptides. 2000;21:543–51.
14. Kitazawa T, Nakagoshi K, Teraoka H, Taneike T. 5-HT(7) receptor and β_2-adrenoceptor share in the inhibition of porcine uterine contractility in a muscle layer-dependent manner. Eur J Pharmacol. 2001;433:187–97.
15. Buxton IL. Regulation of uterine function: a biochemical conundrum in the regulation of smooth muscle relaxation. Mol Pharmacol. 2004;65:1051–9.
16. Franczak A, Ciereszko R, Kotwica G. Oxytocin (OT) action in uterine tissues of cyclic and early pregnant gilts: OT receptors concentration, prostaglandin $F_{2\alpha}$ secretion, and phosphoinositide hydrolysis. Anim Reprod Sci. 2005;88:325–39.
17. Franczak A, Kurowicka B, Oponowicz A, Petroff BK, Kotwica G. The effect of progesterone on oxytocin-stimulated intracellular mobilization of Ca^{2+} and prostaglandin E_2 and $F_{2\alpha}$ secretion from porcine myometrial cells. Prostaglandins Other Lipid Mediat. 2006;81:37–44.
18. Franczak A, Bogacki M. Local and systemic effects of embryos on uterine tissues during early pregnancy in pigs. J Reprod Dev. 2009;55:262–72.
19. Jana B, Jaroszewski JJ, Czarzasta J, Włodarczyk M, Markiewicz W. Synthesis of prostacyclin and its effect on the contractile activity of the inflamed porcine uterus. Theriogenology. 2013;79:470–85.
20. Langendijk P, Bouwman EG, Soede NM, Taverne MA, Kemp B. Myometrial activity around estrus in sows: spontaneous activity and effects of estrogens, cloprostenol, seminal plasma and clenbuterol. Theriogenology. 2002;57:1563–77.
21. Langendijk P, Soede NM, Kemp B. Uterine activity, sperm transport, and the role of boar stimuli around insemination in sows. Theriogenology. 2005;63:500–13.
22. Kurowicka B, Franczak A, Oponowicz A, Kotwica G. In vitro contractile activity of porcine myometrium during luteolysis and early pregnancy: effect of oxytocin and progesterone. Reprod Biol. 2005;5:151–69.
23. Zięcik AJ, Wacławik MM, Kaczmarek A, Blitek B, Moza Jalali B, Andronowska A. Mechanisms for the establishment of pregnancy in the pig. Reprod Domest Anim. 2011;46:31–41.
24. Wasielak M, Głowacz M, Kamińska K, Wacławik A, Bogacki M. The influence of embryo presence on prostaglandins synthesis and prostaglandin E2 and F2alpha content in corpora lutea during periimplantation period in the pig. Mol Reprod Dev. 2008;75:1208–16.
25. Pope WF, Maurer RR, Stormshak F. Intrauterine migration of the porcine embryo-interaction of embryo, uterine flushings and indomethacin on myometrial function in vitro. J Anim Sci. 1982;55:1169–78.
26. Kim BK, Ozaki H, Hori M, Takahashi K, Karaki H. Increased contractility of rat uterine smooth muscle at the end of pregnancy. Comp Biochem Physiol. 1998;121:165–73.
27. Roberts JM, Insel PA, Goldfien RD, Goldfien A. α-adrenoceptors but not β-adrenoceptors increase in rabbit uterus with oestrogen. Nature. 1977;270:624–5.
28. Williams LT, Lefkowitz RJ. Regulation of rabbit myometrial receptors by estrogen and progesterone. J Clinic Invest. 1977;60:815–8.
29. Choppin A, Stepan GJ, Loury DN, Watson N, Eglen RM. Characterization of the muscarinic receptor in isolated uterus of sham operated and ovariectomized rats. Br J Pharmacol. 1999;127:1551–8.
30. Ontsouka EC, Reist M, Graber H, Blum JW, Steiner A, Hirsbrunner G. Expression of messenger RNA coding for 5-HT receptor, alpha and beta adrenoreceptor (subtypes) during oestrus and dioestrus in the bovine uterus. J Vet Med A Physiol Pathol Clin Med. 2004;51:385–93.
31. Rexroad CE Jr, Guthrie HD. Alpha-adrenergic receptors in myometrium of pregnant and nonpregnant pigs until day 19 postestrus. Biol Reprod. 1983;29:615–9.
32. Kennedy TG, Gillio-Meina C, Phang SH. Prostaglandins and the initiation of blastocyst implantation and decidualization. Reproduction. 2007;134:635–43.
33. Herschman HR. Prostaglandin synthase 2. Biochim Biophys Acta. 1996;1299:125–40.
34. Dittrich R, Henning J, Maltaris T, Hoffmann I, Oppelt PG, Cupisti S, et al. Extracorporeal perfusion of the swine utersu: effect of of human seminal plasma. Andrologia. 2012;44:543–9.

7

Cervid herpesvirus 2 and not *Moraxella bovoculi* caused keratoconjunctivitis in experimentally inoculated semi-domesticated Eurasian tundra reindeer

Morten Tryland[1*], Javier Sánchez Romano[1], Nina Marcin[1,4], Ingebjørg Helena Nymo[1], Terje Domaas Josefsen[2,5], Karen Kristine Sørensen[3] and Torill Mørk[2]

Abstract

Background: Infectious keratoconjunctivitis (IKC) is a transmissible disease in semi-domesticated Eurasian reindeer (*Rangifer tarandus tarandus*). It is regarded as multifactorial and a single causative pathogen has not yet been identified. From clinical outbreaks we have previously identified Cervid herpesvirus 2 (CvHV2) and *Moraxella bovoculi* as candidates for experimental investigations. Eighteen reindeer were inoculated in the right eye with CvHV2 (n = 5), *M. bovoculi* (n = 5), CvHV2 and *M. bovoculi* (n = 5) or sterile saline water (n = 3; controls).

Results: All animals inoculated with CvHv2, alone or in combination with *M. bovoculi*, showed raised body temperature, increased lacrimation, conjunctivitis, excretion of pus and periorbital oedema; clinical signs that increased in severity from day 2 post inoculation (p.i.) and throughout the experiment, until euthanasia 5–7 days p.i. Examination after euthanasia revealed corneal oedema, and three animals displayed a corneal ulcer. CvHV2 could be identified in swab samples from both the inoculated eye and the control eye from most animals and time points, indicating a viral spread from the inoculation site.

Conclusions: This study showed that CvHV2 alone and in combination with *M. bovoculi* was able to cause the characteristic clinical signs of IKC in reindeer, whereas inoculation of *M. bovoculi* alone, originally isolated from a reindeer with IKC, did not produce clinical signs. Previous studies have suggested that herding procedures, animal stress and subsequent reactivation of latent CvHV2 infection in older animals is a plausible mechanism for IKC outbreaks among reindeer calves and young animals in reindeer herds. However, further studies are needed to fully understand the infection biology and epidemiology associated with IKC in reindeer.

Keywords: Alphaherpesvirus, Eye disease, IKC, Moraxella, Ophthalmology, Reindeer, Wildlife

Background

Infectious keratoconjunctivitis (IKC) has been reported in semi-domesticated Eurasian tundra reindeer (*Rangifer tarandus tarandus*) in Fennoscandia for more than a century [1], causing outbreaks among calves of the year (<1 year) and young animals particularly [2–4]. The first sign of the disease is increased lacrimation observed as an untidy and miscoloured periocular hair coat followed by conjunctivitis and increasing periorbital and corneal oedema. The oedema is giving the eye an opaque, and whitish to bluish appearance (Fig. 1a), which is how IKC is usually recognized in the field by reindeer herders. In the absence of spontaneous healing, the infection progresses with an increasing severity of conjunctivitis and oedema, corneal ulceration, and panophthalmitis leading to permanent blindness (Fig. 1b). For reindeer, that spend most of the year free-ranging and unattended, this

*Correspondence: morten.tryland@uit.no
[1] Arctic Infection Biology, Department of Arctic and Marine Biology, UiT-The Arctic University of Norway, POBox 6050, Langnes, 9037 Tromsø, Norway

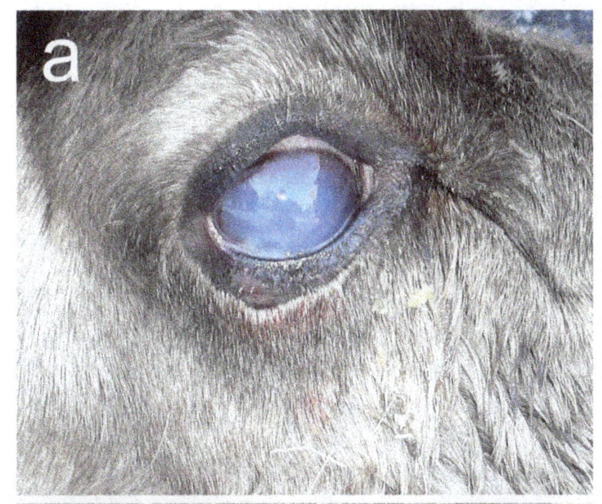

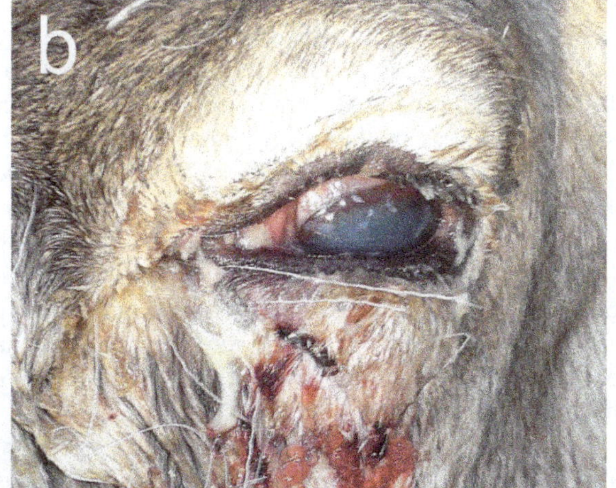

Fig. 1 Infectious keratoconjunctivitis (IKC) during an outbreak among free-ranging Eurasian semi-domesticated tundra reindeer (*Rangifer tarandus tarandus*): **a** corneal oedema indicated by an opaque and discolored cornea. **b** Severe grade of IKC with panophthalimitis, oedema and haemorrhage. This condition often involves corneal ulcer and may lead to permanent blindness

disease represents an important animal welfare issue as well as a potential source of economic loss for the herders [2, 4].

In spite of long-term awareness of IKC in reindeer, a causative agent has not yet been identified and IKC in reindeer is regarded as a multi-factorial disease, similar to infectious bovine keratoconjunctivitis (IBK), commonly referred to as "pinkeye" in cattle. The Gram-negative bacterium *Moraxella bovis* is suggested as the causative agent of IBK [5], although recent studies have shown that *Moraxella bovoculi*, originally identified in 2002 and shown to be distinct from *M. bovis*, may also be associated with IBK [6, 7]. A disease similar to IKC has also been documented in sheep and goats [8, 9], as well as in a wide range of wild animal species, such as moose (*Alces alces*), mule deer (*Odocoileus hemionus*), ibex (*Capra ibex*), chamois (*Rupicapra rupicapra*), roe deer (*Capreolus capreolus*) and red deer (*Cervus elaphus*). Many different infectious agents have been associated with the disease in the different species [10–14], of which the majority have been bacteria, including known potential pathogens such as *Mycoplasma* spp.

Similarly, many different bacteria have been isolated from reindeer with IKC, such as *M. bovoculi*, *M. ovis*, *Pasteurella multocida*, and *Trueperella pyogenes* [2–4, 15, 16]. In a recent study of reindeer in Norway, Sweden and Finland, analyses of swab samples from the conjunctiva of clinically healthy reindeer and of reindeer with clinical IKC, showed that *M. bovoculi* was the bacterial agent that was most prevalent [17].

However, during an outbreak of IKC in reindeer in Troms County, Norway, the reindeer alphaherpesvirus, cervid herpesvirus 2 (CvHV2), was identified as the primary infectious agent based on the finding of this virus during the early clinical stages of the disease. Bacteria such as *M. bovoculi* seemed to dominate during later stages of IKC along with declining virus titers from the swab samples of the conjunctiva of affected animals [4].

In addition, environmental factors such as stress associated with gathering, corralling, handling and transport, reduced body condition or emaciation, exposure to UV light, and a dry and dusty environment may impact the pathogenesis of IKC in reindeer [2, 18, 19]. During natural outbreaks of IKC in reindeer, it is difficult to gain an overview of which potential pathogens are involved. It is also challenging to conduct a controlled sampling regime and to register the onset and development of disease. In addition, it is difficult to control environmental factors. In this study, reindeer calves <1 year old were inoculated with CvHV2 and *M. bovoculi*, which are considered the two most relevant candidates for IKC [4, 17]. The aim of this study was to investigate if experimental inoculation with CvHV2, *M. bovoculi*, or a combination of the two agents, was able to cause clinical IKC in reindeer.

Methods

Animals

Semi-domesticated Eurasian tundra reindeer (n = 27) calves, approximately 11 months old, were gathered from their mountain pastures. They were corralled and physically restrained for ID-tagging (plastic collar) and sampling to check for previous exposure to CvHV2 and *M. bovoculi*. Blood was obtained with a vacutainer system from the jugular vein and serum prepared by centrifugation and stored at −20 °C. For virological investigation, sterile cotton swabs were used to sample the conjunctiva bilaterally, the nostrils and the vagina (females). Swabs were subsequently placed in 1.8 ml cryotubes with 800 µl of Eagle's minimum essential medium (EMEM) containing antibiotics (10,000 U/ml penicillin and 10 mg/ml streptomycin; 1 ml/l of gentamicin, 50 mg/ml and 10 ml/l of amphotericin B 250 μg/ml; EMEMab 10 ml/l) and stored at −80 °C. For bacteriological investigation, a swab (Transwab^R, Medical Wire & Equipment, Wiltshire, UK) was introduced into both conjunctivae, rubbed gently against the mucosal lining and placed in its transport medium container. Blood samples were tested for antibodies against CvHV2. Swab samples from the conjunctiva and nostrils were tested for the presence of CvHV2 DNA (nested polymerase chain reaction [PCR]), whereas swab samples from conjunctiva were tested for *M. bovoculi* (cultivation), as described below. Based on the test results, 21 animals (5 females and 16 males) with no indication of previous exposure to CvHV2 or *M. bovoculi* were recruited to the study. The animals were corralled together in a fence (see below) for a habituation period of four weeks before inoculation. The inoculation experiment lasted for a total of 15 days.

All animals were chemically immobilized and weighed twice during the study, i.e. on day 0 (inoculation) and on the day of euthanasia. Animals were immobilized by darting (Dan-Inject JM Special; Dan-Inject ApS, Børkop, Denmark) using a combination of medetomidine (Zalopine® 10 mg/ml, Orion Corporation Animal Health, Espoo, Finland) and ketamine (Ketalar® 50 mg/ml, Pfizer AS, Oslo, Norway) at a fixed ratio of 1:5 (mg:mg) medetomidine:ketamine. When the inoculation process was completed, sedation was reversed by intramuscular injection of atipamezole (Antisedan™; Atipamezole 5 mg/ml, Zoetis, UK) at a fixed ratio of 5:1 atipamezole:medetomidine and animals were monitored until they were standing. Despite using recommended drugs and doses being reduced to one-third of those recommended for semi-domesticated reindeer [20], three reindeer (one female, two males) died from acute shock-like complications. Similar complications did not occur during the second round of chemical immobilization using the same drugs and doses. When chemically immobilized, body temperature was measured with a digital clinical thermometer (Fluke Thermometer 51/52 II; Fluke Norge, Oslo, Norway), with a sensor positioned 30 cm inside the rectum. Pulse rate and arterial oxyhemoglobin (SpO_2) was measured with a handheld pulse oximeter (Masimo RAD 57; Masimo International Sàrl, Neuchatel, Switzerland) with the clip-sensor applied to the tongue. Respiratory rate was recorded by counting breathing movements of the chest using a stopwatch.

Animals were euthanized at different time points during the experiment using a captive bolt stunning gun followed by bleeding of the jugular vein. Animals R19 (CvHV2-group) and R16 (*M. bovoculi* group) were euthanized on day 2 and 3 respectively, due to fracture of the femur. Animals in the two groups inoculated with CvHV2 (alone or in combination with *M. bovoculi*) were euthanized according to defined animal welfare end-points on days 3–7 post inoculation (p.i.) (Table 1). Remaining animals of the *M. bovoculi* group were euthanized on day 6 (n = 1) and day 13 (n = 3) p.i., whereas the control animals (n = 3) were euthanized on day 15 p.i. Animals with no other clinical symptoms besides those observed in the eyes were sampled in the animal experimental facility, whereas animals with trauma and animals that experienced respiratory distress upon chemical immobilization were subjected to a full necropsy in an attempt to determine the cause of these unexpected complications.

Animal facility, feeding and handling

Animals were introduced to an outdoor field research facility on May 6th, 2014. The corral consists of one large pen (approx. 100 × 80 m) and four smaller pens (approx. 50 × 50 m), all separated from each other and from the surrounding areas by 2.5 m high steel wire fences. The ground inside the pens was covered with a deep layer of snow in the beginning, but due to snow melting and greening in the spring, fresh grass pasture became available. Animals were ID-tagged with an ear tag and by spraying a number on the fur on both sides of the body to ensure easy identification. They were corralled together for the first four weeks (habituation period) to get used to the facility, the feed and the presence of people.

The animals were fed lichen (*Cladina* spp.), which was gradually replaced by commercial pelleted feed for reindeer (Reinsdyrfôr, Felleskjøpet, Trondheim, Norway). 1 week before inoculation and throughout the remaining experiment, the animals were fed pellets ad libitum, supplemented with lichen. Fresh water was provided and changed on a daily basis. Body condition, evaluated by visual inspection and palpation, varied from medium to lean, but increased during the habituation period. On the day of inoculation, the animals weighed 37–59 kg (mean 49.1 kg) and were separated into four groups without further contact (Control, CvHV2, *M. bovoculi* and CvHV2/*M. bovoculi*).

During the entire study, the animals were fed and inspected three times a day by veterinarians licenced for conducting animal experiments. A record was kept describing the behaviour of each animal, condition, food intake and interactions between animals as well as development of clinical signs.

Except for day 0 (inoculation) and on the day of euthanasia at varying time points p.i. when animals were chemically immobilized, all other close inspections and sampling were conducted during physical restraint. However, on days when animals were not handled, the evaluation and development of clinical signs was observed at a distance of a few metres with binoculars.

Table 1 Clinical signs from the right eye of 10 semi-domesticated Eurasian tundra reindeer (*Rangifer tarandus tarandus*) after inoculation with cervid herpesvirus 2 (CvHV2; n = 5) or a combination of CvHV2 and *Moraxella bovoculi* (n = 5) (data from animals inoculated with *M. bovoculi* alone or from control animals are not shown)

Inoculum	ID	Day 0	Day 1	Day 2	Day 3	Day 4	Day 5	Day 6	Day 7
CvHV2	R4	None		Pus (2)[a] P-oedema (1)[b] Conjunctivitis	Pus (2) P-oedema (3)	Lacrimation P-oedema (3)	Pus (3) P-oedema (3) Corneal oedema T: 40.3	Pus (3) P-oedema (3)	*Pus (3)* *P-oedema (3)* *Conjunctivitis* *Corneal oedema* *T: 39.8*
	R5	None		Pus (1) P-oedema (1)	Pus (3) P-oedema (2)	Pus (3) P-oedema (3)	*Pus (3)* *P-oedema (3)* *Corneal oedema* *Corneal ulcer: 12 mm* *T: 40.5*		
	R10	None		Pus (3) P-oedema (1) Conjunctivitis	Pus (3) P-oedema (2)	Pus (3) P-oedema (3)	*Pus (3)* *P-oedema (3)* *Conjunctivitis* *Corneal oedema* *T: 40.0*		
	R19	None		*Lacrimation* *Pus (1)* *P-oedema (1)* [c]					
	R21	None		P-oedema (1)	Lacrimation Pus (2) P-oedema (2)	Lacrimation Pus (2) P-oedema (2)	Pus (2) P-oedema (2) Corneal oedema Corneal ulcer: 4 mm	*Pus (3)* *P-oedema (3)* *Corneal oedema* *Corneal ulcer: 10 mm* *T: 40.1*	
CvHV2 and *M. bovoculi*	R1	None	Pus (1)	Lacrimation Pus (1) P-oedema (1) Red sclera	Lacrimation Pus (2) P-oedema (2)	Pus (2) Lacrimation P-oedema (2)	Pus (3) P-oedema (3) Corneal oedema T: 40.4	Pus (3) P-oedema (3)	*P-oedema (3)* *Conjunctivitis* *Corneal oedema* *Corneal ulcer: 3 mm* *T: 39.1*
	R3	None		Lacrimation P-oedema (1)	Pus (3) P-oedema (3)	Pus (3) P-oedema (3)	P-oedema (3) Adherent pus Blue cornea T: 40.0	*Pus (3)* *Conjunctivitis* *Corneal oedema* *T: 39.8*	
	R7	None		Pus (1)	Pus (2) Lacrimation P-oedema (2)	Pus (2) Lacrimation P-oedema (2)	*Pus (3)* *P-oedema (3)* *Conjunctivitis* *Corneal oedema* *T: 40.3*		
	R13	None		Pus (1) Lacrimation Red sclera P-oedema (2)	Pus (3) Lacrimation P-oedema (2)	*Pus (3)* *P-oedema (3)* *Conjunctivitis* *Corneal oedema* *T: 40.4*			
	R17	None	Dry cornea	Pus (1) Lacrimation P-oedema (2)	*Pus (3)* *P-oedema (2)* *T: 40.9*				

Clinical signs are indicated, relative to the day of inoculation (day 0). Observations during day 1, day 3, day 4 and day 6 were conducted without handling the animals, whereas all animals were captured (physical restraint) and sampled at day 2 and day 5

The time of euthanasia for each animal is indicated with italic text

[a] Pus: (1) small amounts (clots), (2) large amounts, and (3) huge amounts of pus, adherent to eyelids/skin and covering the eye

[b] P-oedema: periorbital oedema: (1) slight swelling of conjunctiva, (2) severe oedema, and (3) extensive oedema, periorbital tissues covering the eyeball

[c] Euthanized due to trauma

Preparation of inocula

CvHV2 was originally isolated from the conjunctiva of a reindeer with clinical IKC [4]. The virus was propagated in Madin-Darby bovine kidney (MDBK) cells (ATCC CCL22) in EMEM supplemented with 10% horse serum (LGC Standards, Middlesex, UK). Virus cultures were harvested when more than 90% of the cells showed cytopathic effect (CPE). Cellular debris was removed by centrifugation (7800g, 30 min) and viral particles in the supernatant were pelleted through a 30% sucrose cushion (20,000 g, 1 h), re-suspended in 5 ml PBS, filtered through a 0.45 μm cellulose filter (Merck Millipore, Darmstadt, Germany) and frozen at −80 °C. The virus titre of the inoculum was 5.8×10^6 $TCID_{50}$/ml.

The *M. bovoculi* strain used for inoculation was originally cultivated from a swab sample from the conjunctiva of a Norwegian reindeer with clinical IKC in 2014. The colonies were 2–3 mm in diameter, yellow/grey, round, with a shiny "fat" appearance, and revealed beta-haemolysis after 24 h growth on blood agar. The colonies grew at 37 °C, but only in aerobic conditions (without CO_2). The bacteria were Gram negative with a coccoid form, and the catalase and oxidase tests were positive. Potential virulence factors were not investigated. The isolate was verified as *M. bovoculi* by 16s rRNA sequencing (data not shown). After storage (−80 °C), the isolate was cultivated on 5% sheep blood agar at 37 °C under aerobic conditions for 24 h prior to inoculation. The bacterium underwent a total of four in vitro passages (from isolation to inoculation).

Inoculation

While the animals were sedated, both eyes were photographed and checked for general clinical signs and for corneal ulcers using the fluorescein test (Fluoresceinnatrium Minims 20 mg/ml; Chauvin, Surrey, UK). Disposable coats and gloves were used by all persons involved in the inoculation and sampling of the animals. For any intervention with the animals (feeding, inoculation, sampling), the control group was visited before the inoculated animals.

Prior to inoculation and at each of the following inspections, eyes were photographed, sampled (swab) and checked for corneal ulcers using fluorescein, followed by thorough flushing of the eyes with sterile water. Local anaesthesia (Oxibuprokain Minims 4 mg/ml; Chauvin) was applied in the right eye 4 min prior to a mild rubbing of the conjunctival mucosa with sterile sandpaper (grade 60).

The virus was inoculated by introducing a small sterile cotton cushion, soaked in PBS/CvHV2, to the conjunctiva under the lower eyelid and keeping it there for 4 min. *M. bovoculi* was inoculated by picking a colony of *M. bovoculi* from the agar plate with a sterile cotton stick and spreading it onto the rubbed area of the conjunctiva. Bacterial colonies from the same plate were subsequently reseeded onto new agar plates to check for viability. These procedures for viral and bacterial inoculations were conducted to allow access of virus and bacteria in excess to slightly scarified mucosal cells of the conjunctiva. When inoculating both CvHV2 and *M. bovoculi* in the same eye, the virus was inoculated first, followed by the bacterium after 10 min. For the animals in the control group, a sterile cotton stick was soaked in sterile water and applied onto the rubbed conjunctiva. The left eye was inspected as described above, but not further manipulated, and served as a control for each animal (all groups).

Bacterial cultivation

Swab samples from the conjunctiva of both eyes, obtained on the day of inoculation (Day 0) and every second day after inoculation, were subjected to cultivation on a 5% sheep blood agar plate. The plates were incubated aerobically at 37 °C and inspected after 24 and 48 h. Bacterial colonies that were yellow to grey of colour, 2–3 mm in diameter, with a shiny "fat" appearance and were beta-haemolytic, were suspected to be *Moraxella* spp. Such colonies were sub-cultured for purity and further characterized (morphology, Gram staining, catalase, oxidase). Selected isolates were subsequently identified to species level (score > 2) by MALDI-TOF mass spectrometry (Microflex; Bruker UK Limited, Coventry, UK).

DNA extraction, PCR and sequencing

To verify that the animals did not harbour CvHV2 viral particles in the conjunctival mucosa prior to the experiment, DNA was extracted from swabs obtained from the conjunctival mucosa (QIAamp® DNA Mini Kit, Hilden, Germany) with a mean output of 8.1 ng/μl (SD = 8.0) and a nested PCR was conducted as described previously [21]. The inner primer set amplified a 294 bp region of the *UL27* gene encoding glycoprotein B (gB), which is a highly conserved gene region among ruminant alphaherpesviruses [22]. CvHV2 (strain Salla 82) [23] and BoHV1 [24] were used as positive controls. PCR amplicons were separated by agarose gel electrophoresis and visualized with ethidium bromide (Sigma-Aldrich Norway AS, Oslo, Norway).

A quantitative real-time Taqman Probe based PCR (qPCR), amplifying a 95 bp fragment in a different region of the *UL27* gene as compared to the nested PCR and shown previously to detect Rangiferine herpesvirus (now designated CvHV2), was performed as described previously [25]. The PCR was conducted with two slight modifications; the annealing temperature was reduced to 58.9 °C (following thermal gradient analysis) and the volume of nuclease-free water was increased from 4.0 to 4.5 μl for a total reaction volume of 25 µl. Samples were run in duplicates. A positive control (CvHV2, used as inoculum) [4], a negative control (DNA extracted from muscular tissue of a CvHV2 seronegative control animal), and a non-template control containing all PCR-components except DNA were included on each plate. This technique was used to analyse all eye swab and plasma samples collected from day 0 and throughout the experiment.

PCR amplicons were prepared for nucleotide sequencing by enzymatic removal of unused dNTP and primers (ExoSAP-IT™; Amersham Pharmacia Biotech, Sweden), after which sequencing was conducted (BigDye® Terminator v3.1 cycle sequencing kit; Applied Biosystems, Norway) in an Applied Biosystems 3130 XL Genetic Analyzer (Applied Biosystems).

Serology

Serum samples were investigated for anti-alphaherpesvirus antibodies using a commercial bovine enzyme-linked immunosorbent assay (ELISA; gB Blocking, LSI Laboratoire Service International, Lissieu, France) based on BoHV1 glycoprotein B (gB) as an antigen. The kit was previously validated against a virus neutralization test (VNT) for analyzing reindeer serum samples for anti-CvHV2 antibodies [26]. All serum samples were tested in duplicate and evaluated against bovine (provided with the kit) and reindeer [27] positive-control sera.

Results

Clinical signs

A thorough clinical examination, including body temperature measurement, was conducted on each animal when they were physically or chemically immobilized, i.e. upon arrival to the fence, on the day of inoculation one month later (day 0), and on days 2, 5, 7, 13 and 15 p.i., as well as upon euthanasia, if euthanized outside this schedule.

Body temperature (n = 18) at the time of inoculation (day 0) varied from 37.8 to 39.5 °C (mean 39.0 °C, SD 0.05). On day 5 p.i., the mean body temperature for all inoculated animals (except the controls) had increased to 39.8–40.6 °C (mean 40.2 °C), and decreased again over the following days. Mean temperature also increased for the control animals (n = 3), from 39.0 °C (day 0) to 39.9 °C (day 7), after which it decreased to 39.6 °C (day 10) and 39.3 °C (day 15).

In the CvHV2 group, no clinical signs were observed on day 1 (Table 1). On day 2, the inoculated eyes of all animals in this group displayed conjunctival oedema, four of the five animals having purulent exudate and two having hyperaemia of the conjunctiva (3). From day 3 to day 5, the severity of the oedema typically increased from mild (grade 1) to severe (grade 3), involving the whole periorbital region by day 5. Similarly, the suppuration increased from mild (grade 1) to severe (grade 3) (Fig. 2). Upon inspection on day 5, two animals (R5 and R10) were euthanized, showing corneal oedema, high grades of periorbital oedema and suppuration, as well as a slightly raised body temperature, 40.5 and 40.0 °C, respectively. Similar clinical signs were observed for R21 and R4, which were euthanized on day 6 and 7, respectively (Fig. 2). Animals R5 and R21 had at the time of euthanasia developed a corneal ulcer, by day 5 and day 6, respectively.

In the *M. bovoculi* group, a grey or whitish exudate was observed associated with the lower eyelid of the

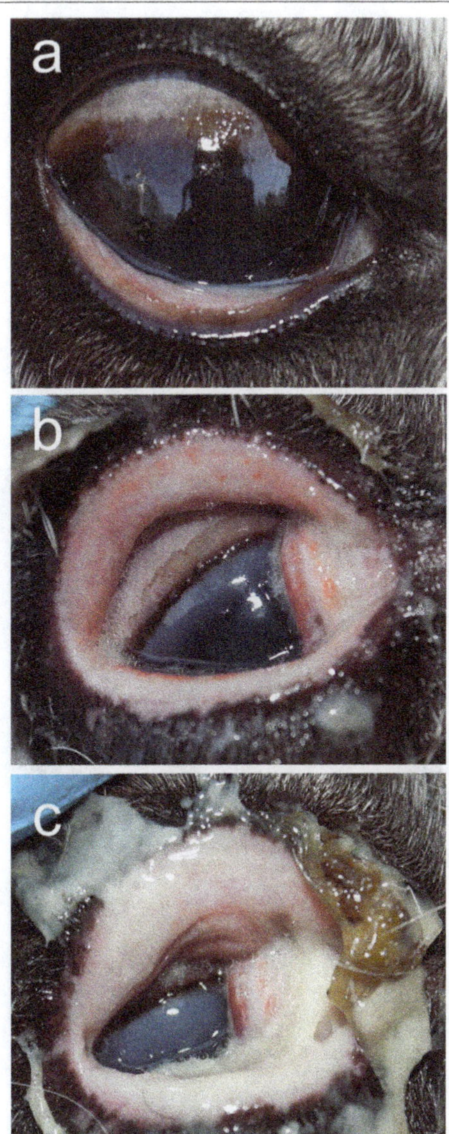

Fig. 2 Semi-domesticated Eurasian tundra reindeer (R21) experimentally inoculated with reindeer alphaherpesvirus (cervid herpesvirus 2; CvHV2). **a** Day 0, i.e. the day of inoculation, **b** day 5 post inoculation (p.i.), and **c** day 6 p.i.

inoculated right eye in two animals (R6 and R8) some hours after inoculation (day 0) and early the following day (day 1), which thereafter disappeared. No clinical signs were observed in this group throughout the remaining period of the experiment (Fig. 3).

The clinical signs observed in the group receiving both CvHV2 and *M. bovoculi* were indistinguishable from those described for the CvHV2 group (Table 1). All animals in this group, except the one euthanized on day 3 (R17), showed suppuration and developed conjunctivitis, and corneal and periorbital oedema (Fig. 4). One animal (R1) developed a corneal ulcer.

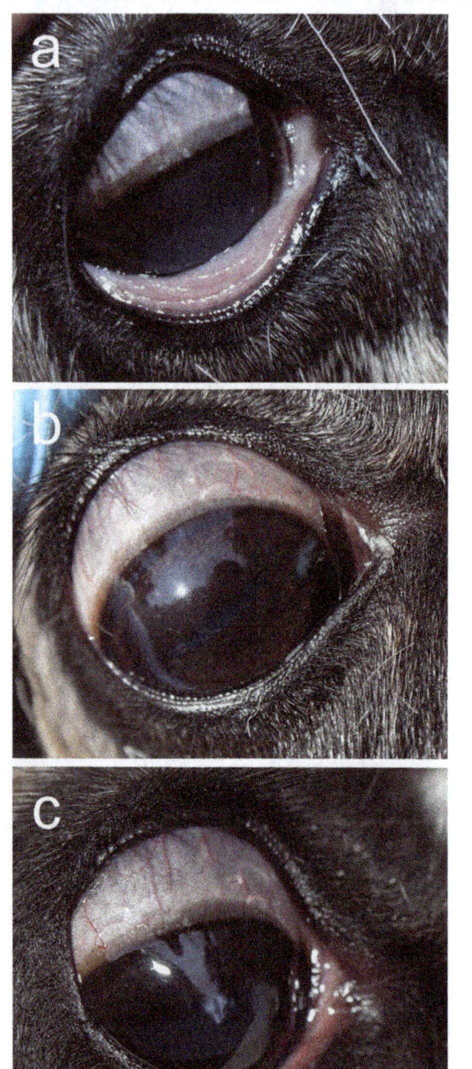

Fig. 3 Semi-domesticated Eurasian tundra reindeer (R15) inoculated with *Moraxella bovculi*. **a** Day 0, i.e. the day of inoculation, **b** day 5 post inoculation (p.i.), and **c** day 10 p.i.

No clinical signs of disease were recorded in the control animals (R2, R18, R20) throughout the experiment (day 0–15).

Bacteriology

On day 0, prior to inoculation, a few colonies of *M. bovoculi* were cultured from the conjunctiva of two animals (R6 and R8) from the group to be inoculated with *M. bovoculi*, and from another two animals (R1 and R17) from the group to be inoculated with CvHV2 and *M. bovoculi*. These isolates were all identified using the MALDI-TOF mass spectrometry. During the experiment, *M. bovoculi* was, at different time points, cultivated from all five animals inoculated with the bacterium. In the group inoculated with CvHV2 and *M. bovoculi*, the bacterium was cultivated from three of five animals. In the group inoculated with CvHV2 alone, *M. bovoculi* was cultivated from four of five animals. No *M. bovoculi* was isolated from the control animals. In most cases, *M. bovoculi* was found with few colonies in a mixed culture.

PCR

In spite of being sero-negative, CvHV2-specific DNA was detected in one eye swab (nested PCR; R21) before the experiment, and this animal was allocated to the CvHV2 group. No CvHV2-specific DNA was detected from conjunctival swab samples from this animal or any other swab samples (both eyes, all animals) taken on day 0 of the experiment, i.e. prior to inoculation. Of the animals inoculated with CvHV2, alone or in combination with *M. bovoculi*, CvHV2 specific DNA was detected (qPCR) in all samples from both inoculated and control eyes, from day 2 until the last sampling of each animal (euthanasia). There were two exceptions: CvHV2 could not be detected in the swab sample from the right (inoculated) eye of animal R3 on day 5 (the day before euthanasia, though detected again upon euthanasia, day 6), nor from the left eye (not inoculated) of animal R21 on day 6 (the day of euthanasia).

From the animals inoculated with only *M. bovoculi*, CvHV2-specific DNA was detected in one sample from the left eye of animal R6 on day 6, but besides this, all samples from animals in this group and the control group were negative for CvHV2. Viral DNA was detected in the plasma of one animal (R7) from the CvHV2-inoculated group on day 2 but not in the plasma of this animal at later time points, and not from plasma samples from any other animal during the experiment.

Serology (CvHV2)

All animals selected for the study were sero-negative for CvHV2 upon arrival and on the day of inoculation (day 0). Animals R21 and R4 from the group inoculated with

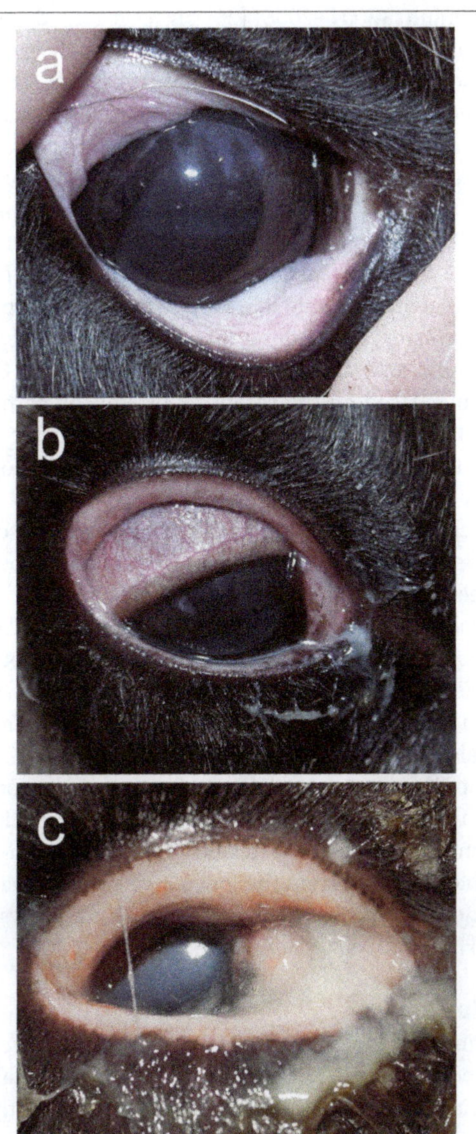

Fig. 4 Semi-domesticated Eurasian tundra reindeer (R1) inoculated with reindeer alphaherpesvirus (cervid herpesvirus 2; CvHV2) and *Moraxella bovculi*. **a** Day 0, i.e. the day of inoculation, **b** day 2 post inoculation (p.i.), and **c** day 5 p.i.

CvHV2 seroconverted on day 6 and 7, respectively, and animal R1 from the group inoculated with CvHV2 and *M. bovoculi* seroconverted on day 7.

Discussion

All animals inoculated with CvHV2, alone or in combination with *M. bovoculi* (Figs. 2 and 4) developed clinical signs characteristic of IKC [2, 4] with a quick onset (day 2) and rapid progression from day 2 to days 5/6/7 (euthanasia). The animals inoculated with *M. bovoculi* alone, and the control animals, remained healthy throughout the experiment. These unambiguous clinical results, generated from an experimental inoculation of one-year-old reindeer with all members of each animal group displaying similar responses, provide powerful support of previous findings during IKC outbreaks [4], that CvHV2 is capable of causing the clinical picture that is characteristic for IKC in reindeer.

The titres of the inoculum of virus and bacteria in this study were probably high as compared to viral and bacterial transmissions under natural conditions, but nevertheless, for the virus, in line with previous reported inoculations of BoHV1 in cattle [28]. It is, however, important to keep in mind that both the virus and the bacterium are replicative agents that, once the infection is established, will multiply in permissive cells, whereas virus and bacteria in excess will be washed away from the surface linings of the eye, rendering the inoculum titres less important.

We gently rubbed a part of the conjunctival mucosa of the lower eye lid to make sure that the infectious agents had access to permissive cells upon inoculation, but we chose not to conduct scarified corneal inoculations as has been done in similar experiments using cattle and *Moraxella* spp. [29]. The rubbing may be somewhat similar to what reindeer may experience when corralled and exposed to sand and dust in the pen. Thus, we think the conditions under which this experiment was carried out were in many ways close to a natural setting, including the fact that animals were young (<1 year) at the time of inoculation, and that they had been exposed to stress by being gathered from their mountain pastures, transported and corralled, and by being exposed to people and handling, all resembling natural herding conditions.

In IBK in cattle, the pathogenicity of *M. bovis* is based on the expression of a pilin protein for attachment [30] and a cytotoxin that damages the corneal epithelial cells [31]. However, *M. bovoculi* has also been associated with IBK. In a retrospective study of *Moraxella* spp. isolated from IBK outbreaks in 282 herds in 30 states of the USA, 701 were identified as *M. bovoculi* and 295 isolates as *M. bovis* [32]. It has also been shown that *M. bovoculi* isolates from cattle may have both putative cytotoxin [33] and pilin [34] genes, similar to those that have been identified in *M. bovis*. However, a randomized blind challenge study to assess the association between *M. bovis* and *M. bovoculi*, and IBK in 31 dairy calves, revealed that nine out of 10 calves inoculated with *M. bovis* developed corneal ulcers consistent with IBK, whereas none of the 10 calves inoculated with *M. bovoculi* did, although the authors stated that the pathogenicity of this particular *M. bovoculi* strain was not yet characterized [29]. This was also the situation for the *M. bovoculi* isolate used in our study, although it was originally isolated and identified as the bacterium that was dominating the bacterial growth from a swab sample obtained from the conjunctiva of a reindeer with clinical signs of IKC. Large genetic differences have recently been reported between isolates of *M. bovoculi* from eyes of cattle with IBK as compared to isolates from the nasopharynx of asymptomatic cattle, suggesting that certain genetically distinct strains of *M. bovoculi* are associated with IBK in cattle [35], which may also be the case for IKC in reindeer.

Throughout our study period, *M. bovoculi* was cultivated from eight of 10 animals that had been inoculated with the bacterium alone or in combination with CvHV2, but no clinical signs were associated with these findings in those inoculated with *M. bovoculi* alone. This might indicate that the isolate of *M. bovoculi* used for inoculation was not pathogenic, or that the duration of the bacterial infection was too short to produce clinical signs. *M. bovoculi* was also cultivated from four animals prior to inoculation (day 0), and from four animals inoculated with CvHV2 alone, from the right eye of all four animals and from both eyes of one individual. This may indicate the transmission of bacteria from other individuals, which means that *M. bovoculi* was transferred from inoculated animals into the other corrals. However, the fact that *M. bovoculi* was not cultivated from any of the control animals at any time (day 0–day 13 p.i.) indicated that *M. bovoculi* was not introduced but rather sporadically present in apparently healthy reindeer without ocular disease. The bacterium may therefore be a commensal in the conjunctiva of reindeer as also indicated from previous bacteriological screenings [17]. Since serology for antibodies against *M. bovoculi* prior to the inoculation was not conducted, it can be argued that a lack of clinical signs in the animals inoculated with *M. bovoculi* alone may be due to a pre-existing immunity against the bacterium, but it remains uncertain if presence of the bacterium on mucosal membranes such as conjunctiva and nasopharynx would elicit a detectable humoral immune response.

Animals R1 (CvHV2 and *M. bovoculi*), and R4 and R21 (CvHV2) had antibodies against CvHV2 on the day of euthanasia (day 6 and 7, respectively), whereas the other animals inoculated with CvHV2 assumingly were euthanized prior to sero-conversion. This is in line with previous inoculation experiments in reindeer with CvHV2 [36], in which a humoral immune response generally was not evident until days 8–10 p.i. Thus, the rapid onset of clinical signs after inoculation of CvHV2 in the conjunctiva indicates that a primary specific immune response will develop too late to be protective against disease in previously unexposed animals. This, and the observation that the seroprevalence among reindeer aged <1 year in Finnmark County, Norway, was only 8% as compared to 77% in adults (2004–2006) [26] suggests a rapid spread of the virus among young and immunologically naïve animals, sometimes resulting in outbreaks of IKC involving hundreds of animals [1, 18]. The hypothesis that stress causes reactivation of CvHV2 in latently infected animals [37] with subsequent viral shedding, exposing young and immunologically naïve animals to the virus, seems to be valid. During later stages of the disease, however, many different bacterial species, including *M. bovoculi*, have been isolated, but their role may be of a more opportunistic character, establishing infection and possibly being pathogenic once the mucosa is impacted by the CvHV2 infection. Based on the recent reports of the pathogenic properties of *M. bovoculi* in cattle, the pathogenic potential of the *M. bovoculi* isolates from reindeer should be further investigated.

No clinical signs were recorded in the three control animals, or in the left eye (control) of the inoculated reindeer (all groups). This lack of clinical signs in the left (control) eyes is in contrast to the detection of CvHV2-specific DNA from the left eyes of all CvHV2-inoculated animals from day 2 until the last sampling day, with the exceptions of animal R21 on day 6. At the same time, we were also unable to demonstrate viremia, since CvHV2-specific DNA was detected in a plasma sample from only one animal (R7) at one time point (day 2) during the experiment. Thus, these results indicate that the virus was able to spread from the inoculated conjunctiva to the conjunctival mucosa of the other eye within 2 days p.i. in all CvHV2- inoculated animals,

Conclusions

Experimental inoculation of semi-domesticated reindeer revealed that CvHV2 is capable of inducing typical clinical signs of IKC within 2–7 days p.i., suggesting that the reindeer alphaherpesvirus, CvHV2, is the transmissible and causative agent of IKC in reindeer. The combined inoculation of CvHV2 and *M. bovoculi* did not change the onset, development, or the character of the clinical signs. Ocular inoculation of *M. bovoculi* alone did not produce clinical signs. *M. bovoculi* and other bacteria may, however, be important as opportunistic pathogens, especially during later stages of the disease. Based on the recent reports of the pathogenic properties of *M. bovoculi* in cattle [35, 38], the pathogenic potential of the *M. bovoculi* isolates from reindeer should be further investigated.

Authors' contributions

MT, TDJ and TM designed the study. MT, JSR, NM, IHN, KKS, TDJ, and TM conducted the preparations, experiment and sampling. TDJ and TM conducted the necropsy of animals and further sampling. The laboratory analyses were conducted by JSR, NM, IHN and KKS. MT drafted the manuscript. All authors contributed to the manuscript and approved the final version. All authors read and approved the final manuscript.

Author details
[1] Arctic Infection Biology, Department of Arctic and Marine Biology, UiT-The Arctic University of Norway, POBox 6050, Langnes, 9037 Tromsø, Norway. [2] Norwegian Veterinary Institute, POBox 6050, Langnes, 9037 Tromsø, Norway. [3] Vascular Biology Research Group, Department of Medical Biology, Faculty of Health Sciences, UiT-The Arctic University of Norway, Tromsø, Norway. [4] Present Address: Clinique vétérinaire de l'abbatiale, 14 bis Rue Thibaut, 52220 Montier En Der, France. [5] Present Address: Faculty of Bioscience and Aquaculture, Nord University, Bodø, Norway.

Acknowledgements
We thank reindeer herders for their help and patience when working with their herd during selection of experimental animals. We also thank the veterinary students Ole Christian Kjenstad and Pauline Birgitte Ulvig Kiær (Norwegian University of Life Sciences) and Trygve Vik and Jørg Vik for help during the experiments, as well as Eva Marie Breines, Ellinor Hareide (UiT-The Arctic University of Norway) and Karin-Elisabeth Holmgren (Norwegian Veterinary Institute, Tromsø, Norway) for excellent help in the laboratory. Marianne Sunde (Norwegian Veterinary Institute, Oslo, Norway) is acknowledged for conducting the 16S rRNA and the MALDI-TOF mass spectrometry on the *M. bovculi* isolates. Sophie Scotter, UiT-Arctic University of Norway, is acknowledged for language corrections.

Competing interests
The authors declare that they have no competing interests.

Funding
The study was funded by grants from the Norwegian Reindeer Development Fund (RUF) and Nordic Council of Ministers (NORDREGIO). The publication charges for this article have been funded by a grant from the publication fund of UiT The Arctic University of Norway.

References

1. Bergman A. Contagious keratitis in reindeer. Scand Vet J. 1912;2:145–77.
2. Rehbinder C, Nilsson A. An outbreak of kerato-conjunctivitis among corralled, supplementary fed, semi-domesticated reindeer calves. Rangifer. 1995;15:9–14.
3. Oksanen A. Keratoconjunctivitis in a corralled reindeer. Proceedings of the seventh Nordic Workshop on Reindeer Research. Rangifer Report. 1993;1:50.
4. Tryland M, das Neves CG, Sunde M, Mørk T. Cervid herpesvirus 2 the primary agent in an outbreak of infectious keratoconjunctivitis in semi-domesticated reindeer. J Clin Microbiol. 2009;47:3707–13. doi:10.1128/JCM.01198-09.
5. Angelos JA. Infectious bovine keratoconjunctivitis (pinkeye). Vet Clin North Am Food Anim Pract. 2015;31:61–79.
6. Angelos JA, Spinks PQ, Ball LM, George LW. *Moraxella bovoculi* sp. nov., isolated from calves with infectious bovine keratoconjunctivitis. Int J Syst Evol Microbiol. 2007;57:789–95.
7. Angelos JA. *Moraxella bovoculi* and infectious bovine keratoconjunctivitis: cause or coincidence? Vet Clin North Am Food Anim Pract. 2010;26:73–8. doi:10.1016/j.cvfa.2009.10.002.
8. Åkerstedt J, Hofshagen M. Bacteriological investigation of infectious keratoconjunctivitis in Norwegian sheep. Acta Vet Scand. 2004;45:19–26.
9. Gupta S, Chahota R, Bhardwaj B, Malik P, Verma S, Sharma M. Identification of *Chlamydia* and *Mycoplasma* species in ruminants with ocular infections. Lett Appl Microbiol. 2015;60:135–9. doi:10.1111/lam.12362.
10. Dubay SA, Williams ES, Mills K, Boerger-Fields AM. Association of *Moraxella ovis* with keratoconjunctivitis in mule deer and moose in Wyoming. J Wildl Dis. 2000;36:241–7.
11. Giacometti M, Janovsky M, Belloy L, Frey J. Infectious keratoconjunctivitis of ibex, chamois and other caprinae. Rev Sci Tech. 2002;21:335–45.
12. Gortázar C, Fernández-de-Luco D, Frölich K. Keratoconjunctivitis in a free-ranging red deer (*Cervus elaphus*) population in Spain. Z Jagdwiss. 1998;44:257–61.
13. Mavrot F, Vilei EM, Marreros N, Signer C, Frey J, Ryser-Degiorgis MP. Occurrence, quantification and genotyping of *Mycoplasma conjunctivae* in wild Caprinae with and without infectious keratoconjunctivitis. J Wildl Dis. 2012;48:619–31.
14. Grymer J. Infektiøs bovin keratokonjunktivitis hos kvæg og rådyr. Dansk Vet Tidsskr. 1984;67:854–6.
15. Kummeneje K. Isolation of *Neisseria ovis* and a *Colesiota conjunctivae*-like organism from cases of kerato-conjunctivitis in reindeer in northern Norway. Acta Vet Scand. 1976;17:107–8.
16. Aschfalk A, Josefsen TD, Steingass H, Müller W, Goethe R. Crowding and winter emergency feeding as predisposing factors for kerato-conjunctivitis in semi-domesticated reindeer in Norway. Dtsch Tierarztl Wochenschr. 2003;110:295–8.
17. Sanchez Romano J, Marcin N, Josefsen TD, Nymo IH, Sørensen KK, Tryland M. Severe transmissible eye infection in reindeer: bacterium or virus? 64th Annual International Conference of the Wildlife Disease Association, Queensland; 2015. p. 26–30 (abstract 45, page 13).
18. Skjenneberg S, Slagsvold L. Reindriften og dens naturgrunnlag. Oslo: Universitetsforlaget; 1968.
19. Tryland M, Stubsjøen SM, Ågren E, Johansen B, Kielland C. Herding conditions related to infectious keratoconjunctivitis (IKC) in semi-domesticated reindeer (*Rangifer t. tarandus*) in Norway and Sweden—a questionnaire-based survey among reindeer herders. Acta Vet Scand. 2016;58:22. doi:10.1186/s13028-016-0203-x.
20. Ryeng KA, Arnemo JM, Larsen S. Determination of optimal immobilizing doses of a medetomidine hydrochloride and ketamine hydrochloride combination in captive reindeer. Am J Vet Res. 2001;62:119–26.
21. Ros C, Belak S. Studies of genetic relationships between bovine, caprine, cervine, and rangiferine alphaherpesviruses and improved molecular methods for virus detection and identification. J Clin Microbiol. 1999;37:1247–53.
22. Ros C, Belak S. Characterization of the glycoprotein B gene from ruminant alphaherpesviruses. Virus Genes. 2002;24:99–105.
23. Ek-Kommonen C, Pelkonen S, Nettleton PF. Isolation of a herpesvirus serologically related to bovine herpesvirus 1 from a reindeer (*Rangifer tarandus*). Acta Vet Scand. 1986;27:299–301.
24. Miller JM, van der Maaten MJ. Reproductive tract lesions in heifers after intrauterine inoculation with infectious bovine rhinotracheitis virus. Am J Vet Res. 1984;45:790–4.
25. Wang J, O'Keefe J, Orr D, Loth L, Banks M, Wakeley P, West D, Card R, Ibata G, Van Maanen K, Thoren P, Isaksson M, Kerkhofs P. Validation of a real-time PCR assay for the detection of bovine herpesvirus 1 in bovine semen. J Virol Meth. 2007;144:103–8.
26. Das Neves CG, Roger M, Yoccoz NG, Rimstad E, Tryland M. Evaluation of three commercial bovine ELISA kits for detection of antibodies against alphaherpesviruses in reindeer (*Rangifer tarandus tarandus*). Acta Vet Scand. 2009;51:9. doi:10.1186/1751-0147-51-9.
27. Das Neves CG, Thiry J, Skjerve E, Yoccoz N, Rimstad E, Thiry E, Tryland M. Alphaherpesvirus infections in semidomesticated reindeer: a cross-sectional serological study. Vet Microbiol. 2009;139:262–9. doi:10.1016/j.vetmic.2009/06.013.
28. Marin MS, Leunda MR, Verna AE, Morán PE, Odeón AC, Pérez SE. Distribution of bovine herpesvirus type 1 in the nervous system of experimentally infected calves. Vet J. 2016;209:82–6. doi:10.1016/j.tvjl.2015.10.034.
29. Gould S, Dewell R, Tofflemire K, Whitley RD, Millman ST, Opriessnig T, Rosenbusch R, Trujillo J, O'Connor AM. Randomized blinded challenge study to assess association between *Moraxella bovoculi* and Infectious Bovine Keratoconjunctivitis in dairy calves. Vet Microbiol. 2013;164(1–2):108–15. doi:10.1016/j.vetmic.2013.01.038.
30. Jayappa HG, Lehr C. Pathogenicity and immunogenicity of piliated and nonpili-ated phases of *Moraxella bovis* in calves. Am J Vet Res. 1986;47:2217–21.
31. Rogers DG, Cheville NF, Pugh GW Jr. Pathogenesis of corneal lesions caused by *Moraxella bovis* in gnotobiotic calves. Vet Pathol. 1987;24:287–95.
32. Loy JD, Brodersen BW. Moraxella spp. isolated from field outbreaks of infectious keratoconjunctivitis: a retrospective study of case submissions from to 2013. J Vet Diagn Invest. 2010;2014(26):761–8.

33. Angelos JA, Ball LM, Hess JF. Identification and characterization of complete RTX operons in *Moraxella bovoculi* and *Moraxella ovis*. Vet Microbiol. 2007;125:73–9.
34. Calcutt MJ, Foecking MF, Martin NT, Mhlanga-Mutangadura T, Reilly TJ. Draft genome sequence of *Moraxella bovoculi* strain 237T (ATCC BAA-1259T) isolated from a calf with infectious bovine keratoconjunctivitis. Genome Announc. 2014;2:e00612–4. doi:10.1128/genomeA.00612-14.
35. Dickey AM, Loy JD, Bono JL, Smith TPL, Apley MD, Lubbers BV, DeDonder KD, Capik SF, Larson RL, White BJ, Blom J, Chitko-McKown CG, Clawson ML. Large genomic differences between *Moraxella bovoculi* isolates acquired from the eyes of cattle with infectious bovine keratoconjunctivitis versus the deep nasopharynx of asymptomatic cattle.
36. Das Neves CG, Mørk T, Godfroid J, Sørensen KK, Breines E, Hareide E, Thiry J, Rimstad E, Thiry E, Tryland M. Experimental infection of reindeer with cervid herpesvirus 2. Clin Vaccine Immunol. 2009;16:1758–65. doi:10.1128/CVI.00218-09.
37. Das Neves CG, Mørk T, Thiry J, Godfroid J, Rimstad E, Thiry E, Tryland M. Cervid herpesvirus 2 experimentally reactivated in reindeer can produce generalized viremia and abortion. Virus Res. 2009;145:321–8. doi:10.1016/j.virusres.2009.08.002.
38. O'Connor AM, Shen HG, Wang C, Opriesnig T. Descriptive epidemiology of *Moraxella bovis*, *Moraxella bovoculi* and *Moraxella ovis* in beef calves with naturally occuring infectious bovine keratoconjunctivitis (pinkeye). Vet Microbiol. 2012;155:374–80.

8

Occurrence of *Salmonella* spp.: a comparison between indoor and outdoor housing of broilers and laying hens

Martin Wierup[1*], Helene Wahlström[2], Elina Lahti[2], Helena Eriksson[4], Désirée S. Jansson[4], Åsa Odelros[3] and Linda Ernholm[2]

Abstract

Background: Outdoor production of poultry is rapidly increasing, which could be associated with increased risks for exposure to different environmental sources of *Salmonella*. We report a comparison on the occurrence of *Salmonella* during 2007–2015 in broilers and laying hens in outdoor and indoor production subjected to the same requirements for the prevention and control of *Salmonella* as applied in Sweden.

Results: Our results give no indication that, during the period studied, the exposure to *Salmonella* in outdoor poultry production was higher than in the indoor production. The annual incidence of *Salmonella* infected flocks in outdoor production remained at a very low and at a similar level as for indoor production. For laying hens the annual proportion of birds in test positive flocks ranged from 0 to 1.3% for indoor production from 0 to 2.0% for outdoor production. For broilers the proportion of *Salmonella* infected flocks (2013–2015) was 0.16% for indoor, and 0% in outdoor production. The difference was not statistically significant and was further reduced when flocks infected due to vertical transmission or from a hatchery source were excluded. It should, however, be considered that the number of outdoor flocks included in this evaluation is very small and continuous evaluation is needed.

Conclusions: New animal production systems, including those driven by consumer and welfare demands, may be associated with a higher risk for the exposure of potential pathogens to food animals and possibly also subsequent outbreaks of food borne infections. In this study no increase in the risk for exposure of flocks to *Salmonella* in outdoor poultry production was found. The situation may well change and the possibility of *Salmonella* contamination in outdoor poultry production requires continuous attention.

Keywords: *Salmonella*, Broiler, Laying hen, Outdoor poultry production, Indoor poultry production, Environmental exposure, Wildlife, Free-range

Background

Salmonella is a major food borne pathogen which globally is estimated to cause 93 million enteric infections and 155,000 diarrheal deaths each year [1]. Poultry products are a significant source which initially was considered to be a consequence of the global introduction of industrialized production of broiler chickens around some 50 years ago [2]. In the late 1980s, the emerging and pandemic spread of *Salmonella* Enteritidis primarily via table eggs also focused attention on the presence of *Salmonella* in the laying hen industry [3]. This pandemic reached alarming proportions and, e.g. in Germany, it was estimated that two million human food-borne *Salmonella* infections occurred annually, of which the majority were caused by serovar Enteritidis [4]. Efforts were therefore made to prevent the spread of *Salmonella* in particular from the poultry industry, and in the EU a significant decreasing trend of human cases of salmonellosis has been observed mainly attributed to successful

*Correspondence: martin.wierup@slu.se
[1] Department of Biomedical Sciences and Veterinary Public Health, Swedish University of Agricultural Sciences, P.O. Box 7028, SE-75007 Uppsala, Sweden

implementation of national *Salmonella* control programs at the preharvest level in poultry populations [5]. Nevertheless, poultry meat remained the food product from which *Salmonella* was most frequently detected and eggs are still the most important source of reported outbreaks of food-borne salmonellosis [5].

Long term experience from Sweden, Finland and Norway has shown that exposure of poultry to *Salmonella* can largely be prevented in indoor production of broiler chickens and in laying hens [6, 7]. In these countries, the prevalence of *Salmonella* of any serovar is extremely low [5]. However, outdoor production of poultry is rapidly increasing in Sweden, which could be associated with increased risks for exposure to different environmental sources of *Salmonell*a, including wildlife [8–10]. It could further be assumed that cleaning and disinfection applied between flocks in indoor production and in particular when outbreaks of *Salmonella* infections have occurred would be less efficient in minimizing the risk for residual *Salmonella* contamination in outdoor conditions.

The objective of this study was to analyze the risk for exposure of *Salmonella* in outdoor poultry production compared to indoor production. The results should also indicate if methods successfully applied for the prevention and control of *Salmonella* in indoor poultry production are equally useful under outdoor production conditions.

Methods

Control measures for *Salmonella*

This study is based on results from the official Swedish control of *Salmonella* and associated testing procedures, which are similar for indoor and outdoor production. A voluntary preventive *Salmonella* control program for poultry has been in place since 1970. In 1984 pre-slaughter testing of broiler flocks became mandatory. In response to the pandemic spread of *Salmonella* Enteritidis during the late 1980s a voluntary control program based on pre-slaughter sampling was initiated for laying hens in 1990. In 1994 sampling of laying hen flocks became mandatory not only before slaughter but also during the production period [11]. The programme was further intensified in 1995 when Sweden joined the European Union. In case of findings of *Salmonella*, regardless of serovar, the affected flocks (epidemiological unit) are euthanized, followed by cleaning and disinfection of the poultry holding premises and repeated *Salmonella* sampling of the environment, which has to be negative before restocking.

Currently, sampling for *Salmonella* in Swedish poultry flocks is performed as described in the EU harmonized regulations (breeders of *Gallus gallus* EU 200/2010, laying hens of *Gallus gallus* 517/2011, broilers EU 200/2012) with some exceptions. All poultry flocks delivering birds to an abattoir, irrespectively of the flock size, are tested 1–2 weeks before slaughter. In addition, all laying hen flocks are tested once during the rearing period and every 15th week during the production period as well as before slaughter, i.e. usually four to five times during the production period. Samples are taken from all sections of the poultry house. For non-cage systems, the test material consists of two pairs of sock samples in production flocks, five pairs of sock samples in breeding flocks, while for flocks housed in enriched cages faecal samples (2 × 75 g) are collected [12]. The results must be available before slaughter and only test negative flocks are allowed to deliver table eggs to egg packing plants and birds for slaughter. Before the above described controls were implemented for broilers and laying hens, specific requirements for control of *Salmonella* were in place for the breeding flocks as well as for the poultry feed [13].

Only accredited laboratories are allowed to perform the analyses. All samples from animals including poultry are analyzed using the MSRV (EN-ISO 6579:2002/A1: 2007: Amendment 1: Annex D) method. Putative isolates of Salmonella are sent for confirmation, serotyping, antimicrobial susceptibility testing and other typing to the National Veterinary Institute (SVA). The results from the control of Salmonella are reported and are presented annually in National Zoonosis Reports and the EU harmonized data is also included in the EFSA/ECDC´s zoonosis reports.

The results of the monitoring of *Salmonella* in laying hens and broilers are based on the testing of flocks i.e. the epidemiological unit of birds defined for each production holding.

Population and study period

The study was limited to chickens (*Gallus gallus* dom.) i.e. laying hens producing table eggs (including the rearing period up to 16 weeks of age) and broiler chickens. In this study a flock was considered to belong to an outdoor system if the birds during any time period had had access to the outdoor environment. Apart from that separation, all indoor laying hens were considered as equal although different housing systems exist as recently have been described [14]. Breeder flocks (grandparent and parent flocks) were not included since outdoor production is not allowed in this population. The study covered 9 years (2007–2015).

Data sources

Data on the numbers of slaughtered broilers were retrieved from official statistics of the Swedish Board of Agriculture. Data on the laying hen population in terms of housing capacity i.e. maximum total number of laying hens at one time in all Swedish laying hen houses were provided by The Swedish Egg Association. The total number of slaughtered broiler flocks (>350 birds) representing the number of *Salmone*lla—tested flocks, was available for 2013–2015 from the Swedish Poultry Meat Association. Information on whether individual laying hen or broiler flocks were reared indoors or outdoors was obtained through the Swedish Egg Association, The Swedish Poultry Meat Association; and from the organization for organic farming KRAV. Data on *Salmonella*—infected flocks of laying hens and broilers was obtained from the official statistics. Further information on the number of birds in each infected flock and if the flock was housed indoors or outdoors were obtained from reports of outbreak investigations by the Swedish Board of Agriculture and the National Veterinary Institute.

Statistical methods

Laying hens

To obtain an estimate of exposure to *Salmonella* that was comparable between indoor and outdoor production, the number of birds in infected flocks was divided by the respective total housing capacity for indoor and outdoor production. These calculations were made on an annual basis and also for the whole period. For the latter, the nominator was the number of birds in test positive flocks during 2008–2015 (for indoor and outdoor production, respectively) and the denominator was the sum of the total of housing capacity each year for indoor and outdoor production. For year 2010, where data on housing capacity was missing, an average of 2009 and 2011 was used.

Broilers

An estimate of the exposure to *Salmonella* that was comparable between the in-and outdoor production was obtained by dividing the number of birds in test-positive flocks, i.e. the unit of concern where sampling is done, by the total number of slaughtered birds raised in the production specific systems. The latter calculations were made annually for years 2007–2015 and for the whole period. A second estimate of exposure was obtained by calculating the proportion of test-positive flocks in indoor and outdoor production. As data on flock level was only available from 2013, calculations were made for the years 2013–2015 and for the whole period. As all flocks were sampled, there is no random variation for the flock prevalence estimates for each of years 2013–2015. However, to estimate the uncertainty, if these flocks are considered to be samples from the population of outdoor broiler flocks, the exact 95% confidence intervals were calculated for the proportion of test positive flocks using binom test, stats package, R version 3.1.1.

Results

Laying hen production

Between 2007 and 2015, the total number of laying hens (Table 1; Fig. 1) increased from 6.0 million birds to 7.4 million birds (24%). The proportion of outdoor production (out of the total production) increased from 5.9% in

Table 1 Flocks of laying hens tested positive for *Salmonella* in indoor and outdoor production in Sweden

Year	Housing capacity[a]		No. test-positive flocks		No. birds in test-positive flocks		No. birds in test-positive flocks/total housing capacity (%)	
	Indoor	Outdoor	Indoor	Outdoor	Indoor	Outdoor	Indoor	Outdoor
2007	5,649,000	351,000	1	2	Nd[b]	Nd[b]	Nd[b]	Nd[b]
2008	5,285,639	413,305	5	0	66,900	0	1.3	0.0
2009	5,457,711	646,930	1	2	20,000	2820	0.4	0.4
2010	5,690,353	708,435	2	0	23,600	0	0.4	0.0
2011	5,922,995	769,939	0	0	0	0	0.0	0.0
2012	6,222,224	816,864	2	0	17,600	0	0.3	0.0
2013	6,312,001	875,437	7	0	69,800	0	1.1	0.0
2014	6,217,685	896,371	1	1	6600	18,000	0.1	2.0
215	6,289,060	1,153,615	2	0	39,399	0	0.6	0.0
Total[c] 2008–2015	47,397,668	6,280,895	20	3	243,899	20,820	0.5	0.3

[a] Maximum total number of laying hens at one time in laying hen houses

[b] Not available

[c] Year 2007 not included since data on number of birds in test-positive flocks was missing

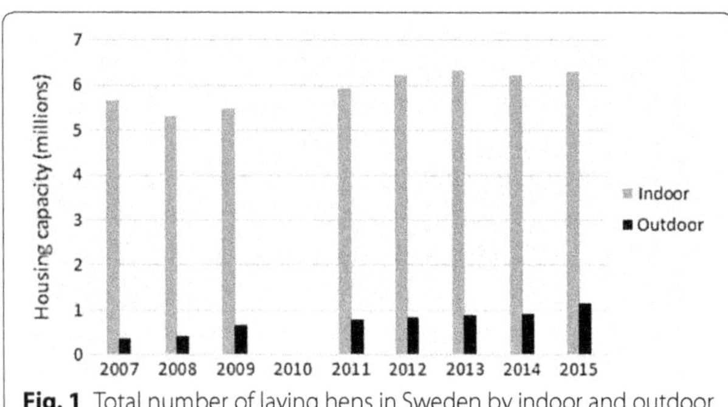

Fig. 1 Total number of laying hens in Sweden by indoor and outdoor production

2007 to 15.5% in 2015. Outdoor production increased both in absolute numbers as a proportion of the total housing capacity.

The results of the control of *Salmonella* in laying hens are presented in Table 1. The numbers of infected flocks ranged from zero to seven flocks annually. In total, 26 flocks were found to be *Salmonella*-infected during the 9-year period (2007–2015) and five of these flocks (19%) were from outdoor production. No rearing flocks were found to be *Salmonella* infected (data not shown). The proportion of birds in test-positive flocks/total housing capacity during the period studied ranged from 0 to 1.3% for indoor production and from 0 to 2.0% for outdoor production on an annual basis. For the whole period the corresponding data was 0.5% for indoor production and 0.3% for outdoor production (Table 1).

Broiler production

The annual production of broiler chickens (no of slaughtered birds) was 94 million in 2015, which represents an increase by 24% since 2007 (Table 2; Fig. 2a). The majority of birds were raised indoors (99.7% in 2015) but the outdoor production increased from 0.06 million 2007 to 0.28 million in 2015 (Fig. 2b).

The results of the control of *Salmonella* are presented in Table 2. The numbers of test-positive flocks were low and ranged from 1 to 17 flocks annually. In total, 61 flocks were found to be infected with *Salmonella* during the 9-year period (2007–2015), of which five flocks (8.2%) were raised outdoors. In 2007 and 2015, three and six of the infected broiler flocks, respectively, could be epidemiologically linked to infected breeding flocks and during 2010, 15 of the infected flocks originated from the same breeding company, hatched very closely in time. For the years when data was available (2013–2015) the proportion of infected broiler flocks was higher in indoor production (0.16%, 95% CI 0.09–0.2%) than in outdoor production (0%, 95% CI 0–2%), but this was not significantly different (Table 2). When excluding the six flocks which during 2015 were linked to infected breeding flocks, the proportion of *Salmonella* test-positive broiler flocks in indoor production during 2013–2015 decreased from 0.16 to 0.10%.

The proportion of the total number of animals in *Salmonella* test-positive flocks out of the total of animals slaughtered, divided by indoor and outdoor production was calculated for the years 2007–2015 (Table 2).

Table 2 Flocks of broilers tested positive for *Salmonella in* indoor and outdoor production in Sweden

Year	No. slaughtered birds		No. slaughtered flocks		No. test-positive flocks		No. birds in test-positive flocks		No. birds in test-positive flocks/no. slaughtered birds (%)		Proportion test-positive flocks (%)	
	Indoor	Outdoor	Indoor	Outdoor	Indoor	Outdoor	Indoor	Outdoor	Indoor	Outdoor	Indoor	Outdoor
2007	75,987,684	62,040	Nd[a]	Nd[a]	10[b]	1	186,500	1400	0.25	2.26	Nd[a]	Nd[a]
2008	76,029,408	79,055	Nd[a]	Nd[a]	8	0	206,700	0	0.27	0.00	Nd[a]	Nd[a]
2009	74,836,094	179,050	Nd[a]	Nd[a]	1	3	35,000	4070	0.05	2.27	Nd[a]	Nd[a]
2010	79,413,074	185,020	Nd[a]	Nd[a]	17[c]	0	320,555	0	0.40	0.00	Nd[a]	Nd[a]
2011	79,193,063	170,030	Nd[a]	Nd[a]	3	1	47,000	400	0.06	0.24	Nd[a]	Nd[a]
2012	77,903,897	170,045	Nd[a]	Nd[a]	1	0	31,000	0	0.04	0.00	Nd[a]	Nd[a]
2013	83,110,440	155,000	3233	43	1	0	61,800	0	0.07	0.00	0.03	0.0
2014	89,504,467	176,500	3232	44	2	0	55,000	0	0.06	0.00	0.06	0.0
2015	93,820,000	280,000	3329	61	13[d]	0	405,574	0	0.43	0.00	0.39	0.0
Total	729,798,117	1,456,740	9794	148	56	5	1,349,129	5870	0.18	0.40	0.16	0.0

[a] Not available

[b] Three of the flocks originated from a *Salmonella*—infected breeding flock

[c] 15 of the flocks originated from a *Salmonella*—contaminated hatchery

[d] Six of the flocks originated from a *Salmonella*—infected breeding flock

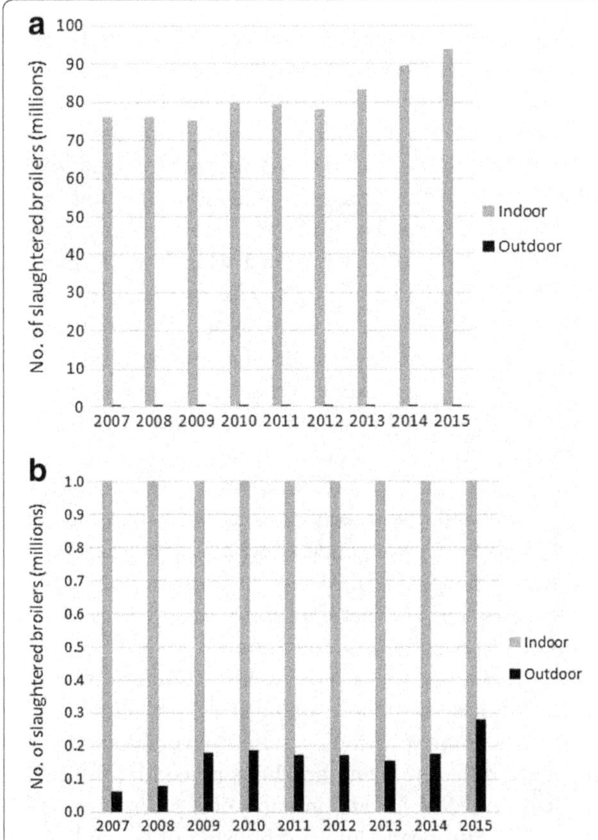

Fig. 2 Total number of broilers slaughtered from indoor and outdoor production in Sweden (**a**) and the outdoor production further visualized using truncated *Y-axis* (**b**)

This proportion was (0.18%) in flocks raised indoors compared to (0.4%) in flocks with access to outdoor conditions.

Isolated *Salmonella* serovars

The isolated serovars of *Salmonella* are listed in Table 3. Only one serovar or subspecies was isolated from each of the 87 infected flocks. In both indoor and outdoor production *Salmonella* Typhimurium was the most common serovar and accounted for 67 and 60% of all the isolates respectively. *Salmonella* Typhimurium was also the only serovar involved in the dissemination of *Salmonella* from parent flocks or hatchery to 24 broiler flocks. All six flocks infected with serovar Agona were recurrently infected broiler flocks housed on the same farm. Infections with serovar Livingstone all involved laying hen flocks at four different farms and in two of these the serovar reoccurred. These reoccurring infections all concerned indoor production.

Table 3 ***Salmonella*** **isolated from laying hens and broilers in indoor and outdoor production in Sweden**

Serovar or subspecies of *Salmonella*	No. isolates/flock 2007–2015[a]	
	Indoor production	Outdoor production
Agona	6[b]	0
Be	0	1
diarizonae (IIIb) serovar O38:r:z	1	1
Epinay	2	0
Goldcoast	0	2
Livingstone	9	0
Mbandaka	3	0
Meleagridis	2	0
Reading	2	0
Typhimurium	52	6
Total	77	10

[a] Only one serovar was isolated from each of the 87 flocks tested positive for *Salmonella*

[b] All six Agona isolates originated from the same farm

Discussion

In this study, the occurrence of *Salmonella* for indoor and outdoor housing of laying hens and broilers was analyzed. The method applied was to compare the occurrence of *Salmonella* test-positive flocks and also the proportion of birds in test-positive flocks (broilers and laying hens) in outdoor and indoor production subjected to similar requirements for the prevention and control of *Salmonella*.

Our results gave no indication that, during the period studied, the exposure to *Salmonella* in outdoor poultry production was higher than in indoor production. In both the outdoor laying hen and broiler production the annual incidence of *Salmonella*-infected flocks remained at a very low level and at a similar level as for indoor production. For laying hens, data at flock level was not available but the proportion of birds in test positive flocks was not higher in outdoor production. For broilers, where data on flock level was available, there was no significant difference between indoor and outdoor production. The proportion of the total number of birds in Salmonella test-positive flocks at slaughter were low, although slightly higher in outdoor production. The overall conclusion was that there is no indication that the risk of Salmonella is much higher in outdoor production in Sweden. It should however be considered that the number of outdoor flocks included in this evaluation is very small and that the risk may vary over time. It is therefore recommended that the situation should be continuously evaluated.

It should be noted that the incidence of *Salmonella* -infected broiler flocks was relatively high for Swedish circumstances and with a substantial variation between years. This variation can largely be explained by vertical transmission from *Salmonella* infected parent flocks in 2007 and 2015 and a *Salmonella*—contaminated hatchery in 2010. Vertical spread of *Salmonella* from the parent stock, which previously has been an extremely rare event in Swedish commercial poultry production, does not reflect the risk for *Salmonella* contamination related to indoor or outdoor production at the production level and this was therefore also considered in the assessment. However, the broilers with outdoor access predominantly originate from the same breeding companies as the indoor broilers. During the period of the study the same genotypes were used for both indoor and outdoor production for both broiler and laying hens respectively. The fact that no outdoor flock was infected by these issues may reflect the small proportion of outdoor production.

The risk for *Salmonella* contamination in outdoor production merits continuous attention, although the results from Sweden so far do not suggest that the current methods for prevention and control of *Salmonella* have to be modified for outdoor production. It should primarily be noted that the period studied represents the early stage of a current trend towards commercial production of poultry outdoors as recently described [14]. In the future, the risk for exposure to *Salmonella* in outdoor production may change. Secondly, an increased risk can follow on infected farms if residual *Salmonella* contamination cannot be eliminated by the sanitary methods that are successfully applied in indoor production. So far, our corresponding knowledge for outdoor production is limited and requires further attention, in particular decontamination of outdoor runs and natural ground surfaces. Methods for preventing contact and contamination from wildlife, mainly passerine birds, are also of importance. Apart from passerine birds and in certain areas hedgehogs, *Salmonella* in wild-life in Sweden is very rare [12, 15] but the situation can be considerably different in other countries [10]. The location of outdoor poultry production in areas with a high density of farm animal populations, particularly in countries with less stringent control of *Salmonella* in pigs and cattle can be an additional factor that may significantly influence the risk for *Salmonell*a -infection in outdoor production. In order to minimize the risk for exposure of *Salmonella* to the outdoor production, basic knowledge on biosecurity, including prevention and control of *Salmonella* is, essential for new producers and farm staff.

The isolated serovars of *Salmonella* included those generally isolated from poultry and animal feed ingredients [12]. Independent of housing conditions, Typhimurium was the most commonly isolated serovar. Further subtyping by e.g. multi-locus variable number tandem repeat analysis (MLVA) can reveal additional epidemiological information on the source of infection [10]. Recurrent infections may thus be linked to certain strains, as was observed in this study for Agona where one farm with indoor broilers had infected flocks recurring six times over a period of two and a half years. Recurrent infections could also be seen for other serovars in our study, but not to the same extent. However, in our study only one outdoor holding has shown a repeated *Salmonella*—infection during the studied period. The test-positive flocks at that holding were of different categories, one in laying hens and one in broilers and were spaced 2 years apart. Both flocks were infected with *S. Typhimurium* but of different phage types, RDNC for broilers and U277 for laying hens, and are therefore more likely to result from separate introductions of infection.

For various reasons it is difficult to compare the result of our studies with those of most others found in the literature. Some previous studies have described the impact of different laying hen housing conditions on the prevalence of *Salmonella*, in particular prior to the 2012 ban in the European Union of housing of laying hens in conventional battery cages. However, due to many different risk factors involved including e.g. flock size, methods for cleaning and disinfection between batches and methods of sampling, it is difficult to draw detailed conclusions concerning risks for *Salmonella* infection in poultry in outdoor conditions [16–18]. A major limiting factor for an evaluation and comparison with the results of our study is that the referred studies generally were performed under what could be called high *Salmonella* prevalence conditions in flocks where active specific control of *Salmonella* was limited or absent as previously observed in studies on *Salmonella* in the pig production [19]. In the absence of such control, the prevalence of *Salmonella* is generally higher, which was demonstrated in a comprehensive EU baseline study based on a harmonized sampling from 5310 poultry holdings in 24 Member States. In the EU study, *Salmonella* was detected in 30.8% of the laying hen holdings [6]. That study also found that in the Member States, the observed flock prevalence of *Salmonella* ranged from 0 to 79.5%. The lowest prevalence figures were observed in countries including Sweden, with a long history of active control of *Salmonella*. However, in an individual country production system with special control measures for *Salmonella* can be applied. Recent data from France reports a decreasing trend of *Salmonella* contamination in outdoor production in the traditional free-range "Label Rouge" broiler production [20]. The prevalence of *Salmonella*—contaminated carcasses decreased from 16 to <2% during 1994–2014, and a prevalence of 1.47–2.65% *Salmonella*—infected flocks was achieved during 2010–2014, although this is higher than in this study.

Interestingly, in the present study, only one serovar of *Salmonella* was isolated from each of the 87 flocks found infected. This fact most likely also reflects that this study was performed in a low prevalence country were the serovar diversity of environmental *Salmonella* contamination, in particular around animal farms, can be expected to be lower than in countries where the implementation of preventive measures and control of *Salmonella* has been more limited. It is here also interesting to compare with *Campylobacter*, another highly important zoonotic poultry associated pathogen. In Sweden a significant difference have been found in the prevalence of *Campylobacter* in caecum of conventionally indoor produced broilers (13%) and broilers produced in organic and other small scale production systems with outdoor access (60%) [21]. Because the epidemiology of *Campylobacter* is different from *Salmonella* and only partly understood, there in contrast to *Salmonella* are currently no identified measures for the reliable control of this organism in free ranged poultry [22].

Conclusions

In summary, new animal production systems, including those driven by consumer and welfare demands may potentially be associated with a higher risk for the exposure of potential pathogens to food animals and possibly also subsequent outbreaks of food-borne infections. In order to prevent such scenarios, new production systems require special attention and monitoring so necessary actions can be taken should such risks incursions occur. In this study, no increase in the risk for exposure of *Salmonella* in outdoor poultry production was found so far, despite the current trend towards such production conditions. However, this situation may well change and opportunity for *Salmonella* -contamination in the outdoor poultry production requires continuous attention.

Authors' contributions

MW initiated and was the main author of the study. The data was compiled and condensed from the data systems of the responsible authorities and industries by HE, LE, DJ, EL and ÅO. HW made the statistical analyses and assessment of the data and coordinated the project together with MW. All authors read and approved the final manuscript.

Author details

[1] Department of Biomedical Sciences and Veterinary Public Health, Swedish University of Agricultural Sciences, P.O. Box 7028, SE-75007 Uppsala, Sweden. [2] Department of Disease Control and Epidemiology, National Veterinary Institute, SVA, SE-751 89 Uppsala, Sweden. [3] Åsa Odelros AB, Österåkersvägen 21, SE-81040 Hedesunda, Sweden. [4] Department of Animal Health and Antimicrobial Strategies, National Veterinary Institute, SVA, Österåkersvägen 21, SE-81040 Hedesunda, Sweden.

Acknowledgements

The authors express their thanks to Dr. Pia Gustafsson, Swedish Poultry Meat Association and Alexandra Jeremiasson, Swedish Egg Association for providing data from the production of broilers and layers respectively and to Dr. Ingrid Hansson, Swedish University of Agricultural Sciences for providing data on *Campylobacter*.

Competing interests

The authors declare that they have no competing interests.

Funding

This study was done without any specific funding.

References

1. Majowicz SE, Musto J, Scallan E, Angulo FJ, O'Brein SJ, Jones TF. The global burden of nontyphoidal *Salmonella* gastroenteritis. Clin Infect Dis. 2010;50:882–9. doi:10.1086/650733.
2. Boegel K. Global cooperation in the control of salmonellosis. In: Snoyenbos GH, editor. Proceedings of the Symposium on the Diagnosis and Control of *Salmonella*, 29 October 1991. San Diego: United States Animal Health Association; Library of Congress Catalog card Number 17-128242; 1992. p. 1–6.
3. Gantois I, Ducatelle R, Pasmans F, Haesebrouck F, Gast R, Humphrey TJ, Van Immerseel F. Mechanisms of egg contamination by *Salmonella* enteritidis. FEMS Microbiol Rev. 2009;33:718–38. doi:10.1111/j.1574-6976.2008.00161.x.
4. Report of WHO consultation on epidemiological emergency in poultry and egg salmonellosis, Geneva, 20–23 March, 1989; WHO/CDS/VPH 89.92; http://apps.who.int/iris/handle/10665/60822 Accessed 27 Oct 2016.
5. EFSA and ECDC (European Food Safety Authority and European Centre for Disease Prevention and Control). The European union summary report on trends and sources of zoonoses, zoonotic agents and food-borne outbreaks in 2013. EFSA J. 2015;13(1):3991. doi:10.2903/j.efsa.2015.3991.
6. European Food Safety Authority. Report of the task force on zoonoses data collection on the analysis of the baseline study on the prevalence of *Salmonella* in holdings of laying hen flocks of *Gallus gallus*. EFSA J. 2007. doi:10.2903/j.efsa.2007.97r.
7. European Food Safety Authority. Report of the task force on zoonoses data collection on the analysis of the baseline study on the prevalence of *Salmonella* in broiler flocks of *Gallus gallus*, Part A. EFSA J. 2007;98:1–85. doi:10.2903/j.efsa.2007.97r.
8. Skov MN, Madsen JJ, Rahbek C, Lodal J, Jespersen JB, Jørgensen JC, Dietz HH, Chriél M, Baggesen DL. Transmission of *Salmonella* between wildlife and meat-production animals in Denmark. J Appl Microbiol. 2008;105:1558–68. doi:10.1111/j.1365-2672.2008.03914.x.
9. Greiga JD, Ravelb A. Analysis of foodborne outbreak data reported internationally for source attribution. Int J Food Microbiol. 2009;130:77–87. doi:10.1016/j.ijfoodmicro.2008.12.
10. Chousalkar K, Gole V, Caraguel C, Rault JL. Chasing *Salmonella* Typhimurium in free range egg production system. Vet Microbiol. 2016;192:67–72. doi:10.1016/j.vetmic.2016.06.013.
11. Wierup M, Engström B, Engvall A, Wahlström H. Control of *Salmonella* enteritidis in Sweden. Int J Food Microbiol. 1995;25:219–26. doi:10.1016/0168-1605(94)00090-S.
12. Surveillance of infectious diseases in animals and humans in Sweden 2015, National Veterinary Institute (SVA), Uppsala, Sweden. 2016; SVA's report 34, ISSN 1654-1798. http://www.sva.se/globalassets/redesign2011/

pdf/om_sva/publikationer/surveillance-2015-w.pdf. Accessed 27 Oct 2016.

13. Wierup M, Häggblom P. An assessment of soybeans and other vegetable proteins as source of salmonella contamination in pig production. Acta Vet Scand. 2010;52:15. doi:10.1186/1751-0147-52-15.
14. Wall HA, Jeremiasson M, Jeremiasson J, Odelros Å, Eriksson H, Jansson DS. Svensk äggnäring efter omställningen, del 1 Inhysning och aktuella trender. [Egg production in Sweden after the change to alternative housing systems, part 1. Housing of laying hens and current trends] (Summary in English). Svensk Veterinärtidning. 2016;68:11–8.
15. Wahlström H, Tysen E, Olsson Engvall E, Brändström B, Eriksson E, Mörner T, Vågsholm I. Survey of *Campylobacter*, VTEC and *Salmonella* in Swedish wildlife. Vet Rec. 2003;153:74–80.
16. Van Hoorebeke S, Van Immerseel F, De Vylder J, Ducatelle R, Haesebrouck F, Pasmans F, et al. Faecal sampling underestimates the actual prevalence of *Salmonella* in laying hen flocks. Zoonoses Public Health. 2009;56:471–6. doi:10.1111/j.1863-2378.2008.01211.x.
17. Van Hoorebeke S, Van Immerseel F, Haesebrouck R, Ducatelle F, Dewulf J. The influence of the housing system on *Salmonella* infections in laying hens: a review. Zoonoses Public Health. 2011;58:304–11.
18. Wales A, Breslin M, Carter B, Sayers R, Davies R. A longitudinal study of environmental *Salmonella* contamination in caged and free-range layer flocks. Avian Pathol. 2007;36:187–97. doi:10.1080/03079450701338755.
19. Opinion of the Scientific Panel on biological hazards (BIOHAZ) related to "Risk assessment and mitigation options of Salmonella in pig production". EFSA J. 2006; 341, 1–131, doi: 10.2903/j.efsa.2006.341.
20. Salvat G, Guyot M, Protino J. Monitoring *Salmonella, Campylobacter, Escherichia* coli and *Staphylococcus* aureus in traditional free-range "Label Rouge" broiler production: a 23-year survey program. J Appl Microbiol. 2016. doi:10.1111/jam.13313.
21. Hansson I, Gustafsson P, Hellquist B, Lahti E, Pudas N, Olsson Engvall E. *Campylobacter* in Swedish small scale chicken production. A comparison with findings in conventionally produced 5 Swedish and European broilers. In: Forbes K, Omar EE, Strachan N, Hold G, editors. 17th International workshop on *Campylobacter, Helicobacter* and related organisms. Spencers Wood: Society for General Microbiology; 2013. p. 113.
22. Humphrey T, O'Brien S, Madsen M. *Campylobacters* as zoonotic pathogens: a food production perspective.

9

Liver morphometrics and metabolic blood profile across divergent phenotypes for feed efficiency in the bovine

Yuri Regis Montanholi[1*], Livia Sadocco Haas[2], Kendall Carl Swanson[3], Brenda Lynn Coomber[4], Shigeto Yamashiro[4] and Stephen Paul Miller[5,6]

Abstract

Background: Feed costs are a major expense in the production of beef cattle. Individual variation in the efficiency of feed utilization may be evident through feed efficiency-related phenotypes such as those related to major energetic sinks. Our objectives were to assess the relationships between feed efficiency with liver morphometry and metabolic blood profile in feedlot beef cattle.

Methods: Two populations (A = 112 and B = 45) of steers were tested for feed efficiency. Blood from the 12 most (efficient) and 12 least feed inefficient (inefficient) steers from population A was sampled hourly over the circadian period. Blood plasma samples were submitted for analysis on albumin, aspartate aminotransferase, γ-glutamyl transpeptidase urea, cholesterol, creatinine, alkaline phosphatase, creatine kinase, lipase, carbon dioxide, β-hydroxybutyrate, acetate and bile acids. Liver tissue was also harvested from 24 steers that were blood sampled from population A and the 10 steers with divergent feed efficiency in each tail of population B was sampled for microscopy at slaughter. Photomicroscopy images were taken using the portal triad and central vein as landmarks. Histological quantifications included cross-sectional hepatocyte perimeter and area, hepatocyte nuclear area and nuclei area as proportion of the hepatocyte area. The least square means comparison between efficient and inefficient steers for productive performance and liver morphometry and for blood analytes data were analyzed using general linear model and mixed model procedures of SAS, respectively.

Results: No differences were observed for liver weight; however, efficient steers had larger hepatocyte (i.e. hepatocyte area at the porta triad 323.31 vs. 286.37 μm^2) and nuclei dimensions at portal triad and central vein regions, compared with inefficient steers. The metabolic profile indicated efficient steers had lower albumin (36.18 vs. 37.65 g/l) and cholesterol (2.62 vs. 3.05 mmol/l) and higher creatinine (118.59 vs. 110.50 mmol/l) and carbon dioxide (24.36 vs. 23.65 mmol/l) than inefficient steers.

Conclusions: Improved feed efficiency is associated with increased metabolism by the liver (enlarged hepatocytes and no difference on organ size), muscle (higher creatinine) and whole body (higher carbon dioxide); additionally, efficient steers had reduced bloodstream pools of albumin and cholesterol. These metabolic discrepancies between feed efficient and inefficient cattle may be determinants of productive performance.

Keywords: Albumin, Carbon dioxide, Cholesterol, Creatinine, Energy metabolism, Hepatocyte dimensions, Histomorphometry, Liver size, Metabolic rate, Residual feed intake

*Correspondence: Yuri.R.Montanholi@gmail.com
[1] Department of Animal Science and Aquaculture, Faculty of Agriculture, Dalhousie University, 58 River Road, Bible Hill, Truro, NS B2N 5E3, Canada
Full list of author information is available at the end of the article

Background

Feed costs are a major expense in the production of beef cattle [1]. An avenue for decreasing feeding costs is the improvement of feed utilization through utilization of cattle with improved feed efficiency. The identification of such cattle is limited by practical phenotypes for feed efficiency with application in commercial herds. The evaluation of physiological aspects underlying feed efficiency has been studied in beef cattle through residual feed intake (RFI) [2, 3]. This feed efficiency measure reflects the variation in feed intake upon adjustment for body size, body weight gain and body composition. Thus, the residual of this determination represents variation in the requirements for basal metabolic processes rather than differences in productivity, constituting a relevant trait in the search of biological indicators for feed efficiency.

Requirements for basal metabolic processes represent a large amount of total energy expenditure of the animal [4]. Cattle raised under the same conditions, at the same physiological state, and with similar genetic composition vary in basal energy requirements [5, 6]. A significant portion of these energy requirements supports the metabolism of visceral organs [7]. Despite the fact that these organs only represent approximately 6–10% of body-weight, about 40–50% of the total basal energy requirements is due to the metabolism of the liver and digestive tract [8]. Liver metabolism accounts for about half of this amount [9], while comprising 1.45% of body weight in beef steers [10].

Variation in feed intake results in changes to the metabolic rate of visceral organs [11], which in turn creates fluctuations in blood flow affecting both organ size and tissue metabolic activity [12]. Johnson et al. [7] found that an increase in the functional workload of the liver through dietary manipulation in cattle and sheep, resulted in an increase in liver weight, which is associated with hepatocyte hypertrophy [13]. Conversely, Zaitoun et al. [14] observed that a decrease in liver metabolism through surgical manipulation in rats resulted in hepatocyte hypotrophy. Interestingly, Montanholi et al. [15] observed an increase in the small intestine crypt cellularity in cattle with improved feed efficiency. Such histological and functional evidence is associated with increased metabolic rate of the digestive tract in snakes [16] and also associated with variation in feed efficiency in beef cattle calves [17].

Besides micro-structural changes, variation in workload of the liver and other metabolic systems is also reflected in blood plasma analytes; such findings were reported by Gonano et al. [18] while evaluating a series of blood analytes over the circadian period and across physiological states in beef heifers; by Bourgon et al. [19] while evaluating blood analytes over the ultradian period in young beef bulls and; by Richardson et al. [20] while evaluating blood analytes over spot sampling in feedlot cattle. Products related to liver function including albumin, cholesterol, urea and bile acids (BA); enzymes related to liver function including alkaline phosphatase (ALP), aspartate aminotransferase (AST), γ-glutamyl transpeptidase (GGT) and lipase; indicators of energetic status including acetate, β-hydroxybutyrate (BHBA) and carbon dioxide (CO_2); and indicators of muscle metabolism including creatinine and creatine kinase (CK) are important analytes to be evaluated over the circadian period due to their relevance in the basal energy requirements [20, 21].

Since variation in feed efficiency results in differences in feed intake and, consequently, impacts the workload placed on visceral organs in which metabolic changes affect tissue microarchitecture and blood metabolic profile, it can be hypothesized that these biological indicators may also indicate variation in feed efficiency. Therefore, our objectives were to characterize: (1) the morphometry of liver tissue; and (2) the circadian metabolic blood profile in beef cattle with divergent feed efficiency.

Methods

Experimental units and animal husbandry

The experiment followed recommendations outlined by the Canadian Council of Animal Care guidelines (2009). A total of 112 (population A) plus 45 (population B) crossbred steers with known dates of birth were fed for 140 days at the Elora Beef Research Centre, Canada. The breed composition of the steers was primarily 57.1% Angus, 29.6% Simmental and 3.5% Hereford for population A, and 33.0% Angus, 27.7% Charolais, and 13.9% Piedmontese for population B. The remaining breed composition was comprised of other European breeds in both populations. Steers were allowed to adjust to the facilities, feed and feeding system for 15 days prior to the start of the feeding and performance evaluation trial. Pens were naturally ventilated, bedded with wood shavings and each held 14–15 steers. Every pen contained four electronic feeding stations (Insentec, B.V., Marknesse, The Netherlands) with access to fresh water. Radio frequency identification tags (Allflex, St. Hyacinthe, Canada) were placed in the right ear of each steer to continuously record individual feeding events. Both populations were fed ad libitum a high moisture, corn-based diet similar to a formulation used elsewhere [23]. The ration was added with 28 mg of monensin (Rumensin®; Elanco, Greenfield, USA) per kilogram of dry matter, which is typical for commercial operations in regions that produce corn in North America. Every 28 days for a period of 140 days, in the morning, steers were weighed using a calibrated livestock scale and ultrasound scanned for body composition by a trained technician. Backfat thickness (BKFT; mm) and rib eye area (RBEA; cm^2) were assessed using real-time ultrasound as described by [3]. Shortly after the end of the productive performance evaluation (10 ± 2.4 days), steers from population A were subjected to blood sampling and then sent to slaughter, steers from population B were sent to slaughter within 2 weeks after the completion of the performance evaluation. The average age of the steers at slaughter was 477 ± 21 days (mean ± standard deviation) for population A and 411 ± 18 days for population B. Both groups of steers were also weighed on the day before and on the day of the slaughter at the research station.

Feed efficiency determination and feed efficiency ranking

Body weight (BW), body composition and feed intake measures were assessed to determine the residual feed intake following the methodology described by Montanholi et al. [3]. Briefly, the individual daily dry matter intake (DMI; kg/day) was computed by combining feeding events within each day. The daily feed intakes were filtered for outliers, which represented less than 2% of the feeding records, and converted to a dry matter basis. Average BW, BKFT and RBEA was calculated by computing the animals' intercept plus the average daily gains of each of these traits times 70. Individual DMI, average BW gain, average BW and ultrasound measurements were used to calculate RFI. The most appropriate model for the population A had a R^2 of 0.63, as presented by Montanholi et al. [24]. Similarly, for population B the best fit model had a R^2 of 0.72, as computed by Montanholi et al. [23]. Steers were then ranked based on residual feed intake and the animals in the extremes for feed efficiency (12 efficient and 12 inefficient) were selected for circadian blood plasma metabolic profile analysis from population A only. In the case of biometry, liver morphometry and productive performance traits, steers from both populations were considered. Thus, the same 12 efficient and 12 inefficient steers from population A, subjected to blood sampling, were added to the 10 efficient and 10 inefficient steers from population B in these datasets based on statistics detailed below.

Blood collection and processing

Steers from population A were blood sampled in six groups of four animals at 6 ± 3.6 days prior to slaughter. The methodology for hourly blood collection over the circadian period and sample processing applied to steers from population A is described in detail by Montanholi et al. [24]. Briefly, the groups of four animals were composed of two efficient and two inefficient steers and offered water and feed for ad libitum consumption over the duration of blood sampling. Steers were blood sampled hourly from noon until 11:00 the following morning. Steers had a heparinized jugular catheter coupled to a tubing placed in between the shoulders to minimize the distress of blood sampling. Blood samples (10 ml) were withdrawn and immediately centrifuged (3000*g* for 25 min at 4 °C), then blood plasma was harvested and stored at −80 °C until further metabolic profile analysis.

Liver biometrics, sampling and microscopic imaging

Liver weights were measured and reported as whole liver weight and as a proportion of the animal's live weight. The body weight used for this proportionate trait was the average of the weights measured the day before slaughter and assessed immediately before transportation to the abattoir. The transportation to the abattoir lasted 25 min and steers were slaughtered without prior fasting. The entire liver was removed, inspected and weighed after excising the gallbladder. All the livers sampled were considered healthy by the federal inspector. Liver fragments, sampled within 42 ± 6 min of stunning, were gently collected from the visceral side of the right lobe and adjacent to the insertion of the portal vein. Samples (1.0 × 1.0 × 0.5 cm) were fixed in 10% neutral phosphate buffered formalin for 24 h under gentle agitation and processed for paraffin embedding (Sakura Tissue Tek VIP 6®: Sakura Finetek; Alphen aan den Rijn, The Netherlands). Paraffin blocks were sectioned at 5 μm thickness using a microtome (Leica 2255®: Leica Biosystems; Wetzlar, Germany). Tissue fragments mounted on glass slides were left to dry overnight on a hot surface (36 °C) and stained with hematoxylin and eosin according to the method described by Carson [25]. Liver tissue slides were first screened by an animal histologist to ensure that all livers were free of any abnormality. Then, liver tissue microscopic images were taken using a Leica DMLB microscope (Leica Microsystems Inc.®, Wetzlar, Germany) equipped with a video camera QICAM Fast 1394 (QImaging®, Surrey, Canada) connected to the computer-based image analysis software QImaging (QImaging®, Surrey, Canada). Images were taken using the portal triad and central vein as histological references [13]. A total of 10 images around each of these two regions were taken from each liver and from a single section at 200× magnification.

Liver histomorphometry analyses

Four measurements performed in both central vein and portal triad regions included the following: hepatocyte area (HA; μm^2), hepatocyte perimeter (HP; μm), hepatocyte nuclei area (NA; μm^2) and percentage of the total hepatocyte area occupied by the nuclei (NH; %).

Hepatocytes were selected and analyzed by an experienced judge, who was blinded to the feed efficiency group of the corresponding animal. Ten hepatocytes where chosen per image of central vein or portal triad, totaling 100 hepatocytes measured per animal in each histological region. The criteria for selecting hepatocytes were established as the following: proximity to the histological landmark (central vein or portal triad), well delimited cellular boundaries, and presence of round shaped nuclei. The same 100 hepatocytes were used to perform each of the four histological assessments. Histological quantifications were performed using ImageJ® (ImageJ, U. S. National Institutes of Health, Bethesda, USA). Both HA and HP were assessed using a free hand drawing tool by outlining the perimeter of the chosen hepatocytes. This was followed by the application of the threshold option, which highlights the area covered by the nuclei, to determine NA. The NH was calculated as the percentage of the HA occupied by the NA. Figure 1 illustrates the histomorphometric measures (HA, HP and NA).

Blood plasma metabolic profile

The blood plasma samples were analyzed through an animal diagnostic service (Animal Health Laboratory, University of Guelph, Guelph, Canada). Briefly, an automated analyzer (Cobas® c311/501 analyzer, Roche Diagnostics GmbH, Indianapolis, USA) [26] was used to measure the following blood plasma metabolic parameters: albumin (g/l), aspartate aminotransferase (AST; U/l), γ-glutamyl transpeptidase (GGT; U/l), urea (mmol/l), cholesterol (mmol/l), creatinine (mmol/l), alkaline phosphatase (ALP; U/l), creatine kinase (U/l) and lipase (U/l). Carbon dioxide (CO_2; mmol/l) levels were determined using an automated analyzer (Cobas® 4000 c311, Roche Diagnostics GmbH, Mannheim, Germany). The determination of β-hydroxybutyrate (μmol/l) was completed using a commercial kit (Randox®, RANDOX Laboratories Ltd., Crumlin, UK). Blood plasma acetate (g/l) was determined via spectrophotometry using a commercial kit (K-ACETRM, Megazyme© International, Wicklow, Ireland) according to the manufacturers' protocol. A colorimetric-based assay was used to determine the concentration of total bile acids (BA; μmol/l) (Diazyme total bile acids, Diazyme©, Poway, USA).

Statistical analyses

Data were analyzed using the SAS® software (SAS Institute, Cary, USA). Data normality was tested using the univariate procedure for each continuous variable. Nonnormal data, based on Anderson–Darling test and kurtosis and skewness out of the −2 and +2 range, were either log or reciprocal transformed and then backtransformed to report the results. Preliminary regression analysis using the general linear model procedure, as was described by Montanholi et al. [3], indicated an absence of significant breed effects ($P \geq 0.10$); therefore, breed effect was not included in the analyses detailed below. Additionally, preliminary analysis indicated substantial increase in statistical power by pooling the two populations for the measurements done in common. Thus, means of the two feed efficiency groups for biometry, productive performance and liver morphometry measures were tested using the general linear model procedure and compared using *T* test, according to the following model:

$$Y_{ijk} = \mu + Population_i + Efficiency_j + \beta(Age_{ijk} - Age_{..}) + \varepsilon_{ijk}$$

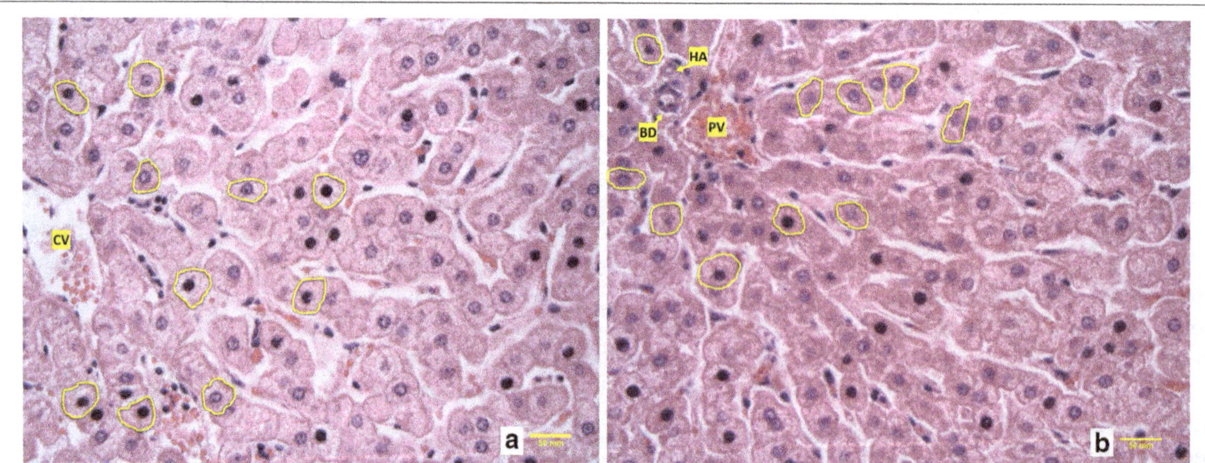

Fig. 1 Liver histomorphometry, example of selected hepatocytes around central vein (**a**) and portal triad (**b**) histological regions for measurements on livers from both populations of steers. *CV* central vein, *PV* portal vein, *HA* hepatic artery and, *BD* bile duct

where Y_{ijk} is the dependent variable measured on the kth steer, belonging to the jth feed efficiency group and sampled in the ith population; μ is the overall mean effect for the measure; $Population_i$ is the fixed effect of ith population (A or B); $Efficiency_j$ is the fixed effect of jth feed efficiency group (efficient or inefficient); $\beta(Age_{ijk}–Age..)$ indicates the inclusion of age at slaughter as a covariate; and ε_{ijk} is the residual random effect associated with the assessment on the kth steer. The interaction between population and efficiency group was tested and due to the lack of significance, it was removed from the model described above.

The repeated measures of blood analytes over the circadian cycle from population A were analyzed through repeated measures using the mixed procedure, according to the following model:

$$Y_{ijk} = \mu + Efficiency_i + Time_{ij} + \varepsilon_{ijk}$$

where Y_{ijk} is the dependent variable, μ is the overall mean, $Efficiency_i$ is the fixed effect of feed efficiency groups (i = efficient or inefficient), $Time_{ij}$ is the fixed effect of sampling time within feed efficiency groups (j = 1,2,...24), and ε_{ijk} is the residual random error. Adjustment for age was tested and revealed unnecessary within population A, thus not included in the repeated sampling analysis. Although not included in the model, the interaction between feed efficiency group and time generated the least square means plotted in Fig. 2. The autoregressive covariance structure was selected based upon maximum likelihood according to the Bayesian information criterion and the bet-within degrees of freedom option was used as repeated measures adjustments. The Scheffé's test was used to compare the least square means of efficient and inefficient steers from the repeated analysis. For all analyses, data were considered statistically significant when $P \leq 0.05$ and were considered a trend towards significance when $0.10 \geq P > 0.05$.

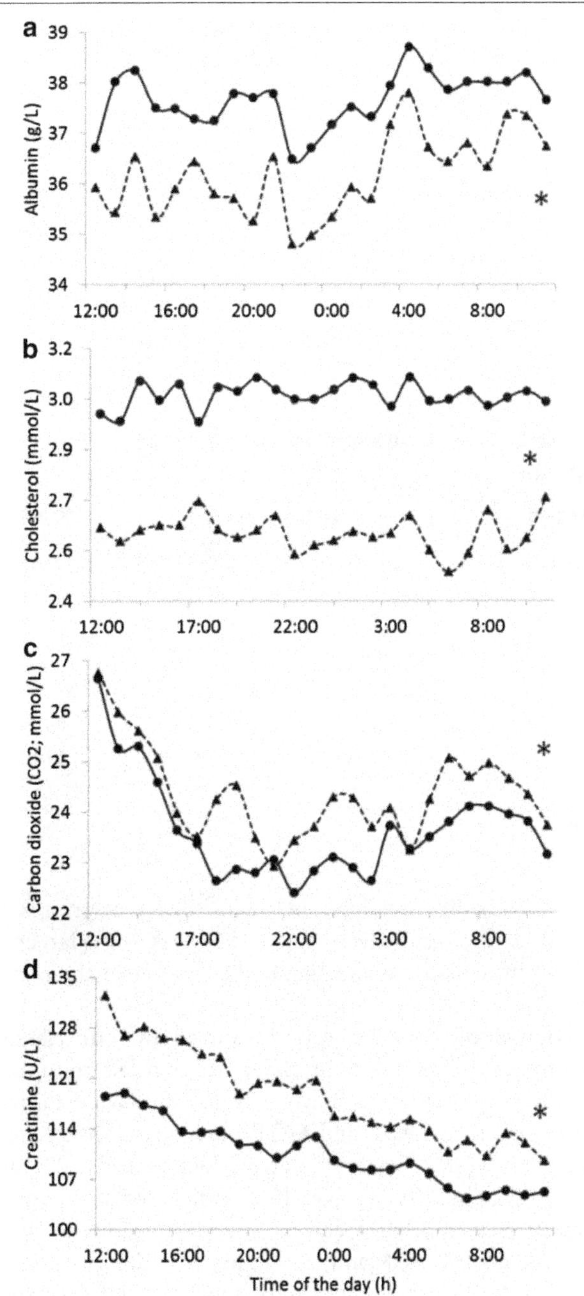

Fig. 2 Circadian profile of **a** albumin, **b** cholesterol, **c** carbon dioxide and **d** creatinine. Feed efficient (*filled triangle*) and inefficient (*filled circle*) beef steers. Presence of asterisk denotes P < 0.05 over the circadian period

Results

The descriptive statistics and least square mean comparisons of indicators of productive performance are presented in Table 1. The efficient and inefficient groups of steers differed in residual feed intake. Efficient steers consumed 1.85 kg/day less feed (dry matter basis) than inefficient steers while achieving a comparable performance in terms of daily weight gain, body weight and body composition, as measured by ultrasonic assessments of back fat thickness and rib eye area. The biometrics of livers assessed at slaughter are listed in Table 1. No differences were observed between feed efficiency groups for liver weight or liver to body weight ratio.

Table 2 presents the descriptive statistics and least square mean comparisons of liver histomorphometric measures by histological region (portal triad and central vein). Consistently across the two histological regions, HA, HP and NA were larger in efficient steers. While the relative size of hepatocyte nuclei in relation to hepatocyte

Table 1 Descriptive statistics and least square means of the productivity and liver biometrics by efficiency groups

Measures (unit)	Mean	Standard deviation	Efficient	Inefficient	P value
Residual feed intake (kg/d)	0.00	0.98	−0.90	0.89	0.001*
Average daily gain (kg/d)	1.77	0.25	1.74	1.76	0.662
Average feed intake (kg/d)	9.54	1.22	8.56	10.41	0.001*
Back fat thickness (mm)	12.17	3.06	12.27	12.09	0.885
Rib eye area (cm^2)	108.77	6.24	109.20	108.41	0.770
Body weight (kg)	535.4	48.86	533.4	545.0	0.361
Liver weight (kg)	7.35	1.09	7.24	7.55	0.363
Liver weight (% body weight)	1.26	0.25	1.26	1.29	0.561

*$P \leq 0.05$

Table 2 Descriptive statistics and least square means of liver histomorphometry by histological regions and efficiency groups

Region	Measures (abbreviation; unit)	Mean	Standard deviation	Efficient	Inefficient	P value
Portal triad	Hepatocyte area (HA; μm^2)	302.66	36.29	323.31	286.37	0.001*
	Hepatocyte perimeter (HP; μm)	66.38	5.13	68.55	63.61	0.001*
	Hepatocyte nuclei area (NA; μm^2)	68.93	14.12	71.73	65.23	0.007*
	Nuclei area by HA (NH; % HA)	4.58	0.78	4.65	4.49	0.232
Central vein	Hepatocyte area (HA; μm^2)	332.16	38.09	357.43	321.26	0.037*
	Hepatocyte perimeter (HP; μm)	69.23	4.40	70.64	67.76	0.024*
	Hepatocyte nuclei area (NA; μm^2)	69.61	11.95	71.92	66.93	0.031*
	Nuclei area by HA (NH; % HA)	7.14	1.33	7.10	7.02	0.759

*$P \leq 0.05$

size (NH) did not differ between efficiency groups in either of the histological regions. NH was 57.3% larger in the central vein region compared to its size at the portal triad.

The blood analytes were organized in four classes; namely, products related to liver function (albumin, BA, cholesterol and urea), enzymes primarily related to liver function (ALP, AST and GGT) and lipase that is primarily secreted by the pancreatic acinar cells [27] but also described in the liver [28], indicators of energetic status (acetate, BHBA and CO_2) and indicators of muscle metabolism (CK and creatinine). The descriptive statistics and mean comparisons between feed efficiency groups for metabolic profile parameters are presented in Table 3. Creatinine and CO_2 levels were greater in blood plasma of efficient steers compared to inefficient steers, while albumin and cholesterol levels were lower in efficient steers. A trend ($P \leq 0.10$) was observed suggesting greater levels of lipase in blood of efficient steers. No differences ($P \geq 0.10$) between efficiency groups were observed for the remaining analytes evaluated, which include BA, urea, ALP, AST, GGT, acetate, BHBA and CK.

The circadian pattern of the blood analytes differing between efficient and inefficient steers are presented in Fig. 2. It is remarkable, the symmetry of the circadian pattern of cattle from distinct feed efficiency groups for albumin and cholesterol levels. It is also noticeable, the similarity of the CO_2 and creatinine patterns, especially during the first hours of blood sampling.

Discussion

Steers were monitored for productive performance during the finishing phase of the beef cattle production cycle; a period which is particularly impacted by major expenses associated with the rich diets fed to ensure fast growth and desirable carcass composition [1]. We observed that during this period of 140 days, each of the efficient steers consumed a total of 259 kg less feed (dry matter basis) to achieve similar growth rate, body weight and carcass composition (as indicated by the ultrasonographic assessments of body fatness and leanness) when compared to the inefficient steers. This phenotypic divergence in feed efficiency has also been reported elsewhere [29] and reinforces the economic and environmental [30] benefits of increasing the efficiency of feed utilization in the bovine. Herein, indicators of metabolic rate and liver function are discussed in the context of feed efficiency, not only to advance our knowledge on physiological mechanisms related

Table 3 Descriptive statistics and least square means for metabolic profile parameters by efficiency groups

Parameter (abbreviation; unit)	Mean	Standard deviation	Efficient	Inefficient	P value
Products related to liver function					
Albumin (g/l)	36.92	1.76	36.18	37.65	0.001*
Bile acids (BA; umol/l)	13.75	5.65	9.79	10.64	0.491
Cholesterol (mmol/l)	2.84	0.47	2.62	3.05	0.008*
Urea (mmol/l)	4.66	0.84	4.56	4.49	0.920
Enzymes related to liver function					
Alkaline phosphatase (ALP; U/l)	98.72	18.36	101.80	99.76	0.816
Aspartate aminotransferase (AST; U/l)	103.31	88.97	77.71	79.68	0.830
γ-glutamyl transpeptidase (GGT; U/l)	23.01	4.46	22.69	23.17	0.558
Lipase (U/l)	7.43	0.80	7.71	7.15	0.082**
Indicators of energetic status					
Acetate (μg/ml)	46.33	15.17	47.62	46.13	0.359
β-hydroxybutyrate (BHBA; umol/l)	369.57	84.18	354.15	379.98	0.222
Carbon dioxide (CO_2; mmol/l)	24.10	1.55	24.36	23.65	0.019*
Indicators of muscle metabolism					
Creatine kinase (CK; U/l)	320.14	180.43	278.57	258.59	0.702
Creatinine (mmol/l)	116.58	15.78	118.59	110.50	0.037*

* $P \leq 0.05$

** $P \leq 0.10$

to energy utilization, but also to identify potential biomarkers that could be applied in the livestock industry to indirectly assess feed efficiency. Such biomarkers could be complementary and of assistance to support molecular approaches of research on gene expression [31] and gene networks [32] as these relate to feed efficiency.

Liver weight appears to increase or decrease in direct proportion to the nutritional plane [33] and across physiological stages [7]. Our results indicated no difference in liver biometrics when efficient and inefficient steers were compared, suggesting that metabolic differences in liver function related to feed efficiency [6] may not be reflected in the liver weight. Gravimetric assessments of organ function are relatively coarse assessments when used to capture diminished structural and functional changes such as those due to variation in feed efficiency. Alternatively, one can assess certain physiological events which result in drastic changes in liver workload and weight. This lack of differences in liver and other visceral organ weights in relation to feed efficiency category is also reported elsewhere [20].

Despite the lack of liver weight differences between feed efficiency groups, the micro-structural evaluation of the liver parenchyma revealed direct associations between hepatocyte and hepatocyte nuclei size with feed efficiency in both histological regions evaluated. Overall, these results indicated that improved feed efficiency is associated with a greater functional workload placed on the liver. It is known that the liver primarily responds to fluctuations in workload through hepatocyte hypertrophy or hypotrophy [7]. For instance, Zaitoun et al. [14] demonstrated that a portacaval shunt resulted in substantial hypotrophy of hepatocytes in rats due to the surgical decrease in liver workload. Compared to other organs that are constantly being renewed (such as the intestine), the hepatic parenchyma is a relatively stable cell population; dividing cells are seldom seen in the normal liver [13]. Thus, the observed enlarged hepatocytes in efficient steers strongly indicates that a higher metabolic pace in liver is consonant with improved feed efficiency. This is further reinforced by the observation of increased mitochondrial enzymatic activity in the liver of cattle with superior feed efficiency [6]. Moreover, the larger hepatocytes found in the efficient steers and the lack of difference in weight when compared to the inefficient steers, suggests an overall reduced number of hepatocytes in the liver of efficient steers, which remains to be evaluated through extensive cellularity studies including other lobes of the liver, combined with cellular turnover assessments [34].

The histomorphometrical findings herein, are also in agreement with observations in the intestine metabolism and structure in the context of feed efficiency and productivity [15], when evaluating the histomorphometry of the small intestine of the steers from population B reported in the present study, found larger cellularity in both the duodenum and ileum, corresponding to a higher functional workload in the small intestine of cattle with superior feed efficiency. Similarly, Steinhoff-Wagner et al. [35] found that breeds of cattle with higher growth rates and superior feed efficiency had greater cellularity in the small intestine compared with the cattle breeds with lower growth rates. Unlike the healthy liver [36], the intestine responds to changes in workload primarily by adjusting its cellularity [11]. In fact, our histomorphometrical results in the liver are in line with findings in the small intestine [15, 35] as both indicate that improved feed efficiency is accompanied by a higher metabolic demand on these visceral organs. Interestingly, a study by Colnot et al. [37] on glucose absorption in the small intestine of neonatal calves demonstrated the primary role of the mucosal growth to trigger the intestinal metabolism of glucose. In another study in calves, Meyer et al. [17] demonstrated the relevance of intestinal growth to the variation in feed efficiency.

Despite the functional differences in hepatocytes neighboring the portal triad and central vein microscopic regions [38], we did not observe histomorphometrical differences between these relating to feed efficiency. However, the relatively larger hepatocyte nuclei area in the central vein region in comparison to the portal triad region is an expected finding [13], and reinforces the soundness of our histomorphometry methodology.

The circadian profile of blood plasma albumin indicated lower concentrations in efficient steers. Gonano et al. [18], also evaluating the circadian cycle, observed no difference in albumin levels according to feed efficiency in beef heifers. Similarly, Bourgon et al. [19] did not find differences on albumin over ultradian sampling in feedlot beef bulls. In another study, Richardson et al. [20] observed a negative correlation between blood plasma albumin and daily feed intake. This observation supports our results, since inefficient steers consumed more feed than efficient steers. Additionally, albumin is solely produced in hepatocytes and is a relatively abundant and large molecule [39] and understanding that the machinery associated with albumin synthesis and secretion represents a large portion of the cytoplasm of hepatocytes [40]. We suggest that the myriad of liver functional differences (i.e., [31, 32]) influencing feed efficiency could be related to the processes involved with production, storage and secretion of albumin by the hepatocytes, which ultimately could influence the histomorphometric differences observed herein. We hypothesize that the secretion of this protein may be enhanced in inefficient animals, resulting in a lower accumulation of albumin in the hepatocytes and partially explaining the diminished cell size in response to lower feed efficiency.

Cholesterol levels exhibited minimal fluctuation throughout the circadian period; this is similar to the findings of Bitman et al. [41] in dairy cows. This relatively stable relationship of cholesterol levels with feed efficiency supports the utilization of cholesterol as a robust indicator of feed efficiency, since fewer blood collections may be sufficient to discriminate groups of cattle by feed efficiency. This result is also supported by the similar findings of Bourgon et al. [19] also studying feedlot cattle. The fact that improved feed efficiency was associated with lower levels of cholesterol, suggests that less lipogenesis, lipid transport and deposition occurs in efficient cattle. The biosynthesis of cholesterol from acetate is an energetically expensive process in the cell [42]; thus, lower cholesterol seems associated with lower basal energy requirements of efficient steers.

These lower levels of cholesterol may also be associated with the suggested increase in levels of lipase in efficient steers. It is known that cholesterol levels are at least partly regulated by pancreatic [43] and hepatic [44] lipases. The hepatic lipase enzyme not only hydrolyzes metabolites in cholesterol, but also stimulates cholesterol ester uptake by hepatocytes [45]. This evidence may also partially explain the enlarged size of the hepatocytes in efficient steers, since liver is the major organ of cholesterol uptake, accounting for 65% of the total [46]. Despite the fact that bile acids are produced in the liver as end products of cholesterol metabolism [47], differences in the size of the cholesterol pool across efficiency groups did not reflect differences in the abundance of bile acids throughout the circadian period; this supports the role of other controlling mechanisms to determine the pool size of bile acids discussed elsewhere [48].

The similarity in the concentration of liver function-related enzymes (ALP, AST and GGT) between efficient and inefficient steers is supported by other studies. Richardson et al. [38] and Bourgon et al. [19] observed no differences for AST and ALP in cattle grouped by feed efficiency. Similarly, Richardson et al. [38] observed no differences for GGT levels in cattle with distinct feed efficiency. On the other hand, Gonano et al. [18] observed increased levels of AST in blood of feed efficient beef heifers. The great variability of these enzymes, potentially due to effects of environment, physiological state and feeding regime, should be addressed in future studies.

Despite the relevance of acetate and BHBA as energy coins in the metabolism of ruminants [42], these parameters did not differ according to feed efficiency classes. Our findings reflect those of Gonano et al. [18], who evaluated acetate over the circadian period for efficient and inefficient beef heifers across different physiological states and noticed no difference between feed efficiency classes, which agrees with the results by Bourgon et al. [19] for acetate. In another study, Richardson et al. [38] found no difference in BHBA between feed efficiency groups of beef steers. The substantial variability of these parameters, even with hourly sampling, is probably the main limitation of the use of these parameters in the characterization of distinct feed efficiency phenotypes.

Conversely, CO_2 was consistently increased throughout the 24 h of sampling in cattle with improved feed efficiency. Since CO_2 serves as a fundamental indicator of metabolic rate [49], our results could be interpreted to suggest the increased metabolic rate is associated with improved feed efficiency. However, this is the opposite of the results reported in a study in beef heifers conducted at a comparable physiological stage and age [18]. An explanation for this divergence may relate to the experimental conditions. In our study, steers were sampled in the warmest period of the year in the Northern hemisphere, with an average barn temperature of 24.9 ± 3.2 °C, while the heifers sampled by Gonano et al. [18] were sampled during the winter, with an average barn temperature of 6.2 ± 1.8 °C, which is within the thermal neutral zone for *Bos taurus* [50], unlike our steers. It is known that blood plasma CO_2 concentration is influenced by heat and cold stress, as evaluated across different breeds of cattle [51]. It is also known that efficient and inefficient cattle differ in their coping styles to stressors, with feed efficient steers being more physiologically capable of dealing with stress [52]. That said, we hypothesize that efficient steers may have a wider range of blood CO_2 tolerance, which allows these animals to increase their CO_2 baseline in response to heat stress without relying extensively on the energetically costly dissipation of heat through evaporative heat loss [49]. Contrarily, the less stress-tolerant, inefficient steers will increase their respiration rate at a lower CO_2 threshold, maintaining their blood CO_2 at a lower level. Further investigations involving circadian patterns of breathe gasses analysis and blood partial pressure of CO_2 and oxygen in different environmental conditions are warranted to elucidate this hypothesis.

Creatine kinase is a clinical marker for muscle protein turnover [53] that has been shown to differ according to feed efficiency class. Gonano et al. [18] observed greater levels of CK in efficient heifers at pubertal age. This relationship was inverted when the same heifers were tested over the circadian period during late gestation, which may be related to changes in CK activity in response to aging [54]. In our study, CK did not differ between feed efficiency groups; the same was observed by Richardson et al. [38], when also evaluating beef steers. This enzyme catalyzes the conversion of creatinine to phosphocreatine, a reversible and energetically demanding reaction occurring mostly in skeletal muscle [22]. Conversely, phosphocreatine spontaneously forms phosphocreatine and creatinine under physiological conditions [55]. In our study, levels of creatinine were increased in efficient steers throughout the circadian period. In another study, creatinine was negatively correlated with feed efficiency [38]. Given the dissociation of our results for CK and creatinine, one may suggest that efficient steers may have a larger proportion of the creatinine metabolism occurring without relying on CK, since these animals had a larger creatinine pool in relation to the pool size of CK across the feed efficiency groups.

Conclusions

Our study provided the first evidence of a relationship between feed efficiency and liver histomorphometry. Improved feed efficiency appears to be associated with enlarged hepatocytes, which may be due to an increased metabolic rate of the liver parenchyma. Further studies utilizing complementary techniques such as microcalorimetry and molecular biology will provide further advances on this subject. Additionally, the evaluation of the metabolic profile across distinct phenotypes for feed efficiency revealed, that improved feed efficiency is associated with increased metabolism of muscle (higher creatinine) and of the whole body (higher CO_2 during heat stress) and reduced bloodstream pools of albumin and cholesterol. In essence, these metabolic discrepancies between feed efficient and inefficient cattle may be determinants of the differences in productive performance and potential phenotypes for indirectly assessing feed efficiency upon extensive validation and refinement for field work applications.

Abbreviations

ALP: alkaline phosphatase; AST: aspartate aminotransferase; BA: bile acids; BKFT: backfat thickness; BW: body weight; BHBA: β-hydroxybutyrate; CK: creatine kinase; CO_2: carbon dioxide; GGT: γ-glutamyl transpeptidase; HA: hepatocyte area; HP: hepatocyte perimeter; NA: hepatocyte nuclei area; NH: percentage of the total hepatocyte area accounted by the nuclei; RBEA: rib eye area; RFI: residual feed intake.

Authors' contributions

YM, KS and SM designed the research trial. YM, BC, SY optimized the histomorphometry evaluation of liver tissue. YM and LH completed the histomorphometry analysis and collected blood from the animals for metabolic profile. YM analyzed the data. All the authors contributed with the article writing and final edits. All authors read and approved the final manuscript.

Author details

[1] Department of Animal Science and Aquaculture, Faculty of Agriculture, Dalhousie University, 58 River Road, Bible Hill, Truro, NS B2N 5E3, Canada. [2] Faculdade de Medicina Veterinária, Universidade Federal do Rio Grande do Sul, Porto Alegre, RS 91540-000, Brazil. [3] Department of Animal Sciences, North Dakota State University, Fargo, ND 58102, USA. [4] Department of Biomedical Sciences, University of Guelph, Guelph, ON N1G 2W1, Canada. [5] Department of Animal Biosciences, University of Guelph, Guelph, ON N1G 2W1, Canada. [6] Angus Genetics Inc, Saint Joseph, MO 64506, USA.

Acknowledgements

We remember Ms. Helen Coates and are grateful for her substantial support with liver tissue processing and histomorphometry. We also would like to thank Ms. Tanya Muggeridge for her support with professional writing.

Competing interests
The authors declare that they have no competing interests.

Funding
We greatly appreciate the financial support of Beef Farmers of Ontario, Ontario Ministry of Agriculture and Rural Affairs, Beef Cattle Research Council and Agriculture Agri-Food Canada. The combined support from these entities enabled the design of the study and collection, analysis, and interpretation of data and in writing the manuscript.

References

1. Field TG. Beef production management and decisions. 5th ed. Upper Saddle River: Prentice Hall; 2006.
2. Koch RM, Swiger LA, Chambers D, Gregory KE. Efficiency of feed use in beef cattle. J Anim Sci. 1963;22:486–94.
3. Montanholi YR, Swanson KC, Palme R, Schenkel FS, McBride BW, Caldwell T, et al. On the determination of residual feed intake and associations of infrared thermography with efficiency and ultrasound traits in beef bulls. Livest Sci. 2009;125:22–30.
4. Ferrell CL. Contribution of visceral organs to animal energy expenditures. J Anim Sci. 1988;66:23–4.
5. Kolath WH, Kerley MS, Golden JW, Keisler DH. The relationship between mitochondrial function and residual feed intake in Angus steers. J Anim Sci. 2006;84:861–5.
6. Lancaster PA, Cartens GE, Michal JJ, Brennan KM, Johnson KA, Davis ME. Relationships between residual feed intake and hepatic mitochondrial function in growing beef cattle. J Anim Sci. 2014;92:3134–41.
7. Johnson DE, Johnson KA, Baldwin RL. Changes in liver and gastrointestinal tract energy demands in response to physiological workload in ruminants. J Nutr. 1990;120:649–55.
8. Webster AJF. The energetic efficiency of metabolism. Proc Nutr Soc. 1981;40:121–8.
9. Baldwin RL. Modeling ruminant digestion and metabolism. London: Chapman & Hall; 1995.
10. Terry CA, Knapp RH, Edwards JW, Mies WL, Savell JW, Cross HR. Yields of by-products from different cattle types. J Anim Sci. 1990;68:4200–5.
11. Helmstetter C, Reix N, T'Flachebba M, Pope RK, Secor SM, Le Maho Y, et al. Functional changes with feeding in the gastro-intestinal epithelia of the Burmese python (*Python molurus*). Zool Sci. 2009;29:632–8.
12. Burrin DG, Ferrell CL, Eisemann JH, Britton RA, Nienaber JA. Effect of level of nutrition on splanchnic blood flow and oxygen consumption in sheep. Brit J Nutr. 1989;62:23–34.
13. Fawcett DW. A textbook of histology. 12th ed. London: Chapman & Hall; 1994.
14. Zaitoun AA, Path FRC, Apelqcist G, Al-Mardini HA, Gray T, Bengtsson F, et al. Quantitative studies of liver atrophy after portacaval shunt in the rat. J Surg Res. 2006;131:225–32.
15. Montanholi YR, Fontoura A, Swanson K, Coomber B, Yamashiro S, Miller S. Small intestine histomorphometry of beef cattle with divergent feed efficiency. Acta Vet Scand. 2013;55:9.
16. Lignot JH, Helmstetter C, Secor MS. Postprandial morphological response of the intestinal epithelium of the Burmese python (*Python molurus*). Comp Biochem Physiol A. 2005;141:280–91.
17. Meyer AM, Hess BW, Paisley SI, Du M, Caton JS. Small intestinal growth measures are correlated with feed efficiency in market weight cattle, despite minimal effects of maternal nutrition during early to midgestation. J Anim Sci. 2014;92:3855–67.
18. Gonano CV, Montanholi YR, Schenkel FS, Smith BA, Cant JP, Miller SP. The relationship between feed efficiency and the circadian profile of blood plasma analytes measured in beef heifers at different physiological stages. Animal. 2014;13:1–15.
19. Bourgon SL, Diel de Amorim M, Miller SP, Montanholi YR. Associations of blood parameters with age, feed efficiency and sampling routine in young beef bulls. Livest Sci. 2017;195:27–37.
20. Richardson EC, Herd RM, Oddy VH, Thompson JM, Archer JA, Arthur PF. Body composition and implications for heat production of Angus steer progeny of parents selected for and against residual feed intake. Aust J Exp Agric. 2001;41:1065–72.
21. Goff JP. Digestion, absorption and metabolism. In: Reece WO, Erickson HH, Goff JP, Uemura EE, editors. Dukes' physiology of domestic animals. 13th ed. Hoboken: Wiley; 2013. p. 467–566.
22. Reece WO. Muscle physiology. In: Reece WO, Erickson HH, Goff JP, Uemura EE, editors. Dukes' physiology of domestic animals. 13th ed. Hoboken: Wiley; 2013. p. 263–86.
23. Montanholi YR, Swanson KC, Palme R, Schenkel FS, McBride BW, Lu D, Miller SP. Assessing feed efficiency in beef steers through feeding behavior, infrared thermography and glucocorticoids. Animal. 2010;4:692–701.
24. Montanholi YR, Palme R, Haas LS, Swanson KC, Vander Voort G, Miller SP. On the relationships between glucocorticoids and feed efficiency in beef cattle. Livest Sci. 2013;155:130–6.
25. Carson FL. Histotechnology: A self-Instructional text. Hong Kong: American Society of Clinical Pathologists; 1997.
26. Ledue TB, Collins MF. Development and validation of 14 human serum protein assays on the Roche Cobas® c 501. J Clin Lab Anal. 2011;25:52–60.
27. Sissons JW. Digestive enzymes of cattle. J Sci Food Agric. 1981;32:105–14.
28. Hameed AM, Lam VWT, Pleass HC. Significant elevations of serum lipase not caused by pancreatitis: a systematic review. HPB (Oxford). 2015;17:99–112.
29. Gerber PJ, Steinfeld H, Mottet A, Opio C, Dijkman J, Falcucci A, et al. Tackling climate change through livestock: a global assessment of emissions and mitigation opportunities. Rome: Food and Agriculture Organization of the United Nations (FAO); 2013.
30. Zarek CM, Lindholm-Perry AK, Kuehn LA, Freetly HC. Differential expression of genes related to gain and intake in the liver of beef cattle. BMC Res Notes. 2017;10:1.
31. Weber KL, Welly BT, Van Eenennaam AL, Young AE, Porto-Neto LR, Reverter A, et al. Identification of gene networks for residual feed intake in Angus cattle using genomic prediction and RNA-seq. PLoS ONE. 2016;11:e0152274. doi:10.1371/journal.pone.0152274.
32. Sainz RD, Bentley BE. Visceral organ mass and cellularity in growth-restricted and refed beef steers. J Anim Sci. 1997;75:1229–36.
33. Marongiu F, Serra MP, Sini M, Marongiu M, Contini A, Laconi E. Cell turnover in the repopulated rat liver: distinct lineages for hepatocytes and the biliary epithelium. Cell Tissue Res. 2014;356:333–40.
34. Zitnan R, Voigt J, Kuhla S, Wegner J, Chudy A, Schoenhusen U, et al. Morphology of small intestinal mucosa and intestinal weight change with metabolic type of cattle. Vet Med Czech. 2008;53:525–32.
35. Steinhoff-Wagner J, Zitnan R, Schönhusen U, Pfannkuche H, Hudakova M, Metges CC, et al. Diet effects on glucose absorption in the small intestine of neonatal calves: importance of intestinal mucosal growth, lactase activity, and glucose transporters. J Dairy Sci. 2014;97:6358–69.
36. Ito N, Tatematsu M, Hirose M, Nakanishi K, Murasaki G. Enhancing effect of chemicals on production of hyperplastic liver nodules induced by n-2-fluorenylacetamide in hepatectomized rats. Gan. 1978;69:143–4.
37. Colnot S, Perret C. Liver zonation. In: Monga SPS, editor. Molecular pathology of liver diseases. New York: Springer; 2011. p. 7–16.
38. Richardson EC, Herd RM, Archer JA, Arthur PF. Metabolic differences in steers divergently selected for residual feed intake. Aust J Exp Agric. 2004;44:441–52.
39. Peters T. All about albumin: biochemistry, genetics, and medical applications. Amsterdam: Elsevier; 1995.
40. Oren R, Dabeva MD, Petkov MP, Hurston E, Laconi E, Shafritz DA. Restoration of serum albumin levels in nagase analbuminemic rats by hepatocyte transplantation. Hepatology. 1999;29:75–81.
41. Bitman J, Wood DL, Lefcourt AM. Rhythms in cholesterol, cholesteryl esters, free fatty acids, and triglycerides in blood of lactating dairy cow. J Dairy Sci. 1990;73:948–55.
42. Van Soest PJ. Nutritional ecology of the ruminant. 2nd ed. Ithaca: Comstock Publishing Associates; 1994.
43. Ricketts J, Brannon PM. Amount and type of dietary fat regulate pancreatic lipase gene expression in rats. J Nutr. 1994;124:1166–71.
44. Perret B, Mabile L, Martinez L, Tercé F, Barbaras R, Collet X. Hepatic lipase: structure/function relationship, synthesis, and regulation. J Lip Res. 2002;43:1163–9.
45. Thruren T. Hepatic lipase and HDL metabolism. Curr Opin Lipidol. 2000;11:277–83.
46. Glass C, Pittman RC, Weinstein DB, Steinberg D. Dissociation of tissue uptake of cholesterol ester from that of apoprotein A-I of rat plasma high

density lipoprotein: selective delivery of cholesterol ester to liver, adrenal, and gonad. Proc Natl Acad Sci. 1993;80:5435–9.
47. Li T, Chiang YL. Bile acid signaling in liver metabolism and diseases. J Lipid. 2012;2012:9.
48. Staels B, Fonseca V. Bile acids and metabolic regulation. Diabetes Care. 2009;32:S237–45.
49. Blaxter KL. The energy metabolism of ruminants. London: Hutchinson Scientific and Technical; 1962.
50. Brown-Brandl TM, Eigenberg RA, Nienaber JA. Heat stress factors of feedlot heifers. Livest Sci. 2006;105:57–68.
51. Srikandakumar A, Johnson EH. Effect of heat stress on milk production, rectal temperature, respiratory rate and blood chemistry in Holstein, Jersey and Australian Milking Zebu cows. Trop Anim Health Prod. 2004;36:685–92.
52. Munro JC, Schenkel FS, Physick-Sheard PW, Fontoura ABP, Miller SP, Tennessesen T, et al. Associations of acute stress and overnight heart rate with feed efficiency in beef heifers. Animal. 2017;11:452–60.
53. Baird MF, Graham SM, Baker JS, Bickerstaff GF. Creatine kinase and exercise-related muscle damage implications for muscle performance and recovery. J Nutr Metab. 2012;2012:1–13.
54. Nuss JE, Amaning JK, Bailey CE, DeFord JH, Dimayuga VL, Rabek JP, et al. Oxidative modification and aggregation of creatine kinase from aged mouse skeletal muscle. Aging. 2009;22:557–72.
55. Iyengar MR, Coleman DW, Butler TM. Phosphocreatinine, a high-energy phosphate in muscle, spontaneously forms phosphocreatine and creatinine under physiological conditions. J Biol Chem. 1985;260:7562–7.

10

A retrospective study of forensic cases of skin ulcerations in Danish pigs

Kristiane Barington*, Kristine Dich-Jørgensen and Henrik Elvang Jensen

Abstract

Background: Ulcerations in pigs, as in other farm animals, are considered to be painful and therefore hampering the welfare. Farmers are obliged to provide an intervention to protect animals against unnecessary suffering and failure to do so is considered negligence. Moreover, animals with severe open wounds are considered unfit for transportation and so are pigs with ulcerations located on hernias. This paper presents a retrospective study of forensic case files concerning ulcerations in Danish pigs from 2000 to 2014. The aim of the study was to clarify the number of cases, the number of pigs, the anatomical localization and size of ulcerations, evaluate changes during years and the age of the lesions.

Results: A total of 209 case files concerning 283 pigs with 459 ulcerations were included. In 2004, 2005, 2007–2009 and 2011, sows with shoulder ulcerations were the most frequently submitted, while in 2014 pigs with ulcerations on umbilical outpouchings dominated. The change in pattern on body location most likely reflects specific national regulations enforced from 2003 to 2009. The ulcerations were estimated to be from 4 h to several months old and the median diameter of ulcerations was 4 cm.

Conclusions: Since 2004, the number of cases per year has declined. However, the number of affected pigs has remained almost constant from 2004 to 2014 (23.8 ± 8.5 pigs per year). The change in pattern on body parts with ulcerations likely reflected specific national regulations.

Keywords: Forensic pathology, Pig, Ulcerations, Welfare

Background

Ulcerations in pigs, as in other farm animals, are considered to be painful and therefore hampering the welfare. If neglected, an ulceration can result in a forensic case, i.e. being reported to the police [1, 2]. Most ulcerations are due to external trauma while others are due to fistulation to the skin surface from an underlying condition [3–7]. However, farmers are obliged to provide an intervention to protect animals against unnecessary suffering no matter the cause of the ulceration. Failure to do so is considered negligence and a violation of the European Union Council Directive concerning the protection of animals kept for farming purposes [8]. In addition, animals with severe open wounds are considered unfit for transportation [9]. It has been specified by the Danish Veterinary and Food Administration that animals with ulcerations larger than 3 cm in diameter are unsuitable for transportation from transit locations or for transport across borders [10]. Moreover, the Danish Animal Welfare Council has stated that transport of slaughter pigs with ulcerations located on hernias is prohibited [11, 12].

Since 2003, special attention has been drawn to shoulder ulcerations on sows in Denmark and other countries (e.g. England and Canada) [1, 2, 4, 13–15]. Consequently, the Danish Animal Welfare Council stated that all shoulder ulcerations involving the subcutaneous tissue or deeper structures are considered a violation of the Danish Animal Protection Act [16–19].

*Correspondence: krisb@sund.ku.dk
Department of Veterinary Disease Biology, Faculty of Health and Medical Sciences, University of Copenhagen, Ridebanevej 3, DK-1870 Frederiksberg C, Denmark

The aim of a veterinary forensic examination requested by the police is to perform a thorough and precise documentation of the lesions with respect to diagnosis, dimensions, anatomical localization, and an assessment of the age of the lesions [20, 21]. Depending on the case, the estimated age of ulcerations is used to interpret the degree of negligence; i.e., ulcerations left untreated for a longer period are legally considered more serious than acute lesions [18].

In Denmark, all veterinary forensic investigations are requested by the police and carried out at the University of Copenhagen. This paper presents a retrospective study of forensic case files concerning ulcerations in Danish pigs from 2000 to 2014 submitted to Department of Veterinary Disease Biology, Faculty of Health and Medical Sciences, University of Copenhagen. The aim of the study was to clarify the number of cases, the number of pigs, the anatomical localization and size of ulcerations, evaluate changes during years and the age of lesions.

Methods

Case files concerning ulcerations in pigs sent for forensic investigation to the University of Copenhagen from 2000 to 2014 were examined retrospectively. A case file was defined as a single police record and included information regarding the number of pigs, the number and anatomical localizations of the ulcerations, the sex and age of the animal, the gross and histological descriptions of the ulcerations and usually photo documentation of lesions.

An ulceration was defined as a breach of the epidermis including the basal membrane [3]. Ulcerations included were due to an external force while case files concerning fistulation to the skin surface from underlying lesions were not included. All ulcerations were originally reported to the police by veterinary enforcement officers, i.e. by The Veterinary Task Force for livestock inspection, at transit locations, or at meat inspection at slaughterhouses.

The gross and histological evaluations of the ulcerations had been carried out by five experienced veterinary pathologist (i.e. professors with more than 10 years of experience with diagnostic pathology). Age estimations stated in the case files were made by the pathologists basing their estimations on the presence and amount of granulation tissue. In a few cases, in which granulation tissue was not grossly visible, the histological inflammatory reaction was used to state the age of the ulcerations. As reference to the estimation of age, studies of wound healing in pigs and humans were used [22–27]. Based on the gross (presence of granulation tissue) and histological descriptions, ulcerations were divided into four age intervals: (1) 0–3 days; (2) 4–7 days; (3) 8–28 days; and (4) >28 days. If granulation tissue was absent the ulceration was estimated to be less than 3 days old. In ulcerations with granulation tissue, the mean thickness was [mean ± standard deviation (SD)]: 4–7 days = 0.5 ± 0.3 cm; 8–28 days = 1.5 ± 1.2 cm; >28 days = 2.7 ± 2.5 cm. In ulcerations in which granulation tissue was not grossly visible, histology was applied to state the age of the ulceration. From these ulcerations new sections were cut and evaluated.

From the information given in the case files, the sex and age of the pigs were registered and pigs were grouped according to the anatomical localization of the ulceration: (1) shoulder, (2) umbilical outpouching (hernias, enterocystoma and preputial diverticula), (3) body (head, neck and back), (4) limb and (5) tail region. A pig with multiple ulcerations at different anatomical localizations was allocated to each of the specified anatomical localizations. For each of the anatomical localizations, measurements of the ulcerations were evaluated for normality and data were found to be nonparametric (SAS Institute 9.4). A Wilcoxon Rank Sum Test was used to compare the medians of the five groups (SAS Institute 9.4), and a P value below 0.05 was interpreted as a significant difference between groups.

Results

The inclusion criteria were fulfilled for 209 case files (Fig. 1). Each case file included 1–10 pigs with an average ($\bar{x}$) ± SD of 1.4 ± 1.2 pigs. Each pig had between 1 and 60 ulcerations (1.7 ± 3.7, $\bar{x}$ ± SD) with a median of 1. In total, tissue from 283 pigs had been submitted in which 459 ulcerations were described. In 40 of the 283 pigs, the exact number of ulcerations was not stated. The pigs were registered as females (53 %), males (5 %) and of unknown sex (42 %). Approximately half of the pigs were sows (51.2 %), while 34.3, 6.7, 0.4 and 7.4 % were slaughter pigs (5–6 months), younger pigs (<5 months), adult boars and pigs of unknown age, respectively.

During 2000–2003, 13 cases were sent for forensic investigation (Fig. 1). In 2004, the number of case files peaked (35 case files) being more than 11 times higher than in 2003 (3 case files). After 2004, the number of case files declined, however, the number of pigs with ulcerations each year showed an almost constant level of 23.5 ± 8.5 ($\bar{x}$ ± SD) pigs per year (Fig. 2). The proportion (%) of pigs submitted in relation to the number of produced pigs in Denmark showed roughly the same tendency as seen in Fig. 3. The pattern of distribution of ulcerations in the five groups of anatomical localization is presented in Fig. 4. In total, 131 out of 283 (46.3 %) of the pigs submitted from 2000 to 2014 were sows with shoulder ulcerations. In slaughter pigs and younger pigs, some ulcerations were located on abdominal outpouchings. In total, 52 out of 283 (18.4 %) of all pigs had an ulcerated

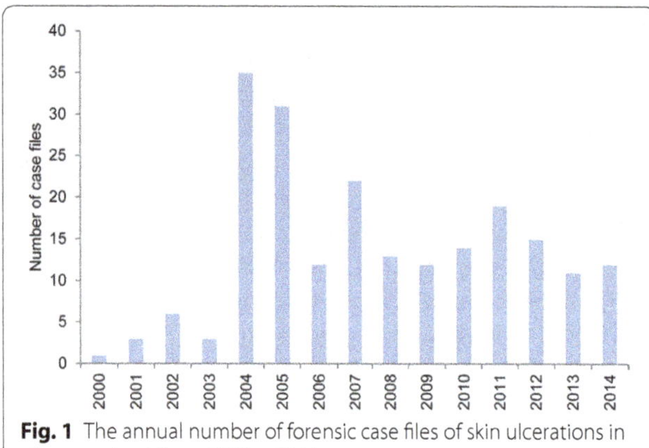

Fig. 1 The annual number of forensic case files of skin ulcerations in pigs examined from 2000 to 2014

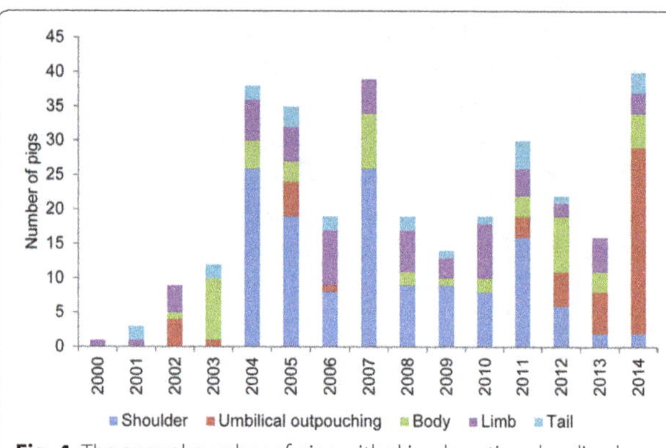

Fig. 4 The annual number of pigs with skin ulcerations localized on the shoulder, umbilical outpouching, body, limbs or tail

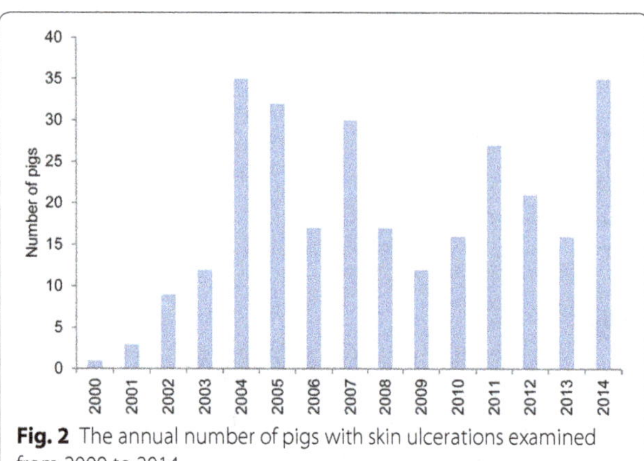

Fig. 2 The annual number of pigs with skin ulcerations examined from 2000 to 2014

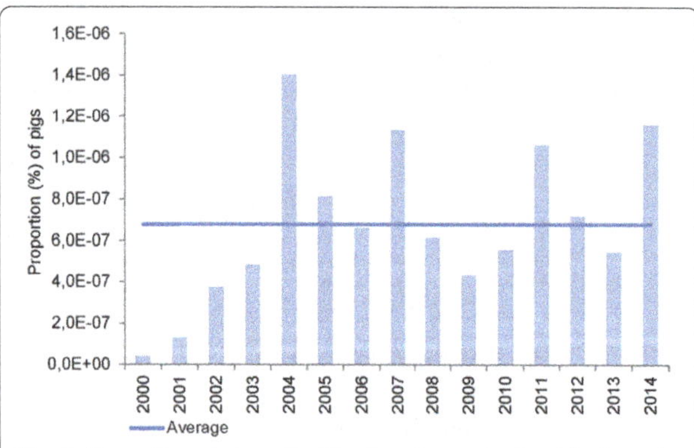

Fig. 3 Proportion of pigs with skin ulcerations submitted for forensic examination in relation to the total number of pigs produced in Denmark annually from 2000 to 2014

outpouching in the abdominal region. Ulcerations on the body and limbs were present in pigs of all ages and were present in 49 out of 283 (17.3 %) and in 61 out of 283 (21.5 %) of pigs, respectively. Ulcerations in the tail region were present in 23 out of 283 pigs (8.1 %). The total sum of the percentages exceeds 100 % as 22 pigs had ulcerations located at more than one location.

In 90.8 % of the ulcerations (417 out of 459), measurements of dimensions were registered. The median diameter of all ulcerations was 4 cm. The median, minimum and maximum values for the diameter of ulcerations in each of the anatomical localizations and totally are presented in Table 1. Differences in the diameter of the ulcerations were highly dependent on the anatomical localization ($P < 0.0001$).

The age had been determined for 65.4 % of the ulcerations (300 out of 459). The ulcerations were evaluated to be: (1) 0–3 days, n = 27; (2) 4–7 days, n = 3; (3) 8–28 days, n = 237; and (4) >28 days, n = 33.

New histological sections were cut in 29 out of 459 (6.3 %) ulcerations because granulation tissue had not been observed at gross evaluation. In a single ulceration, inflammation or granulation tissue was absent at the histological evaluation, and the age was stated as unknown. In another ulceration, in which the amount of granulation tissue could not be determined no estimate of an age was given. Three ulcerations were characterized by the infiltration of neutrophils and stated to be at least 4 h old.

Table 1 The diameter of 417 skin ulcerations in forensic case files (2000–2014)

Anatomical localization	Number of ulcerations	Median diameter (cm)	Minimum diameter (cm)	Maximum diameter (cm)
Shoulder	159	5	1	11
Umbilical outpouching	56	5.8	0.7	21
Body	37	1	0.3	10
Limb	142	1.5	0.2	14
Tail	23	3	1	18
Total	417	4	0.2	21

In nine ulcerations, both neutrophils and macrophages were present and the ulcerations were estimated to be between 6 and 24 h of age. In 15 ulcerations proliferation of fibroblasts was present and in some of the ulcerations newly formed capillaries were also observed. These ulcerations were stated to be 2–3 days old (n = 11) and between 16 and 32 h old (n = 4).

Discussion

Despite the number of case files per year had declined since 2004, the number of pigs affected remained almost constant during the last 10 years suggesting fewer but more serious offenders (Figs. 1, 2). Since 2003, shoulder ulcerations have received increased attention as a reflection of the publication of several papers [1, 2, 4, 14] and statements from the Danish Animal Welfare Council on the subject [17–19]. The development in the number of sows with shoulder ulcerations submitted for forensic investigation reflects the increased attention on the subject (Fig. 4). The first paper addressing the problem with shoulder ulcerations in sows was published in 2003 [14] and already the year after more than 25 cases were received for forensic investigation (Fig. 4). It is also likely that the increase in pigs with ulcerations on umbilical outpouchings from 2011 to 2014 is a consequence of two specific regulations on transportation of animals with ulcerations on umbilical outpouchings enforced by the Danish Animal Welfare Council in 2008 and 2009 [11, 12]. In these regulations, it was deducted that pigs with umbilical outpouching with a diameter of more than 15 cm or with ulcerations were unfit for transportation. Before that time, statements on umbilical outpouching were vaguer; i.e. animals were unfit for transportation if they were hampered by the outpouching.

The median diameter (4 cm) of all ulcerations exceeded the threshold of 3 cm set by the Danish Veterinary and Food Administration regarding ulcerations being too large to allow transportation of the animal. The median diameter of ulcerations on shoulders and umbilical outpouchings both exceeded 3 cm, while the median diameter of ulcerations on the tail, body and limbs did not exceed 3 cm (Table 1).

Estimating the age of ulcerations is central to a forensic investigation, as this in a judicial setting will be used to interpret the degree of negligence or in apportioning blame. In the majority of ulcerations, the age was estimated based on the presence of granulation tissue at gross examination. In order to document the level of violence of animal protection legislations, it is crucial that all cases are examined and filed in a well-documented professional manner. Therefore, in Denmark all requests for forensic examination of porcine ulcerations are taken care of at the University of Copenhagen. Moreover, the filing of cases is also highly important when sending out information material to pig producers, arrangement of courses and communicating with the authorities, e.g. the police and The Danish Welfare Council.

Conclusions

Since 2004, the number of cases per year has declined while the number of affected pigs has remained almost constant. The changes in anatomical localization of the ulcerations during 2000–2014 likely reflected specific national regulations.

Authors' contributions

All authors contributed to the design of the study, the collection of data and interpretation of data. In addition, KB performed the statistical analyses and drafted the manuscript. All authors read and approved the final manuscript.

Acknowledgements

The following Associated Professors are acknowledged for contribution of case files: Jørgen S. Agerholm, Tine Iburg, Pall S. Leifsson and Ole L. Nielsen.

Competing interests

The authors declare that they have no competing interests.

Funding

The authors received no financial support for the research, authorship, and/or publication of this article.

References

1. Herskin MS, Bonde MK, Jørgensen E, Jensen KH. Decubital shoulder ulcers in sows: a review of classification, pain and welfare consequences. Animal. 2011;5:757–66.
2. Larsen T, Kaiser M, Herskin MS. Does the presence of shoulder ulcers affect the behaviour of sows? Res Vet Sci. 2015;98:19–24.
3. Hargis AM, Ginn PE. The integument. In: Zachary JF, McGavin MD, editors. Pathologic basis of veterinary disease. 5th ed. Missouri: Elsevier; 2012. p. 972–1084.
4. Jensen HE. Investigation into the pathology of shoulder ulcerations in sows. Vet Rec. 2009;165:171–4.
5. Mirt D. Lesions of so-called flank biting and necrotic ear syndrome in pigs. Vet Rec. 1999;144:92–6.
6. Petersen HH, Nielsen EO, Hassing AG, Ersbøll AK, Nielsen JP. Prevalence of clinical signs of disease in Danish finisher pigs. Vet Rec. 2008;162:377–82.
7. Schrøder-Petersen DL, Simonsen H. Tail biting in pigs. Vet J. 2001;162:196–210.
8. Commission European. Council Directive (98/58/EC) of 20 July 1998 concerning the protection of animals kept for farming purposes. Off J Eur Commun. 1998;L221:23–7.
9. Commission European. Council Regulation (EC) (No 1/2005) of 22 December 2004 on the protection of animals during transport and related operations and amending Directives 64/432/EEC and 93/119/EC and Regulation (EC) No 1255/97. Off J Eur Commun. 2005;L3:1–44.
10. Anon. Announcement regarding transportation of animals [in Danish]. The Veterinary Food Administration 21.05.2005.
11. Anon. The Danish Animal Welfare Council statement regarding transportation of diseased or injured production animals including horses [in Danish]. The Danish Animal Welfare Council 17.02. 2009.
12. Anon. Statement of the 2 of December 2008 regarding pigs with umbilical or inguinal hernia [in Danish]. The Danish Animal Welfare Council 02.12.2008.

13. KilBride AL, Gilman CE, Green LE. A cross sectional study of the prevalence, risk factors and population attributable fractions for limb and body lesions in lactating sows on commercial farms in England. BMC Vet Res. 2009;5:30.
14. Lund M, Aalbaek B, Jensen HE. Shoulder ulcerations in sows—animal ethics [in Danish]. Dansk Veterinær Tidskrift. 2003;86:8–11.
15. Zurbrigg K. Sow shoulder lesions: risk factors and treatment effects on an Ontario farm. J Anim Sci. 2006;84:2509–14.
16. Anon. The Danish animal protection law LBK nr. 473 af 15.05.2014. [in Danish].
17. Anon. Supplemental statement regarding shoulder ulcerations in sows [in Danish]. The Danish Animal Welfare Council 23.05.2008.
18. Anon. Statement regarding shoulder ulcerations in sows, specific questions [in Danish]. The Danish Animal Welfare Council 18.10.2007.
19. Anon. The Danish Animal Welfare Council statement regarding shoulder ulcerations in sows [in Danish]. The Danish Animal Welfare Council 19.11.2003.
20. Munro R, Munro HMC. Some challenges in forensic veterinary pathology: a review. J Comp Pathol. 2013;149:57–73.
21. Salvagni FA, Siqueira AD, Maria ACBE, Santos CRDS, Ramos AT, Maiorka PC. Forensic veterinary pathology: old dog learns a trick. Braz J Vet Pathol. 2011;5:37–8.
22. Betz P. Histological and enzyme histochemical parameters for the age estimation of human skin wounds. Int J Legal Med. 1994;170:60–8.
23. Heffernan D, Dudley B, McNeil PL, Howdieshell TR. Local Arginine Supplementation results in sustained wound nitric oxide production and reductions in vascular endothelial growth factor expression and granulation tissue formation. J Surg Res. 2006;133:46–54.
24. Kondo T, Ishida Y. Molecular pathology of wound healing. Forensic Sci Int. 2010;203:93–8.
25. Singer AJ, Clark RAF. Cutaneous wound healing. N Engl J Med. 1999;341:738–46.
26. Takamiya M, Fujita S, Saigusa K, Aoki Y. Simultaneous detection of eight cytokines in human dermal wounds with a multiplex bead-based immunoassay for wound age estimation. Int J Legal Med. 2008;122:143–8.
27. van der Laan N, de Leij LF, ten Duis HJ. Immunohistopathological appearance of three different types of injury in human skin. Inflamm Res. 2001;50:350–6.

11

A space–time analysis of *Mycoplasma bovis*: bulk tank milk antibody screening results from all Danish dairy herds

Margarida Arede[1*], Per Kantsø Nielsen[1], Syed Sayeem Uddin Ahmed[1], Tariq Halasa[1], Liza Rosenbaum Nielsen[2] and Nils Toft[1]

Abstract

Background: *Mycoplasma bovis* is an important pathogen causing severe disease outbreaks in cattle farms. Since 2011, there has been an apparent increase in *M. bovis* outbreaks among Danish dairy cattle herds. The dairy cattle industry performed cross-sectional antibody screening for *M. bovis* on four occasions, using the indirect BIO K 302 *M. bovis* enzyme-linked immunosorbent assay (ELISA) (Bio-X, Belgium) in bulk tank milk from all dairy herds between June 2013 and July 2014. The objective of this study was to investigate the evolution of the spatial distribution of *M. bovis* in the Danish dairy herd population throughout the study period. Repeated bulk tank milk samples were used as a proxy for the herd-level diagnosis. Descriptive and spatial analyses were performed for the four screening rounds. Based on a previous diagnostic test evaluation study, the *M. bovis* status for each herd was determined as test-positive or test-negative using a cut-off of 50 optical density coefficient %. The spatial global clustering was evaluated through a modified K-function method, and local clusters were identified by scan statistics.

Results: The results showed that *M. bovis* test-positive herds had a dynamic pattern in space. The global clustering analysis showed that *M. bovis* test-positive herds were spatially correlated in rounds one, three and four. These findings were supported to some extent by the local clustering analysis, which found significant high- and low-risk spatial clusters in rounds one and three in the north and south of the mainland.

Conclusion: The clusters with a high risk of observing test-positive herds did not remain between sampling rounds, indicating that *M. bovis* did not tend to persist upon emergence in dairy herds. In contrast, the clusters with a low risk of observing test-positive herds persisted in the same area throughout the study period.

Keywords: Space–time analysis, *Mycoplasma bovis*, Mastitis, Dairy cattle, Denmark

Background

Mycoplasma bovis causes several production diseases in cattle, such as mastitis and arthritis [1]. Mastitis caused by *M. bovis* has been of increasing concern for farmers and veterinarians throughout the past decades, due to its negative impact on production and welfare. This pathogen is known to have an important economic impact due to the reduction in milk yield [2] and the increase in unplanned culling rates [2, 3]. Furthermore, the associated suffering and pain negatively affect animal welfare [4]. Its prevalence has been rising worldwide [5–7], but whether this is the result of a faster spread of the pathogen or a greater awareness of the pathogenic potential of this microorganism is unknown [3].

The primary route of *M. bovis* transmission is thought to be udder-to-udder in the milking parlour, though the spread of the bacteria to calves via the milk from infected cows, as well as direct contact between animals of all ages are also important transmission routes [1, 2]. The purchase of replacement heifers and cows (which are asymptomatic carriers of this agent) might account for the introduction of the disease and the origin of outbreaks

*Correspondence: marared@vet.dtu.dk
[1] Section for Epidemiology, National Veterinary Institute, Technical University of Denmark, Bülowsvej 27, 1870 Frederiksberg C, Denmark

[8]. Once the infection is established across different age groups in a herd, it can be difficult to eliminate [9]. Other factors counteracting the control and elimination of this disease from dairy herds [9] include: the lack of knowledge about *M. bovis* virulence factors and its mechanisms of pathogenesis [1, 4]; both natural and acquired resistance to most antibiotics in vivo [1, 10], and the absence of an effective vaccine.

The latest report on *M. bovis* herd-level prevalence in Danish dairy herds is out-dated [11]. Therefore, there is a current resurgence in research, due to reports of severe clinical outbreaks associated with this pathogen and the lack of current knowledge about the distribution of the infection in Danish cattle herds. Knowledge of possible space–time patterns of the disease at herd-level would be advantageous in the planning of a potential surveillance programme for *M. bovis*. This type of assessment has the potential to promote the establishment of control and prevention strategies by generating hypotheses of disease causation [12] and enables the planning of test-strategies, including choice of methods and testing frequencies.

Veterinary spatial and temporal epidemiology emerged in the late 1990s, after becoming very popular in the field of human disease epidemiology. The advances made within this area have facilitated the identification and adjustment for confounding factors and the development of new hypotheses regarding disease transmission by researchers and health officials [13]. To optimize spatial analysis, data should be analyzed using more than one technique [12]. This can be seen in many studies of different infectious diseases all over the world, for instance acute respiratory disease in cattle in Norway [14], Highly Pathogenic Avian Influenza (HPAI) in Bangladesh [15] and *Salmonella* Dublin in Denmark [16].

The objective of this study was to investigate the spatio-temporal patterns of *M. bovis* based on four available bulk tank milk (BTM) antibody screenings from all dairy cattle herds in Denmark in 2013–2014.

Methods

Sample collection

The Danish dairy cattle industry performed four full dairy herd population cross-sectional screenings of antibodies directed against *M. bovis* in BTM between 01 June 2013 and 01 July 2014, in order to estimate the apparent prevalence of *M. bovis* infection. Milk truck drivers collected the samples through the Danish milk quality control scheme, using standardized procedures. The farmers were not notified when the sampling would be performed. All samples were tested using the indirect BIO K 302 *M. bovis* ELISA test-kit (BIO-X Diagnostics, Jemelle, Belgium). Diagnostics were performed at the Eurofins Steins A/S Laboratory, Holstebro, Denmark. Based on a previous test-evaluation study, an optical density coefficient (ODC) $\geq$50 % was used to define test results from each herd as test-positive [17]. At that cut-off, the BTM ELISA was estimated to have a sensitivity (Se) = 43.5 % (95 % CI: 21.1–92.5 %) and specificity (Sp) = 99.6 % (95 % CI: 98.8–100 %).

Some herds were tested more than once per round because they participated in parallel projects or requested their own samples. However, only the sample with the highest ELISA-value in each round was kept in the dataset, as this was thought to improve the Se of the analysis without excessively reducing the Sp. All herds located on the island of Bornholm were excluded from the dataset, since their limited number and remote geographical location could introduce bias to the analysis.

Cartesian coordinates (EUREF 89; UTM zone N32) for all dairy herds included in the current study were available for spatial analysis.

Spatial analysis

The spatial analysis of *M. bovis* test-positive herds in Denmark was accomplished in two steps: 1) the global spatial clustering was evaluated with the Monte Carlo simulation of the K-function [18]; 2) the local clustering was assessed using purely spatial scan statistics [19].

Global clustering

The K-function is a widely used method for evaluating global spatial clusters. The complete spatial randomness (CSR) defined by the absence of clustering is tested using a homogenous Poisson process for the null-hypothesis K-function. This assesses the global clustering of test-positive herds relative to the test-negative herds throughout the study region. The function does not identify the location of the clusters, instead it provides a summary of the spatial dependence between test-positive herds as a function of distance [20].

In order to overcome the assumptions connected with this technique and to adapt it to the present data, a Monte Carlo simulation of the K-function was applied [18]. The difference between the empirical K-function and the estimated null-hypothesis version of the K-function (the D-function), with 95 % confidence interval, was plotted against the distance between farms. This was done for each of the four sampling rounds.

Local spatial clusters

Local clusters were estimated with scan statistics [21] for each sampling round. This technique is characterized by a circular window, which is moved in space for each possible geographic location and size [19].

A Bernoulli model was applied in SatScan™ (version 9.4.1, Martin Kulldorff and Information Management

Services Inc.; http://www.satscan.org/), where test-positive and test-negative herds were defined as previously described. The most likely clusters for higher or lower risk were identified by likelihood ratio testing, and their significance estimated through a Monte Carlo simulation consisting of 999 random replications of the dataset. A significance level of 5 % was used.

Results

Summary statistics

Of the total number of participating herds (3700), the majority were tested in all four rounds.

The overall decrease in the number of herds tested in each round throughout time reflects the demographic changes in the dairy herd population (Table 1).

The prevalence of test-positive herds ranged from 1.6 to 5.2 % during the study period (Table 1).

During the first screening round, 186 herds were *M. bovis* test-positive. Of these, 179, 170 and 165 herds were also tested in rounds two, three and four, respectively, and only 18 (10 %), 28 (16 %) and 12 (7 %) retested positive for *M. bovis*.

The majority of the 55 test-positive herds (60 %) in the second round either tested negative or were not tested on the previous round. The third and fourth screening rounds showed a similar pattern, with 70 and 60 % of the test-positive herds for each round testing positive for the first time.

Global clustering

The results of the D-function analyses for each round of sampling are illustrated in Fig. 1. The results indicate significant global clustering in the first and third sampling round, with the D-function rising above the 95 % simulation envelope in the first round at approximately 1–90 and 1–100 km in the third round. The analysis for the fourth round showed a decreased, yet significant global clustering with a modest rise in the D-function above the 95 % simulation envelope at a distance of approximately 40–60 km.

Local clustering

The purely spatial analysis performed with different spatial windows of 50, 25 and 15 % of the population at risk showed consistency in size and location of the clusters. Results relating to the space scan-statistics for 15 % of the population at risk in each round are presented in Table 2. No significant low-risk or high-risk clusters were identified in rounds two or four. Figure 2 shows the location and size of the significant clusters in rounds one and three.

The significant clusters with a high risk of test-positive herds were located to the north of the mainland for round one and to the south of the mainland for round three. The low-risk analysis of *M. bovis* test-positive herds identified two clusters in round one and one cluster in round three, all located in the southeast of Jutland, Funen and Zealand.

A density map of the average herd size of the sampled dairy herds during the study period was obtained using Quantum GIS.

Discussion

The objective of this study was to explore the spatial distribution of *M. bovis* antibody-positive dairy cattle herds in Denmark and to identify temporal patterns and/or spatial persistence of test-positivity between screening rounds. The global cluster analysis showed that *M. bovis* test-positive herds were spatially correlated in screening rounds one, three, and (to a certain extent) four. These findings were confirmed by the local clustering analysis for rounds one and three, which identified significant spatial clusters: some of which were spatial clusters of herds with a higher risk of being test-positive, whilst the remaining clusters were herds with a lower risk than the other herds included in the analysis. The results for the

Table 1 Descriptive data and apparent prevalence for each sampling round

Sampling round	1	2	3	4
Duration[a]	01 June–31 july 2013	01 August–31 december 2013	27 January–18 march 2014	11 June–01 july 2014
No of test-positive[b]	186	55	107	55
No of herds sampled[c]	3578	3583	3446	3379
Apparent prevalence[d] (%)	5.2	1.5	3.1	1.6
(CI 95 %)[e]	(4.5–5.9)	(1.1–1.9)	(2.5–3.7)	(1.2–2.1)

[a] Duration of the sample period

[b] Number of test-positive herds for *M. bovis* in each sampling round

[c] Total number of sampled herds for *M. bovis* in each sampling round

[d] Apparent prevalence of *M. bovis* in each sampling round

[e] Confidence interval for the apparent prevalence of *M. bovis* in each sampling round

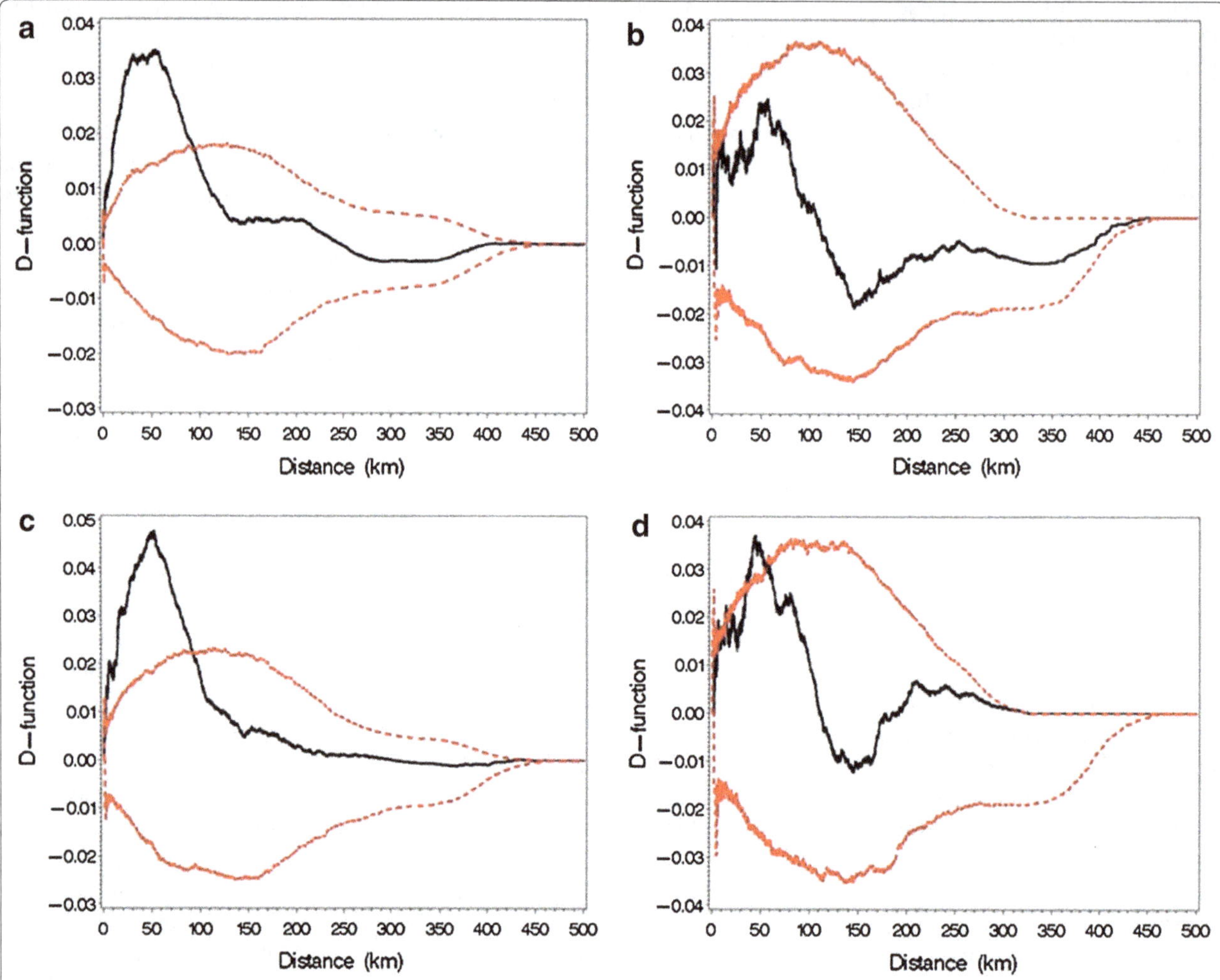

Fig. 1 Global clustering per sampling round. Legend: estimated D-function (*black line*) with 95 % simulation envelope (*red line*) of *Mycoplasma bovis* test-positive herds for round 1 (**a**); round 2 (**b**); round 3 (**c**); and round 4 (**d**), in Denmark

purely spatial analysis are reliable as they were shown to be consistent throughout the different spatial windows.

The local cluster analysis identified high-risk clusters of *M. bovis* test-positive herds to the north and south of the mainland, and low-risk clusters to the southeast of the mainland and islands, as well as central areas. Their locations might be partly explained by the different density of dairy cattle in these areas. The low-risk clusters were established in areas with a lower density of dairy cattle and the high-risk clusters were, to some extent, situated in areas where the density of dairy cattle was higher (Fig. 3). The higher animal turnover rate in larger herds (compared to smaller ones) is known to increase the risk of introducing an infected animal [6, 8]. This has been recognized both directly (by the positive association between presence of *Mycoplasma* sp. in BTM in larger herds [7, 22]) and indirectly (through the positive correlation between the weight of shipped milk per herd and the concentration of *M. bovis* in BTM [8]).

In rounds one and three, the low-risk clusters were located in approximately the same area, which implies the herds located in these regions had a lower risk of being infected by *M. bovis*. In contrast, the most significant clusters for the high-risk analysis differed markedly in location and size between screening rounds. The high-risk clusters were located to the north of the mainland in the first round and to the south of the mainland in the third round, with approximately 200 km between the two regions. This suggests that the occurrence of disease changed considerably in space throughout the study period (Fig. 2).

The cluster identified in the north in the first round was not present in the subsequent rounds. This implies a decrease in infected herds at this location in

Table 2 Statistically significant spatial clusters of high- and low-risk *Mycoplasma bovis* test-positive herds in Denmark, by sampling round

Sampling round	Population[a]	Radius (km)	O[b] (E[c])	RR[d]	LR[e]	*P*[f]
1	334	28.89	41 (17)	2.75	14.33	<0.010
	400	87.05	4 (20)	0.17	11.44	0.035
	356	85.93	3 (18)	0.15	11.13	0.047
3	43	8.73	10 (1)	8.15	12.81	0.011
	380	67.36	0 (11)	0	12.72	0.011

Results relating to the space scan-statistics for 15 % of the population at risk in each round are presented

[a] Number of herds in each cluster

[b] Observed number of test-positive herds in each cluster

[c] Expected number of test-positive herds in each cluster

[d] Relative risk

[e] Likelihood ratio

[f] *P* value for the likelihood ratio test

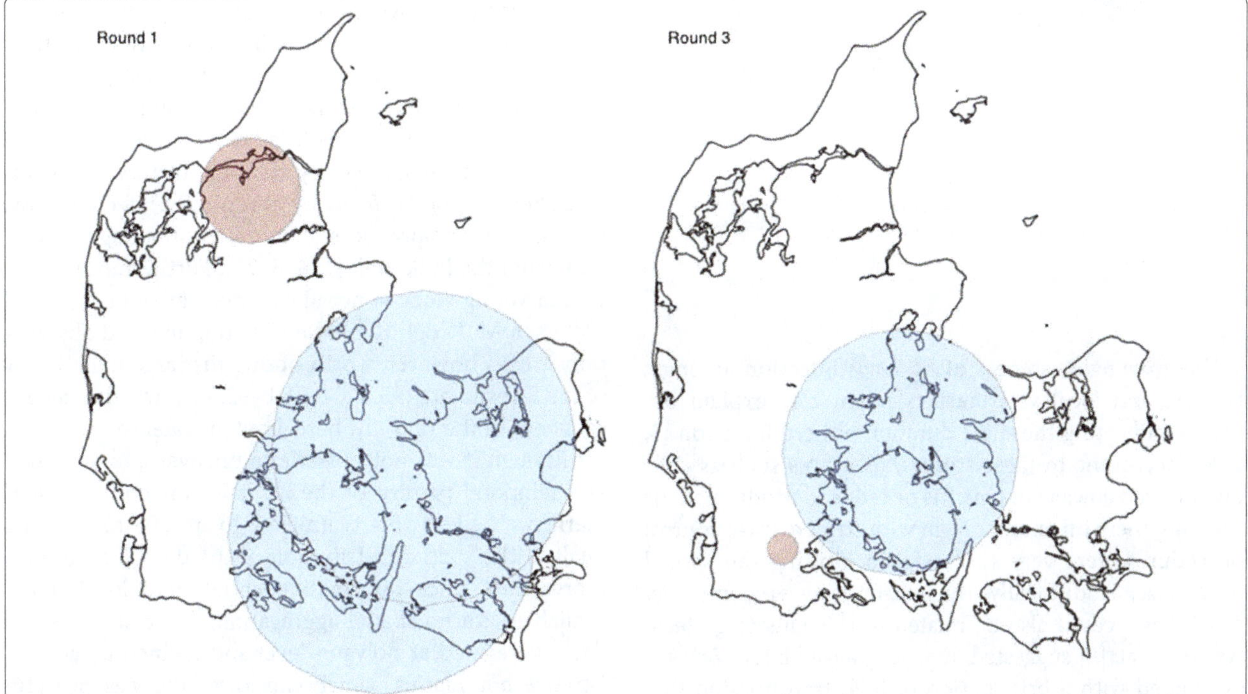

Fig. 2 Map of significant local high-risk and low-risk clusters of *Mycoplasma bovis* infection in Denmark. Legend: location of the significant clusters with a high risk (*red closed circle*) and low risk (*blue closed circle*) of *M. bovis* test-positive herds in Denmark, by sampling round

the months following the first round, assuming that a positive BTM ELISA test result indicates current or recent *M. bovis* infection. The cluster identified in round one contained 41 test-positive herds; of these, only eight herds (20 %) retested positive in the two following rounds, and only three herds (7 %) tested positive in the final round. With a similar pattern, the high-risk cluster identified in the third round had ten test-positive herds, of which only one herd (10 %) retested positive in the fourth round. In general, the test-positive herds in each round did not show a tendency to remain positive in subsequent rounds. In fact, in each round, at least 60 % of the test-positive herds were new. This suggests that the duration of infection in dairy herds is relatively short, an interpretation supported by Bray et al. [23], who found that *M. bovis* bacteria could not be detected in a herd 1 month after a positive diagnosis.

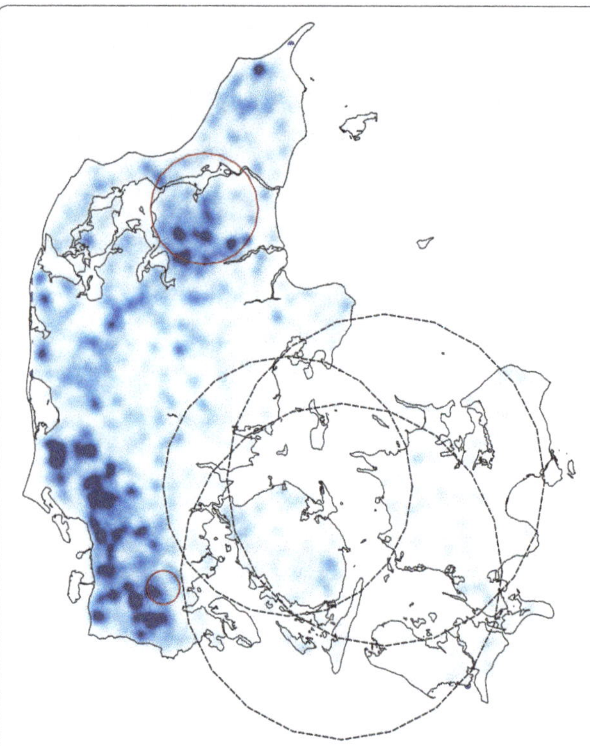

Fig. 3 Density map of the average herd size of the dairy herds sampled during the study period. Legend: Location of the significant clusters with a high risk (*red solid line*) and low risk (*black dashed line*) of *Mycoplasma bovis* test-positive herds in Denmark

The growing awareness of *M. bovis* infection amongst farmers and local veterinarians might also explain the results indicating the short duration of herd infection [3, 7, 8]. According to these studies, measures such as culling infected cows with mastitis or reduced production, or isolating them on another farm with strict disease control procedures were very successful in limiting the spread of disease. Additionally, the self-limiting epidemiology of *M. bovis* could also be related to this cluster pattern. As Fox et al. [8] suggested, mastitis caused by *M. bovis* is associated with a brief period of high transmission that might be followed by a far lower transmission rate that is unable to maintain the presence of the pathogen in the mammary glands of a herd. It is possible that a small number of remaining infected animals excreting lower concentrations of bacteria (and hence producing lower levels of antibodies directed against *M. bovis*) might not be sufficient to elicit a response in the BTM ELISA above 50 ODC % (Petersen M, Krogh K, Nielsen LR; unpublished observations).

Taking into account what is known about *M. bovis* epidemiology, we can hypothesize how an animal may become infected with *M. bovis* in a herd turning test-positive between rounds. The infection could be introduced through a replacement heifer without quarantine or pre-movement testing, by exposure to other animals with pneumonia and arthritis caused by *M. bovis* [1, 2], or through auto-infection by a haematogenous route from other body sites to the mammary gland [6]. As stated previously, after an udder infection is established, the spread within the herd can occur quite rapidly. This is due to the large amount of bacteria shed in the milk before the onset of clinical mastitis infecting several other cows through udder-to-udder transmission at the milking parlour by the milking machines, teat cups or milkers' hands [6].

Regarding the test outcome, false positive results are possible though unlikely, since the Sp of the test at the applied cut-off is close to 100 % [99.6 (95 % CI: 98.8–100)] [17]. False positive tests caused by carry-over between farms during sampling are thought to be negligible since the standardized sampling procedures should minimize this. The low Se of the ELISA test, 43.5 % (95 % CI: 21.1–92.5 %) at the applied cut-off, might have influenced the results and caused an underestimation of the infection. The analysis would probably have underestimated the size of the detected clusters and their significance, and/or have caused the analysis to miss smaller clusters. This could have been caused by dilution factors, intermittent shedding of *M. bovis* by chronically infected cows, or management practices such as withholding mastitic milk from the bulk tank [1, 4, 8, 22]. Furthermore, infection in young stock is not always detectable in the BTM (Petersen M, Krogh K, Nielsen LR; unpublished observations). It is, however, worth noting the large uncertainty of the Se estimate (95 % CI: 21.1–92.5 %), which is a consequence of the very low herd-level prevalence.

Although it was not possible to uncover a clear spatial and temporal pattern of the *M. bovis* infection in Denmark, we believe this is unlikely to be due to the data quality. The spatial distribution of the data is accurately represented since information about herd locations is available with no spatial aggregation. Some studies have data aggregated at polygon level and defined by administrative boundaries, which can lower the variance [16] and influence a false distribution pattern due to the selected boundaries [24]. Whilst in other studies, data are extracted from passive disease surveillance plans and only have information about cases, we had access to diagnostic information from a study population that contained the entire target population. However, the data presented drawbacks in sampling with an irregular timeframe and duration for each screening round.

Further investigation is required to study whether the *M. bovis* strains were the same between high-prevalence clusters in different rounds of sampling, as well as whether the pattern of animal movements between infected and uninfected herds or local short-distance spread (e.g., on pasture) can partially explain the existence of these clusters. It would also be of value to do the same analysis in the future, in order to assess whether the patterns throughout space and time would be similar to the ones reported by this study.

Conclusions

There was no evidence for any *M. bovis* hotspots in Denmark, since the high-risk clusters of *M.bovis* test-positive herds appeared to have a short time span. However, it was verified that the low-risk clusters remained in the same location throughout time, indicating that herds in these geographical areas were at a lower risk of being test-positive for *M. bovis*. Nevertheless, further studies are needed to confirm this, and to elucidate the possible reasons as well as the implications for planning future control efforts.

Abbreviations

BTM: bulk tank milk; CSR: complete spatial randomness; ELISA: enzyme-linked immunosorbent assay; *M. bovis*: *Mycoplasma bovis*; ODC: optical density coefficient; Se: sensitivity; Sp: specificity; UTM: universal transverse mercator coordinate system.

Authors' contributions

MA performed the data management and descriptive statistics, the local spatial analysis in SatScan and drafted the manuscript under supervision by NT, TH and LN. PN participated in the design of the study and assisted in the data management and the draft of the manuscript. SA carried out the global spatial analysis by the K-function method. All authors read and approved the final manuscript.

Author details

[1] Section for Epidemiology, National Veterinary Institute, Technical University of Denmark, Bülowsvej 27, 1870 Frederiksberg C, Denmark. [2] Department of Large Animal Sciences, Faculty of Health and Medical Sciences, University of Copenhagen, Grønnegårdsvej 2, 1870 Frederiksberg C, Denmark.

Acknowledgements

We gratefully acknowledge the Danish Milk Levy fund who funded the sampling, and SEGES who provided the data. Without their participation, this study would not have been possible.

Competing interests

The authors declare that they have no competing interests.

References

1. González RN, Wilson DJ. Mycoplasmal mastitis in dairy herds. Vet Clin North Am Food Anim Pract. 2003;19:199–221.
2. Pfützner H, Sachse K. *Mycoplasma bovis* as an agent of mastitis, pneumonia, arthritis and genital disorders in cattle. Rev Sci Tech. 1996;15:1477–94.
3. Brown MB, Shearer JK, Elvinger F. Mycoplasmal mastitis in a dairy herd. J Am Vet Med Assoc. 1990;196:1097–101.
4. Maunsell FP, Woolums AR, Francoz D, Rosenbusch RF, Step DL, Wilson DJ, et al. *Mycoplasma bovis* infections in cattle. J Vet Intern Med. 2011;25:772–83.
5. Passchyn P, Piepers S, De Meulemeester L, Boyen F, Haesebrouck F, De Vliegher S. Between-herd prevalence of *Mycoplasma bovis* in bulk milk in Flanders, Belgium. Res Vet Sci. 2012;92:219–20.
6. Jasper DE. Bovine mycoplasmal mastitis. Adv Vet Sci Comp Med. 1981;25:121–57.
7. Pinho L, Thompson G, Machado M, Carvalheira J. Management practices associated with the bulk tank milk prevalence of *Mycoplasma* spp. in dairy herds in Northwestern Portugal. Prev Vet Med. 2013;108:21–7.
8. Fox LK, Hancock DD, Mickelson A, Britten A. Bulk tank milk analysis: factors associated with appearance of *Mycoplasma* sp. in Milk. J Vet Med Ser B. 2003;50:235–40.
9. Nicholas R, Ayling R. *Mycoplasma bovis*: disease, diagnosis, and control. Res Vet Sci. 2003;74:105–12.
10. Nicholas R, Ayling R, McAuliffe L. Diseases caused by *Mycoplasma bovis*. In: Nicholas R, Ayling R, McAuliffe L, editors. Mycoplasma diseases of ruminants. Wallingford: CABI; 2008. p. 133–54.
11. Kusiluka LJ, Ojeniyi B, Friis NF. Increasing prevalence of *Mycoplasma bovis* in Danish cattle. Acta Vet Scand. 2000;41:139–46.
12. Ward MP, Carpenter TE. Analysis of time-space clustering in veterinary epidemiology. Prev Vet Med. 2000;43:225–37.
13. Carpenter TE. Methods to investigate spatial and temporal clustering in veterinary epidemiology. Prev Vet Med. 2001;48:303–20.
14. Norström M, Pfeiffer DU, Jarp J. A space-time cluster investigation of an outbreak of acute respiratory disease in Norwegian cattle herds. Prev Vet Med. 2000;47:107–19.
15. Ahmed SSU, Ersbøll AK, Biswas PK, Christensen JP. The space-time clustering of highly pathogenic avian influenza (HPAI) H5N1 outbreaks in Bangladesh. Epidemiol Infect. 2010;138:843–52.
16. Ersbøll AK, Nielsen LR. Spatial patterns in surveillance data during control of *Salmonella* Dublin in bovine dairy herds in Jutland, Denmark 2003–2009. Spat Spatiotemporal Epidemiol. 2011;2:195–204.
17. Nielsen PK, Petersen MB, Nielsen LR, Halasa T, Toft N. Latent class analysis of bulk tank milk PCR and ELISA testing for herd level diagnosis of *Mycoplasma bovis*. Prev Vet Med. 2015;121:338–42.
18. Ersbøll AK, Ersbøll BK. Simulation of the K-function in the analysis of spatial clustering for non-randomly distributed locations-exemplified by bovine virus diarrhoea virus (BVDV) infection in Denmark. Prev Vet Med. 2009;91:64–71.
19. Kulldorff M, Athas WF, Feuer EJ, Miller BA, Key CR. Evaluating cluster alarms: a space-time scan statistic and brain cancer in Los Alamos. Am J Public Health. 1998;88:1377–80.
20. Ripley BD. Statistical Inference for Spatial Processes [Internet]. Cambridge: Cambridge University Press; 1988 [cited 2015 Aug 15]. Available from: http://dx.doi.org/10.1017/CBO9780511624131.
21. Kulldorff M. A spatial scan statistic. Communications in statistics—theory and methods [Internet]. 1997;26:1481–96. Available from: http://www.tandfonline.com/doi/abs/10.1080/03610929708831995.
22. USDA APHIS. Mycoplasma in Bulk Tank Milk on U.S. Dairies [Internet]. USDA APHIS Vet. Serv. Info Sheet. 2003 [cited 2015 Aug 15]. Available from: https://www.aphis.usda.gov/animal_health/nahms/dairy/downloads/dairy02/Dairy02_is_Mycoplasma.pdf.
23. Bray DR, Shearer JK, Donovan CA, Reed PA. Approaches to achieving and maintaining a herd free of Mycoplasma Mastitis. Proc. 36th Annu. Meet Natl Mastit Counc Madison, WI [Internet]. 1997. p. 132–7. Available from: http://dairy.ifas.ufl.edu/dpc/1997/Bray.pdf.
24. Openshaw S. The modifiable areal unit problem. Concepts and techniques of modern geography. Norwich: Geo Books; 1984.

12

Neurophysiological assessment of spinal cord injuries in dogs using somatosensory and motor evoked potentials

Maria Claudia Campos Mello Inglez de Souza[1*], Ricardo José Rodriguez Ferreira[2], Geni Cristina Fonseca Patricio[1] and Julia Maria Matera[1]

Abstract

Somatosensory evoked potentials (SSEPs) and motor evoked potentials (MEPs) are non-invasive neurophysiological tests that reflect the functional integrity of sensory and motor pathways. Despite their extensive use and description in human medicine, reports in veterinary medicine are scarce. SSEPs are obtained via peripheral stimulation of sensory or mixed nerves; stimulation induces spinal and cortical responses, which are recorded when sensory pathways integrity is preserved. MEPs can be obtained via transcranial electrical or magnetic stimulation; in this case, thoracic and pelvic limb muscle responses are captured if motor pathways are preserved. This review describes principles, methodology and clinical applicability of SSEPs and MEPs in companion animal medicine. Potential interferences of anesthesia with SSEP and MEP recording are also discussed.

Keywords: Neurophysiology, Transcranial electrical stimulation, SSEPs, MEPs

Background

Spinal cord injuries may lead to clinical signs ranging from localized pain to paresis or plegia, with or without preservation of conscious pain perception. Along with regenerative therapy, more attention should be given to diagnostic modalities and objective tools designed to monitor neural pathways as a predictor of outcome in veterinary medicine.

Neurophysiological studies involve a range of tests designed to record action potentials along sensory and motor pathways; such tests provide data on injury site and severity and help to assess the progression of spinal cord lesions (i.e., improvement or deterioration) [1, 2]. Some modalities can specifically evaluate the peripheral nervous system, as nerve conduction studies, others will also evaluate the central nervous system, as somatosensory evoked potentials and motor evoked potentials, as described in this review. Intraoperative monitoring during spinal surgery is also possible, with improved prevention of iatrogenic injuries and more accurate prognosis [1, 3]. This review describes basic principles, methodology and clinical applicability of evoked potential tests in small animals.

Search strategy

This overview was provided through searches of Pubmed (http://www.ncbi.nlm.nih.gov/pubmed) and Google Scholar (https://scholar.google.com), using the terms "motor evoked potentials, somatosensory evoked potentials, SSEPs and MEPs". The titles and abstracts were evaluated and pertinent articles related to the current study were identified. Full-text manuscripts were then collected and assessed in detail. Personal archives were used to illustrate SSEPs and MEPs recordings.

Review

Evoked potentials are neurophysiological tests designed to assess, among others, the functionality of neural pathways involved in spinal cord injuries. Somatosensory evoked potentials (SSEPs) correspond to spinal and

*Correspondence: claudiainglez@usp.br
[1] Department of Surgery, School of Veterinary Medicine and Animal Science, University of São Paulo, Cidade Universitária, Prof. Dr. Orlando Marques de Paiva, 87, São Paulo, SP 05508-270, Brazil

cortical sensory responses recorded following electrical stimulation of a peripheral nerve, and reflect the functionality of ascending sensory pathways. In contrast, motor evoked potentials (MEPs) correspond to peripheral muscular responses recorded following motor cortex stimulation and reflect the functionality of descending motor pathways [2, 4].

Neurophysiological techniques are extremely popular in human medicine and are particularly indicated for intraoperative monitoring during spinal surgery; however, reports on neurophysiological assessment of spinal cord injuries in veterinary medicine are scarce. Neurophysiological tests have been employed to record SSEPs [5, 6] and MEPs in healthy animals [7–10] and in cases of cervical spondylomyelopathy [11, 12], intervertebral disk disease [13], lumbosacral stenosis [14], hereditary diseases [15, 16] and traumatic injuries [17]. Their use in evaluation of responses to regenerative therapy [18] and in intraoperative monitoring during cervical spinal surgery [19] has also been reported.

Somatosensory evoked potentials (SSEPs)

Principles

Somatosensory evoked potentials reflect the integrity of large-diameter sensory nerve fibers running through the dorsal funiculus. Potentials generated via stimulation of peripheral nerves are recorded at different levels of the nervous system, such as peripheral nerve, plexus, nerve roots, spinal cord segments and the sensory cortex. The tibial and median nerves are the nerves of choice for stimulation in pelvic and thoracic limbs respectively [2, 5, 6]. Somatosensory evoked potentials correspond to the conscious proprioception pathway; therefore, SSEPs do not represent smaller diameter fibers conveying pain and temperature sensation and may be altered or absent even in individuals with nociception [2].

Methodology

Stainless steel electrode pairs (i.e., cathode and anode) inserted into the subcutaneous tissue over the distal end of the target nerve are used for stimulation. Proximal stimulation can recruit more fibers and then promote larger potentials, but can also cause more muscle reflex activity. Stimulation just above the carpus for the median nerve and just above the tarsus for the tibial nerve can stimulate enough number of fibers avoiding excessive muscle activity [2, 20]. The most negative electrode (cathode) causes axon membrane depolarization, and should be placed 2 cm proximal to the anode, in order to avoid the anodal block of conduction [5, 6]. Surface electrodes are commonly used in humans; however, monopolar needle electrodes are recommended in dogs and cats due to greater skin thickness, larger amounts of subcutaneous fat and the presence of fur [2, 5]. Continuous stimuli applied to one limb at a time help to assess lesion lateralization. Pulse duration of 0.1 ms is most widely used. Stimulus intensity is related to recruitment of nerve fibers and the larger is the diameter of a fiber nerve, more easily it is stimulated. Moreover, with increasing stimulus intensity, more nerve fibers are recruited [20]. Therefore, pulse intensity (mA) is adjusted until a barely visible distal limb contraction is elicited indicating proper stimulation of motor fibers in mixed nerves such as the tibial and median nerves, and this is subject to individual variation. Once a good motor twitch is obtained, increasing the stimulus intensity further does not increase SSEPs amplitudes [20, 21].

Stimulus rates usually range from 2 to 5 Hz [4–6, 13], as amplitudes of scalp-recorded SSEPs can be modified by pulse rates above 2 Hz and spine recorded SSEPs by rates above 4 Hz [20]. Electrodes connected to the stimulator cause axons depolarization, with centrally (also peripherally) propagation, and SSEPs can be recorded from the spinal cord ascending tracts and finally in the scalp.

Filters are used to avoid activity not related to the generator under study that would interfere with the recordings. Commonly, a window from 10 to 4000 Hz in spine recorded SSEP and 10–3000 Hz for the scalp-recorded SSEP is used [5, 6, 17]. As signals under study are of very small magnitude, "Signal averaging" is applied to differentiate signals of interest from other interferences. This signal is time-locked to the stimulus, while noise is a random event. With averaging of repeated responses, noise is averaged out and the signal is averaged in [20].

As mentioned before, the sensory pathway may be further subdivided and topographed using electrode pairs placed at different spinal segments [5, 14, 17]. For spinal cord SSEPs, the active recording electrodes are placed in the dorsal midline parallel to the edges of adjacent to spinous process, aiming the center of the interarcuate ligament. The reference electrode is positioned in the paraspinal muscles 1–3 cm lateral to the recording electrode, at the same level. The active recording electrode can be advanced cranially to study different spinal cord segments, and also adjacent to a lesion, so that is possible to delimit the injury site. Ground electrode can be inserted subcutaneously preferably over a bone prominence, as these are electrically inactive regions [5, 13, 14, 17]. Along the spine, four contributions to SSEP recording can be identified. They are the root component (at L7–S1 level), the cord dorsum potential (in the caudal lumbar area), the ascending evoked potential (at more rostral levels) and the medullary component (at the level of the cisterna magna) [5, 20].

The root component is a potential that originates in the cauda equina nerve roots and can be detected on the three most caudal intervertebral spaces.

The cord dorsum potential is a triphasic potential that originates in the region of the spinal cord segments that receive input from sensory and mixed peripheral nerves. Therefore, it assess integrity of proximal sensory nerves, dorsal nerve roots, and spinal cord dorsal horn gray matter [22].

The ascending evoked potential is a compound action potential of small amplitude that can be difficult to detect in cranial thoracic and cervical areas due to the difficulty of inserting the electrodes properly. Finally, the medullary component possibly originates in the cervical and medullary nuclei [20].

Another feature of spine-recorded SSEP is the evoked injury potential, which is the spinal evoked response obtained by volume recording after injury to the cord, and represent the action potentials ascending the cord tracts up to the site of injury but not passing it. It has also been used as an intraoperative localizing tool for acute spinal cord injury [20, 23].

For scalp recording, the active (also called recording or different) electrode can be placed in the central zone, subcutaneously [5, 13, 17, 19]. Corkscrew (spiral) needle electrodes can be used for better adherence and minimization of external interferences [2, 5]. In the scalp, electrode position reflects the somatosensory area. A reference electrode placed centrally/frontally on the median plane and a ground electrode in the neck or on the forelimb position are also employed [2, 5].

Electrode pairs are connected to preamplifiers, then to specific channels in the equipment [4, 5]. Graphical representations of digitally recorded latency and amplitude data are used to investigate conduction disturbances along the sensory spinal tract [2, 4, 5].

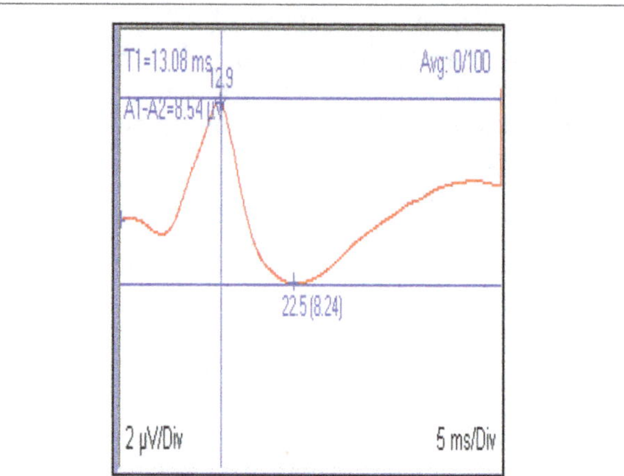

Fig. 1 Somatosensory evoked potentials (SSEPs) recorded from scalp following median nerve stimulation in a dog. Latency (T1 = 13.08 ms; *vertical bar*) and peak-to-peak amplitude (A1–A2 = 8.54 μV; *horizontal bars*) measurements are displayed. Gain = 2 μV/div; sweep speed = 5 ms/div

Recordings

Somatosensory evoked potential recordings are displayed on a computer screen; recordings and waves corresponding to each limb are shown in different windows, which can be adjusted for improved visualization. Figure 1 shows an example of SSEPs recorded from thoracic limb in a dog. Manually managed cursors are used to measure wave amplitude and latency [2, 4–6].

Clinical applicability

Somatosensory evoked potentials reflect sensory pathway conductivity and integrity in areas that cannot be accessed using other electrodiagnostic tests and may therefore be used for investigation of central and peripheral neurological conditions [5]. The method is thought to be sensitive and specific for detection of peroperative complications, is user-friendly and can be combined with other neurophysiological diagnostic modalities [24, 25]. Thoracolumbar spinal cord injuries are expected to generate normal thoracic limb recordings and deteriorated pelvic limb recordings, with the magnitude of changes reflecting injury severity (i.e., the more severe the injury, the longer the latency and the lower the amplitude); alternatively, SSEPs may not be recorded [26]. In lateralized lesions such as lateral intervertebral disk extrusion, evidence of lateralization should be apparent in recordings (Fig. 2). In human medicine, these modalities include monitoring many neurosurgical or orthopedic spine surgeries, such as embolization or tumor resections, aneurysm repairs, peripheral nervous system surgeries, thus helping the safe surgical approach [2].

Observations

Somatosensory evoked potentials may be influenced by mechanical factors, ischemic conditions, systemic hypotension, hypothermia, injectable anesthetics such as thiopental sodium, pentobarbital and ketamine hydrochloride, and volatile agents such as isoflurane, sevoflurane and nitric oxide [2, 24]. Latency changes >10% and drops in amplitude of more 50% are alarming signs in intraoperative monitoring of human patients and should be reported to the surgeon in charge [27]. Somatosensory evoked potentials reflect the functional integrity of the dorsal columns and therefore do not represent motor pathways, which may be individually compromised [2, 24, 27].

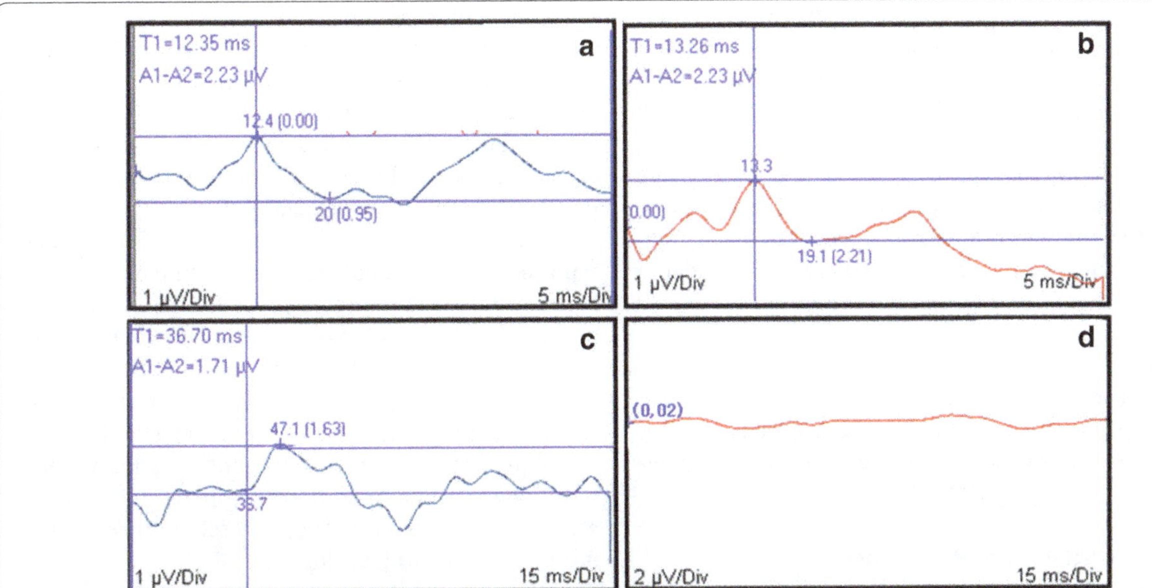

Fig. 2 Somatosensory evoked potentials (SSEPs) recorded from a dog presenting with thoracolumbar spinal injury. Tracings obtained following left (**a**) and right (**b**) median nerve and left (**c**) and right (**d**) tibial nerve stimulation. Lack of SSEP following right pelvic limb stimulation reflects a spinal lesion caudal to right-sided cervical enlargement. Latency (ms; *vertical bar*) and peak-to-peak amplitude (µV) measurements are displayed. Gain = 1 µV/div (**a**, **b** and **c**) or 2 µV/div (**d**); sweep speed = 5 ms/div (**a**, **b**) or 15 ms/div (**c**, **d**)

Motor evoked potentials (MEPs)

Principles

Motor evoked potentials assess motor pathway integrity from the cerebral cortex to the muscles and can be generated via transcranial magnetic [8, 10–12] or electrical stimulation [3, 7, 28]. While electrical stimulation is based on direct stimulation via subcutaneous electrodes inserted into the scalp, in transcranial magnetic stimulation a coil is used to generate magnetic fields that are then converted into electric potentials. Both methods induce depolarization and trigger action potentials that propagate along descending pathways related to the pyramidal and extrapyramidal systems; the first fibers descending from the cortex to the spinal cord form the corticospinal system [2, 10]. Extrapyramidal pathways correspond primarily to the rubrospinal, reticulospinal, tectospinal and vestibulospinal tracts and are particularly relevant in dogs [29]. The need for anesthesia is a major downside of transcranial electrical stimulation, as muscle contractions are painful, besides anticipated pain can occur [7].

In contrast, transcranial magnetic stimulation can be performed in sedated animals [8, 12] and does not require special preparation in humans [10]. However, electrical stimulation is less impacted by anesthetic drugs and is therefore the method of choice for intraoperative monitoring [2]. Also, motor responses induced via transcranial magnetic stimulation are easier to capture following voluntary movements of the target limb made upon request, which is not applicable to animal patients [2].

Methodology

For magnetic stimulation, a coil of wire generates the magnetic field, and it is positioned over the motor cortex, with the purpose to create a pulsed electric current [10]. For electric stimulation, cork screw electrodes provide better attachment to the scalp for proper transcranial stimulation and should be inserted centrally and above the left and right hemispheres, then connected to the stimulator. Active electrodes connected to the anode are expected to elicit better responses on the contralateral side. Multi pulses of 0.05 ms duration, individually adjusted to supramaximal intensity and frequency of 250 Hz are used [2]. Potentials are captured via needle electrodes inserted into target muscles, particularly those caudal to the injury site, although cranially located muscles may be employed as sentinels. The extensor carpi radialis and cranial tibial muscles (thoracic and pelvic limbs respectively) are the muscles of choice for MEP capture in dogs [11, 12, 18].

Recordings

As with SSEPs, MEP wave latency and amplitude values are displayed and measured on a computer screen (Fig. 3); SSEPs and MEPs should not be recorded simultaneously due to potential stimulation artifact interferences [4].

Clinical applicability

Motor evoked potentials have similar clinical applicability to SSEPs; however, motor pathways are reflected instead, and therefore a different system with specific functions and anatomical location [2]. Normal thoracic limb MEPs with altered pelvic limb MEP latency and amplitude should be expected in thoracolumbar spinal injuries. As with SSEPs, recording abnormalities are consistent with lesion severity [30, 31], (i.e., the more severe the injury, the grater the latency and the lower the amplitude), although they do not seem to correlate with prognosis for recovery. MEPs may not be recorded caudal to the injury site [32, 33] (Fig. 4).

Observations

Motor evoked potential changes occur more rapidly than SSEP changes under ischemic conditions; therefore this technique is more sensitive for detection of intraoperative spinal injuries [4, 24, 32, 33].

Anesthesia in SSEP and MEP assessment

Chemical restriction is required for SSEP and MEP recording in veterinary medicine; however, common sedating and anesthetic agents may attenuate or even suppress motor and somatosensory responses. Hypnotic-opioid combinations such as intravenous propofol and remifentanil are routinely used in human patients [25, 28, 34] submitted to electrical stimulation. The hyperpolarization (i.e., creation of a more negative resting potential in cell membranes) induced by volatile anesthetic agents such isoflurane decreases neuronal excitability and may prevent action potentials from reaching motor cortex and motor neuron depolarization thresholds [27, 34–36]. Several anesthetic protocols have been described in veterinary medicine. The use of drugs such as xylazine and dexamedetomidine, midazolam, sufentanil [5, 12, 37–39], ketamine, methohexital and isoflurane [37, 40] has been reported; anesthetic induction and maintenance through constant rate infusion of propofol [15, 35] has also been proposed. While MEPs can be obtained via transcranial magnetic stimulation in sedated patients, strong contraction of masticatory muscles induced by electrical stimulation dictates the need for general anesthesia and the use of protectors to prevent tongue laceration when this technique is employed. Body temperature oscillations may interfere with recordings; therefore, this parameter must be monitored [10, 19].

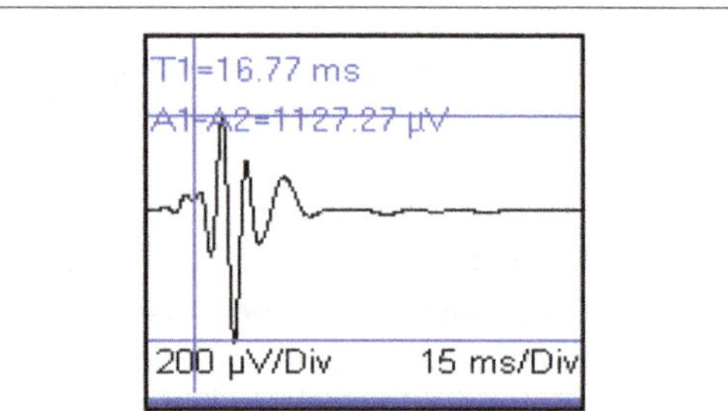

Fig. 3 Motor evoked potentials recorded from the extensor carpi radialis muscle following transcranial electrical stimulation in a dog. Latency (T1 = 16.77 ms; *vertical bar*) and peak-to-peak amplitude (A1–A2 = 1127.27 µV; *horizontal bars*) measurements are displayed. Gain = 200 µV/div; sweep speed = 15 ms/div

SSEPs and MEPs in veterinary medicine

Application of these diagnostic modalities in veterinary medicine is still limited, and two major limiting factors should be mentioned. First, different anesthetic protocols, mainly with substances that strongly suppress cortical activity, can definitely impair proper recordings. Second, mild clinical signs due to spinal cord injury can drastically influence, or even prevent recordings. More investigation and standardization should be determinant for better and more trustable results, and more information extracted from human medicine should be of great benefit to application in animals. SSEPs and MEPs have been used alone or in combination to complement neurological examination, as well as for disease characterization and functional classification of spinal cord injuries [15–17, 20, 26, 31, 37, 40–42]. Several aspects need to be further investigated and defined before results can be compared between studies. Electrode insertion sites, particularly of scalp electrodes used for SSEP capture or MEP induction via transcranial magnetic or electric stimulation, must be standardized. In dogs, extensive anatomical variability in head shape (e.g., brachycephalic vs. dolichocephalic

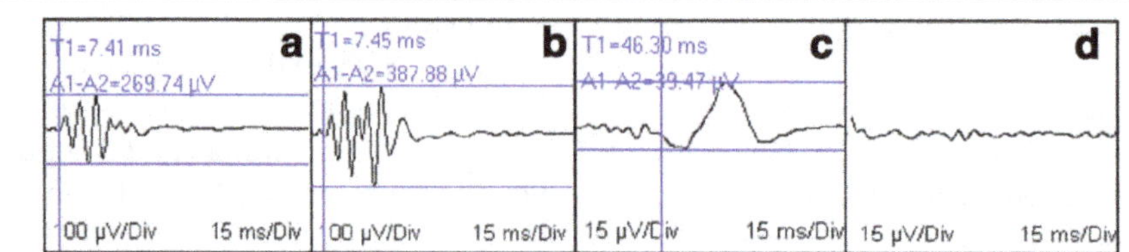

Fig. 4 Motor evoked potential recordings (MEPs) in a dog presenting with thoracolumbar spinal injury. Tracings obtained following left (**a**) and right (**b**) extensor carpi radialis and left (**c**) and right (**d**) cranial tibial muscle stimulation. MEP capture in **a**, **b** and **c** and absence in **d** is consistent with right-sided spinal lesion. Latency (ms; *vertical bar*) and peak-to-peak amplitude (µV) measurements are displayed. Gain = 100 µV/div (**a**, **b**) or 15 µV/div (**c**, **d**); sweep speed = 15 ms/div

breeds) is likely to interfere with correct location of stimulation and signal capture sites. Latency and amplitude reference values are also open to question, given the wide variability even between individuals of the same breed [11, 31]. A single study describes the use of SSEPs for intraoperative monitoring of dogs with spinal cord dysfunction [19]. The value of evoked potentials possibly resides in the contribution of such tests to objective assessment of recovery or deterioration of neurological conditions via paired or serial comparisons of recordings obtained from the same animal. Also, intraoperative monitoring significantly increases procedure safety (i.e., prevention of iatrogenic lesions) and prognostication accuracy. Just as human patients, dogs and cats would certainly benefit from intraoperative neurophysiological monitoring during spinal surgery [43, 44].

Conclusions

Somatosensory and motor evoked potentials reflect the functional integrity of ascending (sensory) and descending (motor) pathways and therefore have diagnostic and prognostic value. Somatosensory and motor evoked potentials constitute promising tools for assessment and follow up of neurological conditions and provide significant contributions to intraoperative monitoring of spinal procedures.

Authors' contributions

MCCMIS created the idea and structure of the review and performed the writing process. RJRF made contributions when describing SSEPs and MEPs and performed the recordings of dogs demonstrated in the figures. GCFP drafted the Anesthesia section, and performed the anesthetic procedure in dogs demonstrated in the figures. JMM had coordinated all the process and was a major contributor in the writing the manuscript. All authors read and approved the final manuscript.

Author details

[1] Department of Surgery, School of Veterinary Medicine and Animal Science, University of São Paulo, Cidade Universitária, Prof. Dr. Orlando Marques de Paiva, 87, São Paulo, SP 05508-270, Brazil. [2] Orthopedic and Traumatology Institute, School of Medicine, University of São Paulo, Rua Dr. Ovídio Pires de Campos, 333, São Paulo, SP 05403-010, Brazil.

Authors' information

MCCMIS is a Ph.D. Student at University of São Paulo, School of Veterinary Medicine and Animal Science, Department of Surgery. Her thesis is about SSEPs and MEPs description in healthy and paraplegic chondrodystrophic dogs.

RJRF is a neurophysiologist and associate physician at Orthopedic and Traumatology Institute, School of Medicine, University of São Paulo. He works with intraoperative neurophysiology monitoring since 1995 and has published within this area.

GCP is an anesthetist at University of São Paulo, School of Veterinary Medicine and Animal Science, Department of Surgery, and she has also experience in anesthetic procedures during SSEPs and MEPs in dogs.

JMM is a Full Professor at the University of São Paulo, School of Veterinary Medicine and Animal Science, Department of Surgery, and works with Neurosurgery and Small Animal Surgery.

Acknowledgements

We are thankful for CNPq for the financial support.

Competing interests

The authors declare that they have no competing interests.

Funding

This study was financially supported by CNPq.

References

1. Langeloo DD, Journée HL, De Kleuver M, Grotenhuis JA. Criteria for transcranial electrical motor evoked potential monitoring during spinal deformity surgery: a review and discussion of the literature. Neurophysiol Clin. 2000;37:431–9.
2. Simon MV. Intraoperative neurophysiology: a comprehensive guide to monitoring and mapping. Ed. New York: Demos Medical; 2009.
3. Szelényi A, Kothbauer KF, Deletis V. Transcranial electric stimulation for intraoperative motor evoked potential monitoring: stimulation parameters and electrode montages. Clin Neurophysiol. 2007;118:1586–95.
4. Ferreira RJR. Monitoramento neurofisiológico intraoperatório nas cirurgias espinais. In: Tratado de medicina e reabilitação. Rio de Janeiro: Guanabara Koogan; 2010. p. 24–39.
5. Pellegrino FC, Sica REP. Potenciales evocados somatosensitivos (PESS) obtenidos por estimulación del nervio mediano (registros espinal y craneano) en caninos. InVet. 2005;7:107–18.
6. Vanderzant CW, Schott RJ, Natale JE, Pondo CA, D'alecy LG. Somatosensory evoked potentials of the dog: recording techniques and normal values. J Neurosci Methods. 1989;27:253–63.
7. Strain GM, Prescott-Mathews JS, Tedford BL. Motor potentials evoked by transcranial stimulation of the canine motor cortex. PVN. 1990;1:321–31.
8. Amendt HL, Siedenburg JS, Steffensen N, Söbbeler FJ, Schütter A, Tünsmeyer J, et al. Transcranial magnetic stimulation with acepromazine or dexmedetomidine in combination with levomethadone/fenpipramide in healthy beagle dogs. Vet J. 2016;217:40–2. doi:10.1016/j.tvjl.2016.06.006.
9. Ferreira R, Oliveira AR, Barros Filho TEP. Padronização da técnica para captação do potencial evocado motor em ratos através da estimulação elétrica transcraniana. Acta Ortop Bras. 2005;13:112–4.
10. Nollet H, Van Ham L, Deprez P, Vanderstraeten G. Transcranial magnetic stimulation: review of the technique, basic principles and applications. Vet J. 2003;166:28–42.
11. Da Costa RC, Poma R, Parent JM, Partlow G, Monteith G. Correlation of motor evoked potentials with magnetic resonance imaging and neurologic findings in Doberman Pinschers with and without signs of cervical spondylomyelopathy. Am J Vet Res. 2006;67:1613–20.
12. Martin-Vaquero P, Da Costa RC. Transcranial magnetic motor evoked potentials in Great Danes with and without clinical signs of cervical spondylomyelopathy: association with neurological findings and magnetic resonance imaging. Vet J. 2014;201:327–32.
13. Poncelet L, Michaux C, Balligand M. Somatosensory potentials in dogs with naturally acquired thoracolumbar spinal cord disease. Am J Vet Res. 1993;54:1935–41.
14. Meij BP, Suwankong N, Van Den Brom WE, Venker-Van Haagen AJ, Hazewinkel HA. Tibial nerve somatosensory evoked potentials in dogs with degenerative lumbosacral stenosis. Vet Surg. 2006;35:168–75.
15. Vanhaesebrouck AE, Van Soens I, Poncelet L, Duchateau L, Bhatti S, Polis I, et al. Clinical and electrophysiological characterization of myokymia and neuromyotonia in Jack Russell Terriers. J Vet Intern Med. 2010;24:882–9.
16. Harcourt-Brown TR, Belshaw Z, Parker JE, Jeffery ND, Granger N. Effects of syringomyelia on electrodiagnostic test results in Cavalier King Charles Spaniels. Am J Vet Res. 2011;72:595–600.
17. Şenel OO, Şirin YS, Önyay T, Beşalti O. Evaluation of spinal somatosensory evoked potentials in cats with traumatic spinal cord injury without deep pain perception. Ank Üniv Vet Fak Derg. 2012;59:41–5.
18. Granger N, Blamires H, Franklin RJ, Jeffery ND. Autologous olfactory mucosal cell transplants in clinical spinal cord injury: a randomized double-blinded trial in a canine translational model. Brain. 2012;135:3227–37.

19. Okuno S, Nakamura A, Kobayashi T, Orito K. Effectiveness of intraoperative somatosensory evoked potential monitoring during cervical spinal operations on animals with spinal cord dysfunction. J Vet Med Sci. 2005;67:719–22.
20. Poncelet L. Electrophysiological assessment of spinal cord function through somatosensory evoked potentials in dogs. Vet Neurol Neurosurg J. 1999;1:1.
21. Cozzi P, Poncelet L, Michaux C, Balligand M. Effect of stimulus intensity on spinal cord somatosensory evoked potential in dogs. Am J Vet Res. 1998;59:217–20.
22. Cuddon PA, Delauche AJ, Hutchison JM. Assessment of dorsal nerve root and spinal cord dorsal horn function in clinically normal dogs by determination of cord dorsum potentials. Am J Vet Res. 1999;60:222–6.
23. Schramm J, Krause R, Shigeno T, Brock M. Experimental investigation on the spinal cord evoked injury potential. J Neurosurg. 1983;59:485–92.
24. Pelosi L, Lamb J, Grevitt M, Mehdian SM, Webb JK, Blumhardt LD. Combined monitoring of motor and somatosensory evoked potentials in orthopaedic spinal surgery. Clin Europhysiol. 2002;113:1082–91.
25. Costa P, Bruno A, Bonzanino M, Massaro F, Caruso L, Vincenzo I, et al. Somatosensory and motor evoked potential monitoring during spine and spinal cord surgery. Spinal Cord. 2007;45:86–91.
26. Shores A, Redding RW, Knecht CD. Spinal evoked potentials in dogs with acute compressive thoracolumbar spinal cord disease. Am J Vet Res. 1998;59:217–20.
27. Gavaret M, Jouve JL, Péréon Y, Accadbled F, André-Obadia N, Azabou E, et al. Intraoperative neurophysiologic monitoring in spine surgery. Developments and state of the art in France in 2011. Orthop Traumatol Surg Res. 2013;99:319–27. doi:10.1016/j.otsr.2013.07.005.
28. Tsutsui S, Yamada H, Hashizume H, Minamide A, Nakagawa Y, Iwasaki H, et al. Quantification of the proportion of motor neurons recruited by transcranial electrical stimulation during intraoperative motor evoked potential monitoring. J Clin Monit Comput. 2013;27:633–7.
29. Lorenz MD, Coates JR, Kent M. Handbook of veterinary neurology. Missouri: Elsevier Saunders; 2011.
30. Kanchiku T, Taguchi T, Kaneko K, Fuchigami Y, Yonemura H, Kawai S. A correlation between magnetic resonance imaging and electrophysiological findings in cervical spondylotic myelopathy. Spine. 2001;26:E294–9.
31. Sylvestre AM, Cockshutt JR, Parent JM, Brooke JD, Holmberg DL, Partlow GD. Magnetic motor evoked potentials for assessing spinal cord integrity in dogs with intervertebral disc disease. Vet Surg. 1993;22:5–10.
32. Owen J, Laschinger J, Bridwell K, Shimon S, Nielsen C, Dunlap J, et al. Sensitivity and specificity of somatosensory and neurogenic-motor evoked potentials in animals and humans. Spine. 1988;13:1111–8.
33. Hilibrand AS, Schwartz DM, Sethuraman V, Vaccaro AR, Albert TJ. Comparison of transcranial electric motor and somatosensory evoked potential monitoring during cervical spine surgery. J Bone Joint Surg Am. 2004;86:1248–53.
34. Tamkus AA, Rice KS, Kim HL. Differential rates of false-positive findings in transcranial electric motor evoked potential monitoring when using inhalational anesthesia versus total intravenous anesthesia during spine surgeries. Spine J. 2014;14:1440–6.
35. Van Soens I, Struys MM, Polis IE, Tshamala M, Nollet H, Bhatti SF, et al. Effects of sedative and hypnotic drug combinations on transcranial magnetic motor evoked potential, bispectral index and ARX-derived auditory evoked potential index in dogs. Vet J. 2009;181:163–70.
36. Kalkman CJ. Motor evoked potentials. Semin Anesth. 1997;16(1):28–35. doi:10.1016/S0277-0326(97)80005-0.
37. Van Oostrom H, Doornenbal A, Schot A, Stienen PJ, Hellebrekers LJ. Neurophysiological assessment of the sedative and analgesic effects of a constant rate infusion of dexmedetomidine in the dog. Vet J. 2011;190:338–44.
38. Van Ham LM, Nijs J, Mattheeuws DR, Vanderstraeten GG. Sufentanil and nitrous oxide anaesthesia for the recording of transcranial magnetic motor evoked potentials in dogs. Vet Rec. 1996;138:642–5.
39. Van Ham LM, Nijs J, Vanderstraeten GG, Mattheeuws DR. Comparison of two techniques of narcotic-induced anesthesia for use during recording of magnetic motor evoked potentials in dogs. Am J Vet Res. 1996;57:142–6.
40. Vanhaesebrouck AE, Bhatti SF, Polis IE, Plessas IN, Van Ham LM. Neuromyotonia in a Dachshund with clinical and electrophysiological signs of spinocerebellar ataxia. J Small Anim Pract. 2011;52:547–50.
41. Poma R, Parent JM, Holmberg DL, Partlow GD, Monteit G, Sylvestre AM. Correlation between severity of clinical signs and motor evoked potentials after transcranial magnetic stimulation in large-breed dogs with cervical spinal cord disease. J Am Vet Med Assoc. 2002;221:60–4.
42. De Decker S, Van Soens I, Duchateau L, Gielen IM, Van Bree HJ, Binst DH, et al. Transcranial magnetic stimulation in Doberman Pinschers with clinically relevant and clinically irrelevant spinal cord compression on magnetic resonance imaging. J Am Vet Med Assoc. 2011;238:81–8.
43. Van Soens I, Van Ham LM. Assessment of motor pathways by magnetic stimulation in human and veterinary medicine. Vet J. 2011;187:174–81.
44. Lall RR, Lall RR, Hauptman JS, Munoz C, Cybulski GR, Koski T, et al. Intraoperative neurophysiological monitoring in spine surgery: indications, efficacy, and role of the preoperative checklist. Neurosurg Focus. 2012;33:E10.

13

Detection and molecular characterization of porcine reproductive and respiratory syndrome virus in Lithuanian wild boar populations

Arunas Stankevicius[1*], Jurate Buitkuviene[1,2], Virginija Sutkiene[1], Ugne Spancerniene[1], Ina Pampariene[1], Arnoldas Pautienius[1], Vaidas Oberauskas[1], Henrikas Zilinskas[1] and Judita Zymantiene[1]

Abstract

Background: Porcine reproductive and respiratory syndrome virus (PRRSV) is recognized worldwide as an important and economically devastating pathogen in pig production. Although PRRSV is widespread in domestic swine, there is a lack of information regarding PRRSV infection in European wild boars (*Sus scrofa*). Currently available information does not provide conclusive evidence that wild boars are a reservoir of PRRSV. Nevertheless, wild boars may be likely to become infected by domestic swine through occasional direct or indirect contact. Furthermore, wild boars can act as a reservoir for infectious diseases of domestic pigs. Therefore, the objectives of the present study were to determine the virus prevalence and further explore the epidemiology and diversity of PRRSV strains present in Lithuanian wild boars over a 5-year period. A total of 1597 tissue and serum samples from wild boars inhabiting 44 districts and ten counties in Lithuania were analysed using conventional nested reverse transcription polymerase chain reaction (RT-PCR) and real-time Taqman RT-PCR for the detection of PRRSV-specific open reading frame (ORF) 1 and 6 sequences.

Results: PRRSV was highly prevalent in Lithuanian wild boar populations, with an average rate of 18.66 % using conventional RT-PCR and 19.54 % using real-time RT-PCR. PRRSV was detected in 36.71 and 41.77 % of 237 hunting grounds tested by conventional RT-nPCR and real-time RT-PCR, respectively. No statistically significant differences in PRRSV prevalence were observed by geographic area in the ten Lithuanian counties. Animals infected with PRRSV were identified in all age groups; however, significantly higher prevalence rates were identified in subadult and adult wild boars than in juveniles up to 12 months old. No positive results were obtained using conventional PCR with Type 2 specific primers. Phylogenetic analysis of the partial ORF5 region revealed that ten wild boars harboured virus sequences belonging to genetic subtypes 3 and 4 and may therefore pose a serious threat to Lithuanian pig farms in which only subtype two strains are circulating.

Conclusions: The results of virus prevalence and phylogenetic analyses strongly support the role of wild boars as a possible natural reservoir for PRRSV in Lithuania.

Keywords: PRRSV, Wild boar, RT-PCR, Real-time RT-PCR, Virus prevalence, ORF5 sequences

*Correspondence: arunas.stankevicius@lsmuni.lt
[1] Faculty of Veterinary Medicine, Lithuanian University of Health Sciences, Tilzes st. 18, LT-47182 Kaunas, Lithuania
Full list of author information is available at the end of the article

Background

Porcine reproductive and respiratory syndrome virus (PRRSV) is globally regarded as an important and economically devastating pathogen in pig production characterized by respiratory disease in piglets and reproductive failure in sows. PRRSV, a member of the family *Arteriviridae* in the order *Nidovirales,* is a small, enveloped virus with a single-stranded positive-sense RNA genome approximately 15 kb in length that encodes at least nine open reading frames (ORF), including ORF1a, 1b, 2a, 2b, and 3–7 [1, 2]. ORFs 2a, 2b, 3, 4, and 5 encode envelope glycoproteins, while ORFs 6 and 7 encode the matrix and nucleocapsid proteins, respectively. The largest and most conserved genes are ORF1a and ORF1b, which encode the viral RNA polymerase. ORF5 encodes the major envelope protein and is often used for phylogenetic analysis and molecular characterization, mainly because of its high variability and large number of available sequences [3, 4]. A novel PRRSV ORF5a protein encoded in an ORF that overlaps the major envelope glycoprotein GP5 ORF has recently been identified [5], and a—two ribosomal frame-shifting has recently been identified for the expression of nonstructural proteins nsp2TF in the nsp2-coding region. The nsp2TF coding sequence is conserved in the PRRSV genome [6].

Based on genetic differences, PRRSV has been divided into two genotypes: Type 1, mainly comprising viruses from Europe, and Type 2, mainly comprising of viruses from North America and Asia. The two types are 55–70 % identical at the nucleotide level. These two PRRSV genotypes have emerged almost simultaneously on their respective continents since the late 1980s. Publications describing the ORF5 PRRSV sequences have shown that the genetic diversity of Type 1 is higher than that of Type 2 [7–9]. A unique cluster of Type 1 PRRSV was thought to be closely related to the common ancestors of the European and American strains was detected in Lithuania [10]. Investigations in ORF5 and ORF7 regions of PRRSV conducted in Belarus and Russia have shown that nucleotide sequences in virus isolates from these countries also differ significantly from those in PRRSV strains circulating in Western Europe [8, 9]. Based on ORF5 and ORF7 sequences, Type 1 East European PRRSV strains were divided into four genetic subtypes representing PRRSV strains prevalent in Belarus, Lithuania and Latvia [11].

Although PRRSV is widespread in domestic swine, there is a lack of information regarding PRRSV infection in European wild boars (*Sus scrofa*). The seroprevalence of antibodies against PRRSV in wild boars has been determined to range from 0.3 to 3.6 % in several countries [12–19]; however, in the Campania Region of Italy, a seroprevalence of 37.8 % was detected [17]. Many other studies have reported negative PRRSV seroprevalence results [20–24]. PRRSV has also been detected using reverse transcription polymerase chain reaction (RT-PCR) methods in the lung tissue of wild boars in Italy [25], Germany [26] and Lithuania [27] as well as in the lung tissue of hybrid wild boars, known as "special wild pigs" in China [28].

Currently available information does not provide conclusive evidence that wild boars are a reservoir of PRRSV [26, 29]. Nevertheless, wild boars may be likely to become infected by domestic swine through occasional direct or indirect contact. Furthermore, wild boars have been found to act as a reservoir for other infectious diseases of domestic pigs, and interactions between wide and domestic pig populations can potentially result in transmission of these diseases [13, 29]. In this case, PRRSV transmission would be favoured within dense wild boar populations, but the lack of infection in many wild boar populations in various European countries suggest that the initial transmission from domestic swine to wild boar does not occur or occurs very sporadically. Therefore, the objectives of the present study were to determine virus prevalence and further explore the epidemiology and diversity of PRRSV strains prevalent in Lithuanian wild boars over a 5-year period.

Methods

Wild boar samples

Samples were collected from wild boars (n = 1597) hunted in forested areas (21,740 km^2) of all 44 districts and 10 counties of Lithuania during the 2011–2015 hunting seasons. Wild boars were numbered and categorized according to age (teeth method) and weight into three age groups: juveniles (n = 335), subadults (n = 652) and adults (n = 610). Lung (n = 755), lymph node and tonsil (n = 264), spleen (n = 143), or serum (n = 435) samples were collected from hunted wild boars within 2–3 h after death from public or private hunting grounds (n = 237) and stored at −20 °C until analysis.

Pig samples

Lung samples from dead weaned pigs (n = 32) were collected from PRRSV-positive farms (n = 5) located near the sites where wild boars were shot. RNA was obtained from PRRSV-positive samples, and ORF5 sequences were used for phylogenetic analysis. All lung samples were transported at 5 °C and then stored at −20 °C until analysis.

RNA isolation and cDNA synthesis

RNA was extracted from tissue samples using the GeneJET RNA purification kit (Thermo Fisher Scientific, Waltham, USA). For each extraction, 30–50 mg of tissue sample was ground thoroughly with a mortar and pestle. Lysis buffer (300 μl) supplemented with β-mercaptoethanol was added. The remaining steps were performed following the manufacturer's instructions. Extracted RNA was eluted in 100 μl nuclease-free water. Total RNA was extracted using the GeneJET Viral DNA and RNA Purification Kit (Thermo Fisher Scientific), designed for rapid and efficient purification of high quality viral nucleic acids from various human and animal liquid samples such as plasma, serum, whole blood. Wild boar serum (200 μl) was used for RNA extraction according to manufacturer protocol. Extracted RNA samples were stored at −80 °C until further analysis.

Reverse transcription (RT) was performed on extracted RNA. Five microlitre RNA was mixed with 1 μl Oligo(dT)18 primer (Thermo Fisher Scientific); 6.5 μl DEPC-treated water; 4 μl 5× reaction buffer (Thermo Fisher Scientific); 0.5 μl (20 U) Thermo Scientific RiboLock RNase Inhibitor; 2 μl dNTP Mix (10 mM each); and 1 μl (200 U) RevertAid reverse transcriptase (Thermo Fisher Scientific). A total volume of 20 μl reaction mixture was incubated for 60 min at 42 °C, and the reaction was then terminated by heating at 70 °C for 10 min. The obtained cDNA was then used for PCR and real-time PCR.

PCR and real-time PCR

A 25 μl PCR mixture containing 5 μl cDNA; 1× Taq polymerase reaction buffer (Thermo Fisher Scientific); 2.5 mM $MgCl_2$; 0.2 mM dNTP Mix; 0.6 U Taq polymerase (Thermo Fisher Scientific); and 20 pmol of each primer was used for amplifying ORF1 258 bp sequences [26] (see Additional file 1). According to a previous study [26], conventional RT-PCR targeting ORF1 has been performed to detect the Type 1 or Type 2 PRRSV in wild boar samples. PCR primers were designed based on ORF 1b and found to be more conserved within and between the two PRRSV virus genotypes than those of other genes.

The nested PCR contained the same reagents as the first PCR except primers were used to amplify ORF1 186 bp sequences for Type 1 PRRSV and 108 bp sequences for Type 2 PRRSV strains [26] (see Additional file 1) and 2.5 μl of the PCR product was used as a template for the nested PCR assay. The positive samples in the ORF1 RT-nPCR and ORF6 real-time RT-PCR were further analysed by amplifying the ORF5 sequences used for phylogenetic analysis of PRRSV. For the ORF5 region, amplification PCR and nested PCR in a final volume of 25 μl were performed using 20 pmol of each primer specific for this region [10]. Details of primers used are displayed in Additional file 1. All reactions were performed in a Mastercycler personal thermocycler (Eppendorf, Hamburg, Germany). Thermal cycling consisted of initial denaturation at 95 °C for 3 min, 40 amplification cycles of 95 °C for 30 s, annealing at 55 °C for 30 s and extension at 72 °C for 60 s followed by final extension at 72 °C for 10 min. For ORF5 region amplification, thermal cycling was performed using 35 cycles of 94 °C for 60 s, 55 °C for 60 s and 72 °C for 90 s with final extension at 72 °C for 10 min. The nested PCR product was separated in 1.5 % agarose gel and visualized with UV light after ethidium bromide staining.

As an alternative to conventional RT-nPCR, real-time RT-PCR was performed using ORF6 region primers and a probe coding for the conserved structural membrane protein M [30]. The 25 μl real-time RT-PCR mixture consisted of 8.5 μl nuclease-free water; 12.5 μl TaqMan Universal Master Mix II with UNG (Applied Biosystems, Foster, USA); 1.0 μl each of the forward and reverse primers (20 μM), 1 μl probe (10 μM) (see Additional file 1); and 2.5 μl cDNA template. Real-time RT-PCR was performed with StepOnePlus (Applied Biosystems) Thermal Cycler using the following program: UNG incubation at 50 °C for 2 min; initial incubation at 95 °C for 10 min; and 40 cycles of 95 °C for 15 s and 60 °C for 60 s.

Sequencing and phylogenetic analysis

Positive ORF5 nested PCR products were excised from the gels, purified using a GeneJET PCR Purification Kit (Thermo Fisher Scientific) and sequenced in both directions using the BigDye Terminator Cycle Sequencing Kit v3.1 (Applied Biosystems) and 3130× Genetic analyzer (Applied Biosystems). Sequences from both strands of the ORF5 PCR products were determined using the same primers used for nested PCR amplification. The sequences were submitted to Genbank under accession numbers KT828652-KT828665.

The obtained partial ORF5 sequences were compared with the reference set of sequences selected from GenBank to represent a full range of genetic diversity and geographic locations of Type 1 PRRSV. The sequences were aligned using the Clustal W software from MegAlign (Lasergene software package, DNASTAR Inc, Madison, USA). Bootstrap values were calculated using CLC Gene Free Workbench software, with bootstrap values based on 100 analysis replicates (v4.0.01, CLC bio A/S, Aarhus, Denmark).

Statistical analysis

Descriptive statistics were calculated using Microsoft Excel 2007 and IBM SPSS Statistics (Version 21.0). Z-tests for proportions were used to estimate the apparent prevalence confidence intervals (95 % CI), and χ^2-tests for equality of two proportions were used to determine significant differences in prevalence between sampling periods, age groups, and counties. The results were considered statistically significant if P values were <0.05.

Results

A total of 1597 samples (lung, lymph node, tonsil, spleen or serum samples) from wild boars inhabiting 44 districts and 10 counties in Lithuania were analysed using conventional nested RT-PCR and real-time Taqman RT-PCR for detection of PRRSV-specific ORF1 and ORF6 sequences, respectively. PRRSV was detected in 18.66 % (298/1597) of wild boars tested using RT-nPCR and 19.54 % (312/1597) of samples tested using real-time RT-PCR (Table 1). Differences in PRRSV prevalence during the sampling period (2011–2015) were not significant (P > 0.05) irrespective of PCR method.

PRRSV Type 1-specific amplicons were detected with both RT-PCR methods in all 10 Lithuanian counties and 36 of 44 districts (data not shown). PRRSV was detected in 87 (36.71 %; 95 % CI 30.57–42.85 %) and 99 (41.77 %; 95 % CI 35.49–48.05) of the 237 hunting grounds tested by conventional RT-nPCR and real-time RT-PCR, respectively (Fig. 1). The highest PRRSV prevalence was detected in Telsiai County at 62.5 % (95 % CI 28.95–96.05 %) by RT-nPCR and 75 % (95 % CI 44.99–105.01 %) by real-time RT-PCR. The differences between PRRSV prevalence by geographic area in all ten Lithuanian counties were also not significant (P > 0.05) irrespective of PCR method.

The PRRSV prevalence for different age groups of wild boars is presented in Table 2. Animals infected with PRRSV were found in all age groups; however, the highest prevalence rates were found in adults and subadults (Table 2). Subadults and adults were twice as likely to be PCR positive than the juvenile boars (P < 0.05).

PRRSV Type 2 was not detected using conventional RT-nPCR with ORF1-specific primers in 1597 tested wild boars from 237 hunting grounds.

For genetic comparison of circulating PRRSV strains in Lithuanian wild boars, ten amplification products of partial ORF5 region were sequenced. All obtained sequences showed the highest similarity to PRRSV Type 1 sequences. Phylogenetic analysis of the partial ORF5 region revealed that wild boar sequences belonged to genetic subtypes 3 and 4 (Fig. 2). The wild boar PRRSV sequences formed well-defined clusters within these subtypes and were aligned with PRRSV ORF5 published reference sequences from domestic pigs in Belarus and Latvia. Interestingly, these subtypes have never been detected in domestic pigs in Lithuania. ORF5 sequences obtained from Lithuanian pig farms clustered in subtype 2 of the phylogenetic tree along with reference sequences previously obtained from Lithuanian, Belarus and Russian Federation pig farms.

Discussion

The study shows that PRRSV infections are prevalent in Lithuanian wild boar populations with an average detection rate of 18.66 % using conventional ORF1 RT-nPCR and 19.54 % tested using real-time RT-PCR. This proportion appears to be quite higher than that indicated in a previous investigation, which found that PRRSV by RT-nPCR was detected in 15.9 % of wild boar samples in Germany [26]. Surveys of wild boars from eastern Slovakia have revealed that PRRSV was present in 1.6 % of samples when tested by nested RT-PCR [31], and PRRSV Type 1 was accidentally identified in a road killed wild boar in Italy [25]. Contrary to our results, Kukushkin et al. [20] failed to detect PRRSV in tissue samples from wild boars in Russia using RT-PCR, while a study in Poland found that PRRSV infections were not prevalent in wild boars [32]. The sera and tissues from wild boars in south-central Spain were also found to be negative by conventional and real-time RT-PCR assays [18].

Throughout Lithuania, the prevalence of PRRSV infection was higher in wild boars from hunting grounds (36.71 and 41.77 % depending on PCR used) than in the general porcine population. The presence of PRRSV-positive wild boars in all Lithuanian counties may be explained by the favourable conditions for wild boars that have developed throughout Lithuania. The population density of wild boars in Lithuanian forests has increased considerably from 1.84 wild boars per km^2 in 2011 to 2.66 wild boars per km^2 in 2015 [33]. Furthermore, these findings could be explained by migration of wild boars from neighbouring countries and their ability to colonize new habitats through abundant supplementary feeding. Supplementary feeding of wild boars during winter has been practised in Lithuania for many years as a dissuasive measure aimed to reduce crop damage by wild boars or an attractive measure during hunting season. Supplementary feeding brings animals closer together near feeding locations, leading to increased level of aggregation among and contact between wild boars. The results of our investigation revealed as unexpectedly high prevalence of PRRSV in wild boars; however, additional studies of wild boar populations in neighbouring Latvia, Belarus, and Kaliningrad Region of Russian Federation are necessary to investigate this further.

The highest prevalence of infected wild boars (19.84 to 22.24 %) was identified in the subadult and adult age groups, a finding that may be explained by an age-dependent higher risk of virus exposure.

This study demonstrated that wild boars can harbour different genetic lineages of PRRSV strains than those

Table 1 Data from RT-nPCR and real-time RT-PCR assays of wild boar samples obtained from 2011 to 2015

Sampling year	Number of hunting grounds tested	Number of wild boars tested	RT-nPCR			Real-time RT-PCR		
			Number of positive wild boars	Percentage of positive wild boars	95 % confidence interval (%)	Number of positive wild boars	Percentage of positive wild boars	95 % confidence interval (%)
2015	37	187	32	17.11	11.71–22.51	34	18.18	12.65–23.71
2014	55	268	43	16.04	11.65–20.43	47	17.54	12.99–22.09
2013	45	290	52	17.93	13.52–22.34	54	18.62	14.14–23.10
2012	52	489	101	20.65	17.06–24.24	104	21.27	17.64–24.90
2011	48	363	70	19.28	15.22–23.34	73	20.11	15.99–24.23
Total	237	1597	298	18.66	16.75–20.57	312	19.54	17.60–21.48

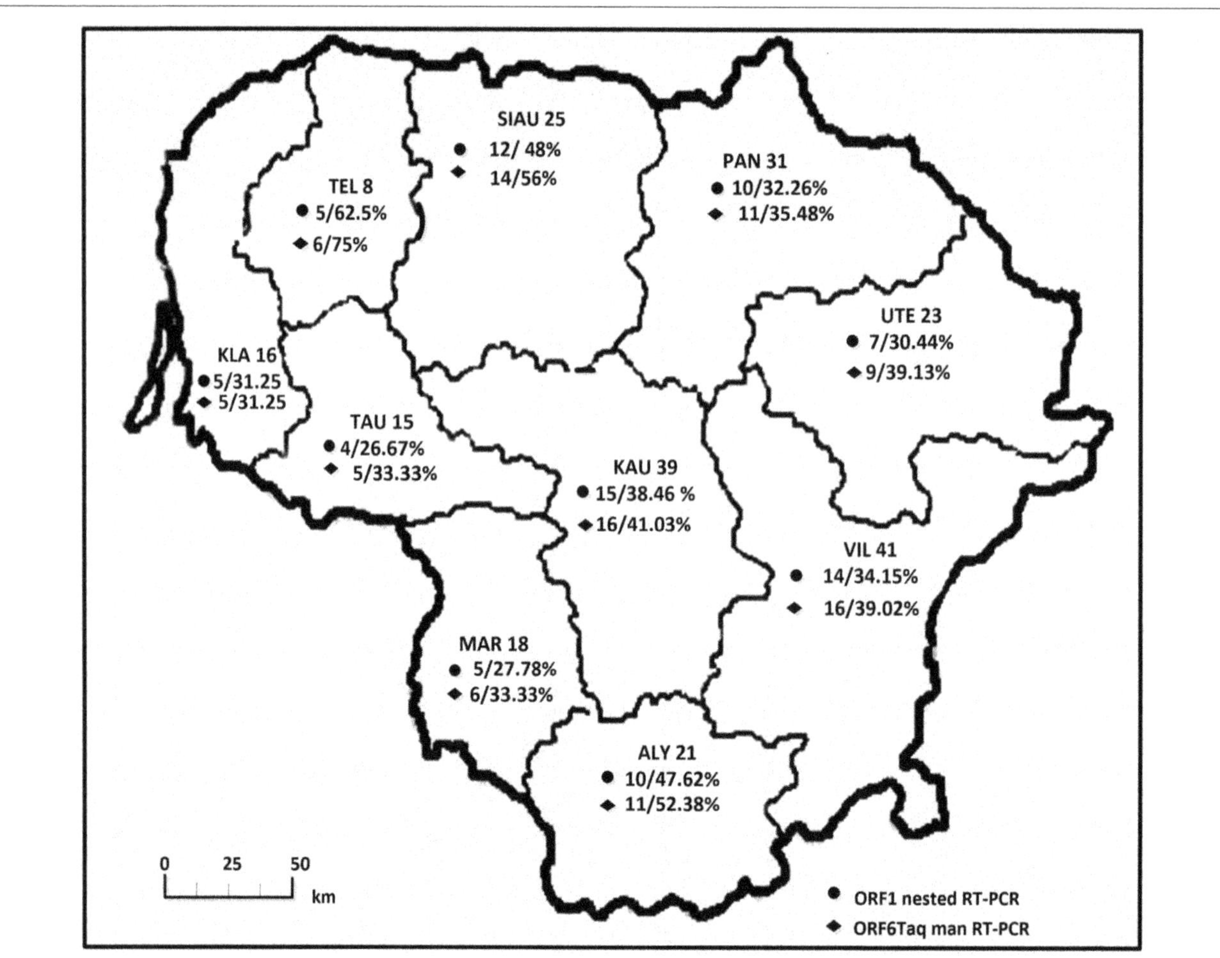

Fig. 1 PRRSV prevalence distribution by hunting grounds in different Lithuanian counties. *Bold letters* indicate counties: *ALY* Alytus, *MAR* Marijampole, *VIL* Vilnius, *KAU* Kaunas, *TAU* Taurage, *KLA* Kaipeda, *TEL* Telsiai, *SIAU* Siauliai, *PAN* Panevezys, *UTE* Utena. The *numbers* indicate tested hunting grounds in each county. *Percentage in the second line* indicates prevalence rate determined by nested and real-time RT-PCR

Table 2 Prevalence of PRRSV infection in wild boars detected by nested and real-time RT-PCR by age group

Age group	Number of wild boars tested	RT-nPCR			Real-time RT-PCR		
		Number of positive wild boars	Percentage of positive wild boars	95 % confidence interval (%)	Number of positive wild boars	Percentage of positive wild boars	95 % confidence interval (%)
Juveniles (up to 12 months)	335	38	11.34	7.94–14.74	39	11.64	8.21–15.07
Subadults (12-24 months)	652	139	21.32	18.18–24.46	145	22.24	19.05–25.43
Adults (over 24 months)	610	121	19.84	16.68–23.00	128	20.98	17.75–24.21
Total	1597	298	18.66	16.75–20.57	312	19.54	17.60–21.48

found in domestic pigs in Lithuania. This may pose a serious threat to the Lithuanian pig industry, where only subtype 2 strains are circulating. Contemporary investigations have found that subtype 3 strains identified in Belarus pig farms [8] may be highly virulent [34]. The most striking finding is detection of the subtype four

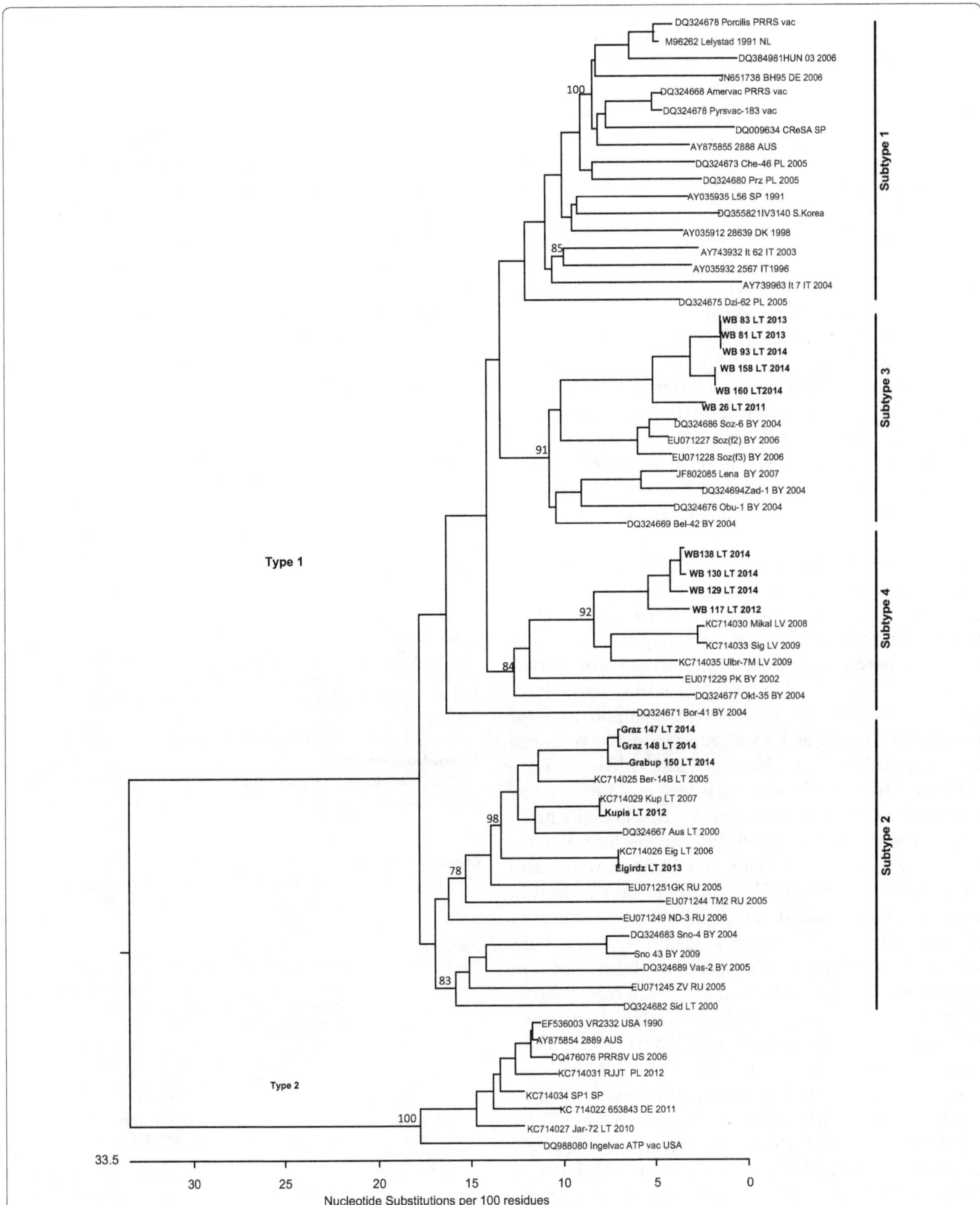

Fig. 2 Phylogenetic analysis of Lithuanian wild boar ORF5 sequences. Clustal W algorithm was used for sequence alignment. *Numbers* adjacent to main branches indicate bootstrap values for different genetic subtypes within the European type of PRRSV. The reference sequences are marked as follows: Gen Banks Access No., name of the sequence, country (up to three letters sign), and years of detection. Sequences determined in this study are indicated in *bold* (GeneBank accession numbers KT828652-KT828665)

strain in wild boars. Previously, this subtype had only been identified in pigs in Belarus and Latvia [8, 11].

In the present study, PRRSV ORF5 partial sequences were obtained only after amplification of highly ORF5 PCR-positive samples. Many ORF5 weak positive samples were not suitable for sequencing or resulted in sequences of poor quality. A possible explanation for this result might be a level of RNA copies in the samples that could only be detected by ORF1 RT-nPCR or by ORF6 real-time RT-PCR. Moreover, Reiner et al. [26] failed to amplify ORF5 as well as ORF7 sequences from wild boars with three PCR-systems that were applied in routine diagnostics of domestic pig samples.

The presence of different PRRSV subtypes in wild boars and pigs suggests that PRRSV infection may be an endogenous infection of wild boars that can serve as a reservoir for infection of domestic pigs. Wild boars have been identified as reservoirs for other viruses, such as those causing classical swine fever and Aujeszky's disease [13]. Therefore, wild boars should be considered important source of viral infections in domestic pigs.

Detection of the highly diverse PRRSV subtypes 3 and 4 in Lithuanian wild boars may also indicate the emergence of PRRSV in domestic pigs. Shi et al. [4] suggested that ancestors of PRRSV subtype 3 may have been present in Eastern Europe before the emergence of subtype 1 PRRSV in Western European pig farms. By molecular clock analysis, the most recent common ancestor for PRRSV Types 1 and 2 existed at least 100 years ago [35]. Although it is possible that PRRSV diverged from other arteriviruses, the pre-emergence evolutionary history of this virus remains a mystery. If wild boars had a longer history of hosting PRRSV strains than domestic pigs, greater viral diversity in wild boars would also be expected. PRRSV ORF5 partial sequences from wild boars obtained in this study exhibited levels of diversity similar to findings in domestic swine population in Lithuania, Latvia, Belarus and European and Asian regions of the Russian Federation [8–10] but different from subtype 1 strains circulating in Central and Western Europe and worldwide. The exceptionally high diversity of PRRSV ORF5 in Eastern Europe indicates that this genotype was established there before establishment in Western Europe; a finding that favours the hypothesis that PRRSV Type 1 emerged in Eastern Europe [4, 6]. Phylogenetic analyses of ORF1 viral sequences from wild boars in Germany [26] presented two highly homologous groups clustered within the diversity of PRRSV Types 1 and 2; however, amplification of ORF5 or ORF7 sequences was not successful. ORF5 encodes the major envelope protein and is often used for phylogenetic analyses mainly because of its high variability; therefore, it has been proposed for subtype definition of PRRSV Type 1 strains [11].

Conclusions

Wild boars may act as a natural reservoir for PRRSV in Lithuania. PRRSV was highly prevalent in Lithuanian wild boar populations, with an average prevalence rate of 18.66 % using conventional RT-PCR and 19.54 % using real-time RT-PCR. PRRSV was detected in 36.71 and 41.77 % of 237 hunting grounds tested by conventional RT-nPCR and real-time RT-PCR, respectively. Phylogenetic analysis of the partial ORF5 region revealed that 10 wild boars harboured virus sequences belonging to genetic subtypes 3 and 4 and may therefore pose a serious threat to Lithuanian pig farms in which only subtype 2 strains are circulating.

Authors' contributions

AS, JB and JZ developed the study design and coordinated the experiment. JB, VS, US, and IP collected samples and performed the PCR analyses. AS, AP, and HZ analysed data and conducted the literature review. AS performed sequence alignments and drafted the manuscript. AP and VO performed the statistical analyses and participated in critical revision of the manuscript. All authors read and approved the final manuscript.

Author details

[1] Faculty of Veterinary Medicine, Lithuanian University of Health Sciences, Tilzes st. 18, LT-47182 Kaunas, Lithuania. [2] National Food and Veterinary Risk Assessment Institute, J. Kairiukscio st. 10, LT-08409 Vilnius, Lithuania.

Acknowledgements

This study was funded by a grant (Project No. MIP-065/2012) from the Research Council of Lithuania.

Competing interests

The authors declare that they have no competing interests.

References

1. Meulenberg JJ, Hulst MM, Demeijer EJ, Moonen PL, Denbesten A, Dekluyver EP, Wensvoort G, Moormann RJ. Lelystad virus, the causative agent of porcine epidemic and respiratory syndrome (pears), is related to Ldv and Eav. Virol. 1993;192:62–72.
2. Wu WH, Fang Y, Farwell R, Steffen-Bien M, Rowland RR, Christopher-Hennings J, Nelson EA. A 10-kDa structural protein of porcine reproductive and respiratory dyndrome virus encoded by ORF2b. Virol. 2001;287:183–91.
3. Murtaugh MP, Stadejek T, Abrahantea JE, Lamc TT, Leung FC. The ever-expanding diversity of porcine reproductive and respiratory syndrome virus. Virus Res. 2010;154:18–30.
4. Shi M, Lam TT, Hon CC, Hui RK, Faaber KS, Wennblom T, Murtaugh MP, Stadejek T, Leung FC. Molecular epidemiology of PRRSV: a phylogenetic perspective. Virus Res. 2010;154:7–17.
5. Jonson CR, Griggs TF, Gnanandarajah J, Murtaugh MP. Novel structural protein in porcine reproductive and respiratory syndrome virus encoded by an alternative ORF5 present in all arteriviruses. J Gen Virol. 2011;92:1107–16.
6. Fang Y, Treffers EE, Li Y, Tas A, Sun Z, van der Meer Y, de Ru AH, van Veelen PA, Atkins JF, Snijder EJ, Firth AE. Efficient 2 frameshifting by mam-

malian ribosomes to synthesize an additional arterivirus protein. PNAS. 2012;109:2920–8. doi:10.1073/pnas.1211145109.

7. Pesch S, Meyer C, Ohlinger VF. New insights into the genetic diversity of European porcine reproductive and respiratory syndrome virus (PRRSV). Vet Microbiol. 2005;107:31–48.
8. Stadejek T, Oleksiewicz MB, Potapchuk D, Podgorska K. Porcine reproductive and respiratory syndrome virus starins of exeptional diversity in Eastern Europe support the definition of new genetic subtypes. G Gen Virol. 2006;87:1835–41.
9. Stadejek T, Oleksiewicz MB, Scherbakov AV, Timina AM, Krabbe JS, Chabros K, Potapchuk D. Definition of subtypes in the European genotype of porcine reproductive and respiratory syndrome virus: nucleocapsid characteristics and geographical distribution in Europe. Arch Virol. 2008;153:1479–88.
10. Stadejek T, Stankevicius A, Storgaard T, Oleksiewicz MB, Belak S, Drew TW, Pejsak Z. Identification of radically different variants of porcine reproductive and respiratory syndrome virus in Eastern Europe: towards a common ancestor for European and American viruses. J Gen Viro. 2002;83:1861–73.
11. Stadejek T, Stankevicius A, Murtaugh M, Oleksiewicz MB. Molecular evolution of PRRSV in Europe: current state of play. Vet Microbiol. 2013;165:21–8.
12. Albayrak H, Ozan E, Cavunt A. A serological survey of selected pathogens in wild boar (*Sus scrofa*) in northern Turkey. Eur J Wildl Res. 2013;59:893–7.
13. Albina E, Mesplede A, Chenut G, Le Potier MF, Bourbao G, Le Gal S, Leforban Y. A serological survey on classical swine fever (CSF), Aujeszky's disease (AD) and porcine reproductive and respiratory syndrome (PRRS) virus infections in French wild boars from 1991 to 1998. Vet Microbiol. 2000;77:43–57.
14. Boadella M, Ruiz-Fons F, Vicente J, Martin M, Segales J, Gortazar C. Seroprevalence evolution of selected pathogens in Iberian wild boar. Transb Emerg Dis. 2012;25:136–42.
15. Closa-Sebastia F, Casas-Diaz E, Cuenca R, Lavin S, Mentaberre G, Marco I. Antibodies to selected pathogens in wild boar (*Sus scrofa*) from Catalonia (NE Spain). Eur J Wildl Res. 2011;57:977–81.
16. Kaden V, Lagen E, Hanel A, Hlinak A, Mewes L, Hergarten G, Irsch B, Deken J, Bruer W. Retrospective serological survey on selected viral pathogens in wild boar populations in Germany. Eur J Wildl Res. 2009;55:153–9.
17. Montagnaro S, Sasso S, De Martin L, Lango M, Iovane V, Ghiumino G, Pisanelli G, Nava D, Baldi L, Pagnini U. Prevalence of antibodies to selected viral and bacterial pathogens in wild boars (*Sus scrofa*) in campania Region. Italy. J Wildl Dis. 2010;46:316–9.
18. Rodriguez-Prieto V, Kukielka D, Martinez-Lopez B, DelasHeras AI, Barasona JA, Gortazar CH, Sanchez-Vizcaino JM, Vincente J. Porcine reproductive and respiratory syndrome (PRRS) virus in wild boar and Iberian pigs in south-central Spain. Eur J Wildl Res. 2013;59:859–67.
19. Saliki J, Rodgers S, Eskew G. Serosurvey of selected viral and bacterial diseases in wild swine from Okklahoma. J Wildl Dis. 1998;34:834–8.
20. Kukushkin S, Kanshina A, Timina A, Baybikov T, Mikhalishin V. Investigation of wild boar (*Sus scrofa*) for porcine reproductive and respiratory syndrome in some territories of Russia. Eur J Wildl Res. 2008;54:515–8.
21. Ruiz-Fons F, Vicente J, Vidal D, Holfe U, Villanua D, Gauss C, Segales J, Almeria S, Montoro V, Gortazar C. Seroprevalence of six reproductive pathogens in European wild boar (*Sus scrofa*) from Spain: the effect on wild boar female reproductive performance. Theriogenol. 2006;65:731–43.
22. Vengust G, Valencak Z, Bidovec A. Serological survey of selected pathogens in wild boar in Slovenia. J Vet Med B. 2006;53:24–7.
23. Vincente J, Leon-Vizcaino L, Gortazar C, Jose Cubero M, Gonzalez M, Martin-Atance P. Antibodies to selected viral and bacterial pathogens in European wild boars from southcentral Spain. J Wildl Dis. 2002;38:649–52.
24. Zupacic Z, Jukic B, Lojki M, Cac Z, Jemersic L, Staresina V. Prevalence of antibodies to classical swine fever, Aujieszky's disease, porcine reproductive and respiratory syndrome, bovine viral diarrhoea viruses in wild boars in Croatia. J Vet Med B Infect Dis Vet Public Health. 2002;49:253–6.
25. Bonilauri P, Merialdi G, Dottori M, Barbieri I. Presence of PRRSV in wild boar in Italy. Vet Rec. 2006;158:395–404.
26. Reiner G, Fresen C, Bronnert S, Willems H. Porcine reproductive and respiratory syndrome virus (PRRSV) infection in wild boars. Vet Microbiol. 2009;136:250–8.
27. Stankevicius A, Buitkuviene J, Valanciute J, Cepulis R, Stadejek T. Porcine reproductive and respiratory syndrome virus (PRRSV) infection in Lithuanian wild boar (*Sus scrofa*) population. Proceedings of the EuroPRRS2011, Novi Sad, Serbia. 2011;54–9.
28. Wu J, Liu S, Zhou S, Wang Z, Li K, Zhang Y, et al. Porcine reproductive and respiratory syndrome in hybrid wild boars, China. Emer Infec Dis. 2011;17:1071–3.
29. Ruiz-Fons F, Segales J, Gortazar C. A review of viral diseases of the European wild boar: effects of population dynamics and reservoir role. Vet J. 2008;176:158–69.
30. Revilla-Fernandez S, Wallner B, Truschner K, Benczak A, Brem G, Schmoll F, Mueller M, Steinborn R. The use of endogenous and exogenous reference RNAs for qualitative detection of PRRSV of PRRSV in porcine semen. J Virol Methods. 2005;126:21–30.
31. Vilcek S, Molnar L, Vlasakova M, Jackova A. The first detection of PRRSV in wild boars in Slovakia. Berl Munch Tierarztl Wochenschr. 2015;128:31–3.
32. Fabisiak M, Podgorska K, Skrypiec E, Szotka A, Stadejek T. Detection of porcine circovirus type 2 (PCV2) and porcine reproductive and respiratory syndrome virus (PRRSV) antibodies in meat juice samples from Polish wild boar (*Sus scrofa*). Act Vet Hung. 2013;61:529–36.
33. Ministry of Environment of the Republic of Lithuania official reports (2012–2015). http://www.am.lt/VI/index.php#r/966, http://www.amvmt.lt/index.php/leidiniai/misku-ukio-statistika. Accessed 19 Feb 2016.
34. Karniychuk UU, Geldhof M, Vanhee M, Van Doorsselaere J, Saveleva TA, Nauwynck HJ. Pathogenesis and antigenic characterization of new East European subtype 3 porcine reproductive and respiratory syndrome virus isolate. BMC Vet Res. 2010;6:30.
35. Forsberg R. Divergence time of porcine reproductive and respiratory syndrome virus subtypes. Mol Biol Evol. 2005;22:2121–34.

14

Herding conditions related to infectious keratoconjunctivitis in semi-domesticated reindeer: a questionnaire-based survey among reindeer herders

Morten Tryland[1*], Solveig Marie Stubsjøen[2], Erik Ågren[3], Bernt Johansen[4] and Camilla Kielland[5]

Abstract

Background: Infectious keratoconjunctivitis (IKC) in Eurasian semi-domesticated reindeer (*Rangifer tarandus tarandus*) is a multifactorial disease, associated to infectious agents such as Cervid herpesvirus 2 (CvHV2) and various species of bacteria, but environmental factors may also be necessary to initiate the disease. Little effort seems to have been invested in addressing the herder`s experience with this disease. An information letter with a link to an online questionnaire was sent to 410 herding community representatives in Norway and Sweden.

Results: Sixty-three herders responded, 76 % of these having reindeer in Norway and 24 % in Sweden. Thirty-three herders (55 %) responded that they had seen this disease during the preceding year (2010) and 23 (38 %) that they had seen it in previous years (2009 or earlier). The majority (67 %) claimed that only 1–5 animals in their herd were affected at one time, whereas three herders (7 %) responded that more than 30 animals had been affected. No environmental factor could be singled out as significantly associated with the appearance of IKC, but when categorizing the number of contact herds for each herd (i.e. sharing pastures, corrals etc.), IKC was observed more often in herds with many (>25) contact herds. The questionnaire revealed that a veterinarian is not always available for reindeer herders, but also that a veterinarian seldom is contacted for this disease. None of the herders practiced isolation of a diseased animal from the rest of the herd when IKC was observed. Slaughter was the action most commonly initiated by the herders in response to IKC, whereas the veterinarian usually prescribed antibiotics, usually an ophthalmic ointment, alone or combined with systemic treatment. The herders claimed that IKC and other diseases had less importance than predators concerning loss of animals.

Conclusions: IKC is to be considered a common disease, observed in 55 % of the herds (2010), typically affecting 1–5 animals, although larger outbreaks (>30 animals) occur. The herders usually slaughtered affected animals rather than consulting a veterinarian for medical treatment.

Keywords: Eye disease, IKC, Keratoconjunctivitis, Ocular disease, Reindeer, Risk factors, Traditional knowledge, Questionnaire

Background

Infectious keratoconjunctivitis (IKC), known as infectious bovine keratoconjunctivitis in cattle (IBK), is a contagious eye disease and the most important eye disease in cattle worldwide [1]. The disease also occurs in other livestock [1, 2] and wildlife [3–5] and is generally regarded as a multifactorial disease. In cattle, the Gram negative bacterium *Moraxella bovis* is regarded as the main cause of the disease. Also, *Moraxella bovoculi* and a range of other bacteria, viruses, and environmental conditions seem to be involved [1, 6].

*Correspondence: morten.tryland@uit.no
[1] Arctic Infection Biology, Department of Arctic and Marine Biology, UiT-Arctic University of Norway, Stakkevollveien 23, 9010 Tromsø, Norway

IKC has been reported in Eurasian semi-domesticated reindeer (*Rangifer tarandus tarandus*) in Norway, Sweden, and Finland since the late 19th century [7]. Increased lacrimation and discoloration of the fur below the affected eye(s) is an early sign of IKC in reindeer. Although neither keratitis nor conjunctivitis may be prominent at this stage, reindeer owners, especially those who have experienced outbreaks in their herd, often notice these initial symptoms. Conjunctivitis and keratitis is usually present, accompanied by corneal oedema, giving the eye a cloudy and bluish appearance. When the disease progresses, periorbital oedema becomes prominent, often followed by corneal ulcers, panophthalmitis and loss of the lens and other structures of the eye, leading to permanent blindness (Fig. 1). Animals may recover spontaneously from the early stages of the disease [8], but sometimes, in severe outbreaks affecting many animals in a herd, IKC cause mortalities with severe losses for the herders [9, 10].

In reindeer, a variety of bacteria, such as *Trueperella pyogenes*, *Staphylococcus* spp., *Escherichia coli*, *Moraxella ovis* and others have been isolated from reindeer with IKC, although most of the studies have addressed agents present at late clinical stages of disease [9, 11–15]. In early stages of IKC, we identified the reindeer alphaherpesvirus (Cervid herpesvirus 2; CvHV2) as the primary cause of an outbreak in 2009 [10], a virus that is considered enzootic in herds of semi-domesticated reindeer in Fennoscandia (for a review, see [16]). Thus, other factors than the presence of infectious agents may be decisive of whether the disease occurs or not.

Reindeer herders live very close to nature and are therefore to a great degree exposed to the potential effects of climate change [17]. With the documented changes of the global climate [18], it is expected that temperature and precipitation will increase in the arctic and sub-arctic regions, including the reindeer herding regions of Fennoscandia. An increase in rain-on-snow and freeze–thaw

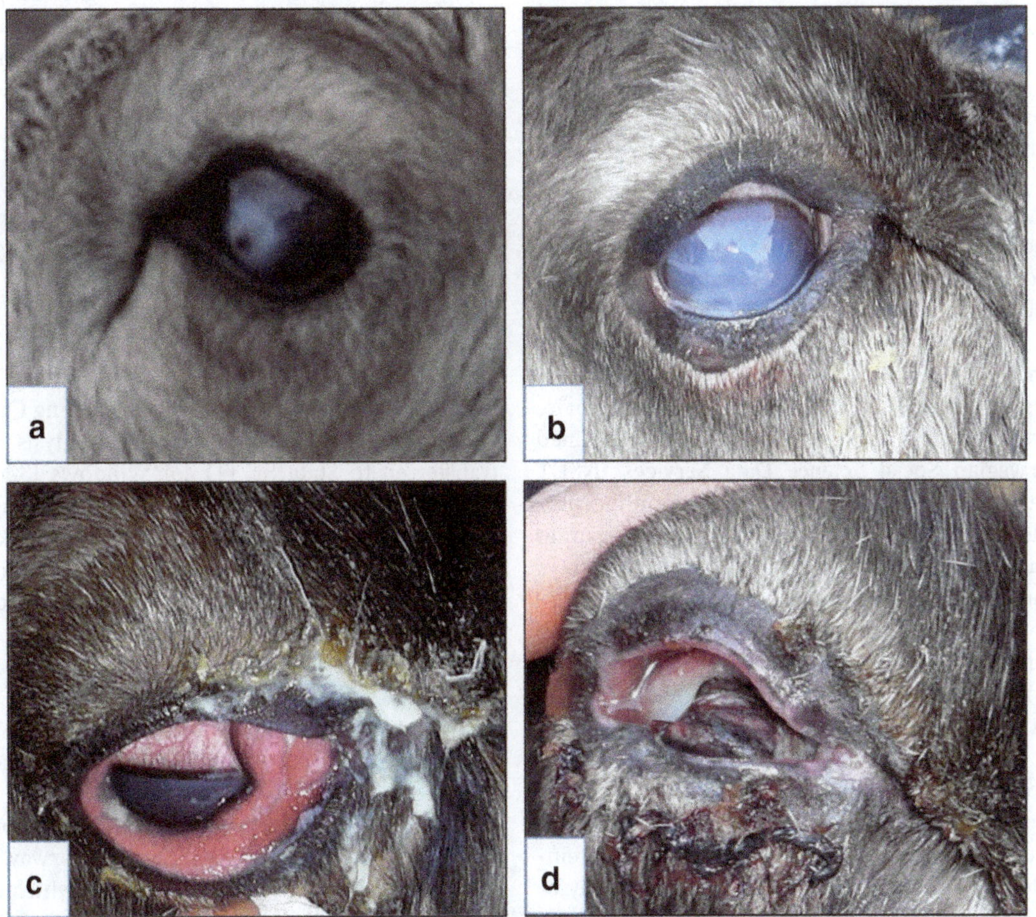

Fig. 1 Clinical symptoms representing different stages of eye disease in reindeer, developing into infectious keratoconjunctivitis and a total destruction of the eye and permanent blindness (see text for further descriptions)

events during winter, may make the winter pastures less available for reindeer, being covered under heavy, hard-crusted snow or ice [17]. One way to mitigate challenging winter pasture conditions is to conduct supplementary feeding of the animals, either by bringing feed to the reindeer pastures, or by feeding the animals in corrals. Corralling and feeding animals will, however, expose the herd to stress which may affect their immunological competence and contribute to the animals being more susceptible to infections. At the same time, the transmission of infectious agents between animals are facilitated due to increased animal-to-animal contact and shared feed and water [15, 19, 20]. Previous outbreaks of IKC, both in Sweden [9] and Norway [10, 15] have indeed occurred in corrals during supplementary feeding. Climate change and mitigation by increased feeding may thus contribute to increased prevalence of diseases, such as IKC.

The aim of this questionnaire survey was to gather traditional knowledge and experience from reindeer herders in Norway and Sweden regarding IKC in reindeer, and identify herding conditions and management factors that might be associated to IKC.

Methods

Subjects

Registered reindeer herders (n = 410), were invited through their reindeer herding unit representatives (siida leaders; Norway, sameby chairperson; Sweden) to participate in this study. The questionnaire was made available to the participants by sending a letter that provided information on the survey and a web address with access to the online questionnaire.

Questionnaire

A permission to conduct an anonymous questionnaire survey among Sami reindeer herders were obtained from Norwegian Social Science Data Services (NSD). The questionnaire was designed using the online program Questback® and translated from Norwegian to Swedish and Sami (Northern Sami). Data from each of the responders were anonymously stored in a database on a web-server. After completing the survey, data were exported to Stata SE/111 for Windows (Stata Corp., College Station, TX, USA) where primary processing of data and quality check was conducted.

Demographics and management

Demographic data collected from the reindeer owners were gender, age and years of experience as a reindeer herder. Herd data consisted of country (Norway or Sweden), herding district, herd size and number of contact herds, the latter defined as how many other herds the actual herd shared pastures, corrals, and transport vehicles with during the year. Herders were also asked about pasture conditions in 2010, which was the year before the survey was sent out, and to evaluate and grade the importance of weather conditions, such as precipitation (summer and winter) and winter temperatures. In addition, methods and time used for translocation of animals between seasonal pastures and the use of supplementary feeding were addressed. Additionally, owners were asked about important causes of loss of animals, other diseases than IKC, prophylactic anti-parasitic treatment, and their access to veterinary expertise.

Appearance and severity of IKC

Specific questions about IKC were related to when the disease normally appeared (season). Pictures of eye infections and IKC in reindeer were provided (Fig. 1), grossly representing four categories of severity; A: a stage which can represent a trauma or a condition developing into IKC, with increased lacrimation and discoloration of the cornea, B: corneal oedema, with severely discoloration (bluish/whitish) of the cornea, increased lacrimation, moderate periorbital oedema C: progressed periorbital oedema and shedding of pus, and D: inflammation with perforation and destruction of the eye resulting in permanent blindness. Herders were asked if they had seen similar conditions, which stage of the disease they had seen the most, how often, and their estimation of how many animals that were affected at a time. They were also asked about how the disease was managed, if a veterinarian generally was available for the herding district, and the choice of treatment, initiated either by the herder or by the veterinarian.

Statistical analysis

Primary data analysis was undertaken using Questback®. For further statistical and graphical analysis, data were transferred to Stata SE/111 for Windows (Stata Corp.). Demographic data was tabulated and percentages calculated. Simple Chi square test was used to look for associations between IKC and possible risk factors. In all analyses, statistical significance was considered with a P value <0.05.

Results

Demographic data of the questionnaire survey

From the 410 reindeer herders in Norway and Sweden that received the letter with the link to the questionnaire, 63 (16 %) responded (Table 1). The majority of the respondents (76 %) had reindeer in Norway, and only Norwegian herders informed about which reindeer-herding district they represented (Fig. 2). Most of the respondents were male herders aged between 31 and 50 years old, and 40 % of the respondents had a herd size

Table 1 General demographic data of the questionnaire survey among Norwegian and Swedish reindeer herders regarding the disease infectious keratoconjunctivitis in reindeer

Parameter	Category	Number	Percentage[a]
Country (herders/animals)	Norway	48	76
	Sweden	15	24
Gender	Male	52	78
	Female	8	22
Age (years)	<30	4	6
	31–40	19	31
	41–50	19	31
	51–60	13	21
	>60	7	11
Experience as reindeer herder (years)	<10	9	15
	10–20	10	16
	21–30	16	26
	31–40	15	24
	>40	12	19
Herd size (approximate number of animals)	1–250	9	15
	251–500	23	38
	501–750	15	25
	751–1000	2	3
	1001–1250	6	10
	1251–1500	2	3
	>1500	4	7
Number of contact herds (shared pastures, corrals, transport etc.)	0	2	3
	1–5	14	23
	6–10	10	16
	11–15	8	13
	16–20	7	11
	21–25	3	5
	>25	18	29

[a] Since decimals are omitted, the sum (percentage) is not always 100 for each question

between 251 and 500 animals. Almost 30 % of the herds were in contact with more than 25 other herds during a year of herding (summer and winter pastures, shared corrals and transports etc.).

Appearance of IKC

Regarding the last time herders saw clinical symptoms resembling IKC (Fig. 1), 11 herders (18 %) answered that they had never observed this, 26 (43 %) answered that they had observed it during the previous year (2010) and 23 (38 %) said they had seen it 2 years ago or in previous years (but not in 2010) (Table 2).

Most of the respondents that had seen IKC among their animals (49 %) claimed that September–November was the most common season of occurrence during the year, whereas 26 % answered June–August, 17 % September–February, and 9 % March–May.

When IKC was observed in the herd, 31 herders (67 %) answered that typically 1–5 animals were affected, 7 (15 %) answered that 6–10 animals were usually affected, whereas 8 (17 %) had experienced that IKC could affect more than 10 animals in their herd. Only three herders reported that more than 30 animals had been affected by IKC at one time (Table 2). There was no significant association between the occurrence of IKC in a herd and the number of contact herds. However, when categorizing the number of contact herds into four groups, a visual trend appeared, since among the herds with >25 contact herds, 35 % reported that they had seen IKC, whereas only 10 % report that they had not seen IKC (Fig. 3).

Based on the responding herder`s experience from 2010, the severity of the IKC disease symptoms was categorized as mild, with 17 % as A and 45 % as B (Fig. 1). Only three had seen the category C, and none of the herders had seen category D, except for three herders that reported to have seen all categories. IKC in reindeer was mainly detected when animals were gathered, corralled and handled for identification, slaughter or other purposes (89 %).

Most of the reindeer herders responding to the survey (n = 35, 58 %) said they had access to a veterinarian, whereas 19 (31 %) said that they had access to a veterinarian some times, and 6 (10 %) claimed that they had no access to a veterinarian in their region. When animals were observed with IKC in a herd, a majority of the herders (56 %) chose slaughter instead of medical treatment (Table 3). The most common treatment against IKC in reindeer initiated by a veterinarian (according to the herders) was the use of ophthalmic ointment containing antibiotics (41 %). Other types of treatment are listed in Table 4.

Environmental conditions and pasture

Of all the respondents, 55 % answered that weather and climatic conditions had a crucial impact on herding on a daily basis, whereas 42 % answered that weather and climate conditions sometimes were of importance. Only 3 % answered that such conditions were not important for their herding. The amount of precipitation as rain was regarded as important, both in the summer (37 %) and in winter (40 %). Regarding temperature fluctuations, 42 % of the respondents thought that large changes of temperature during winter have an impact on their herd, whereas wind, coldness, heat and dry periods were regarded as less important. A vast majority of the respondents characterized their summer and winter pastures as good or very good, for the year of 2010 (Fig. 4).

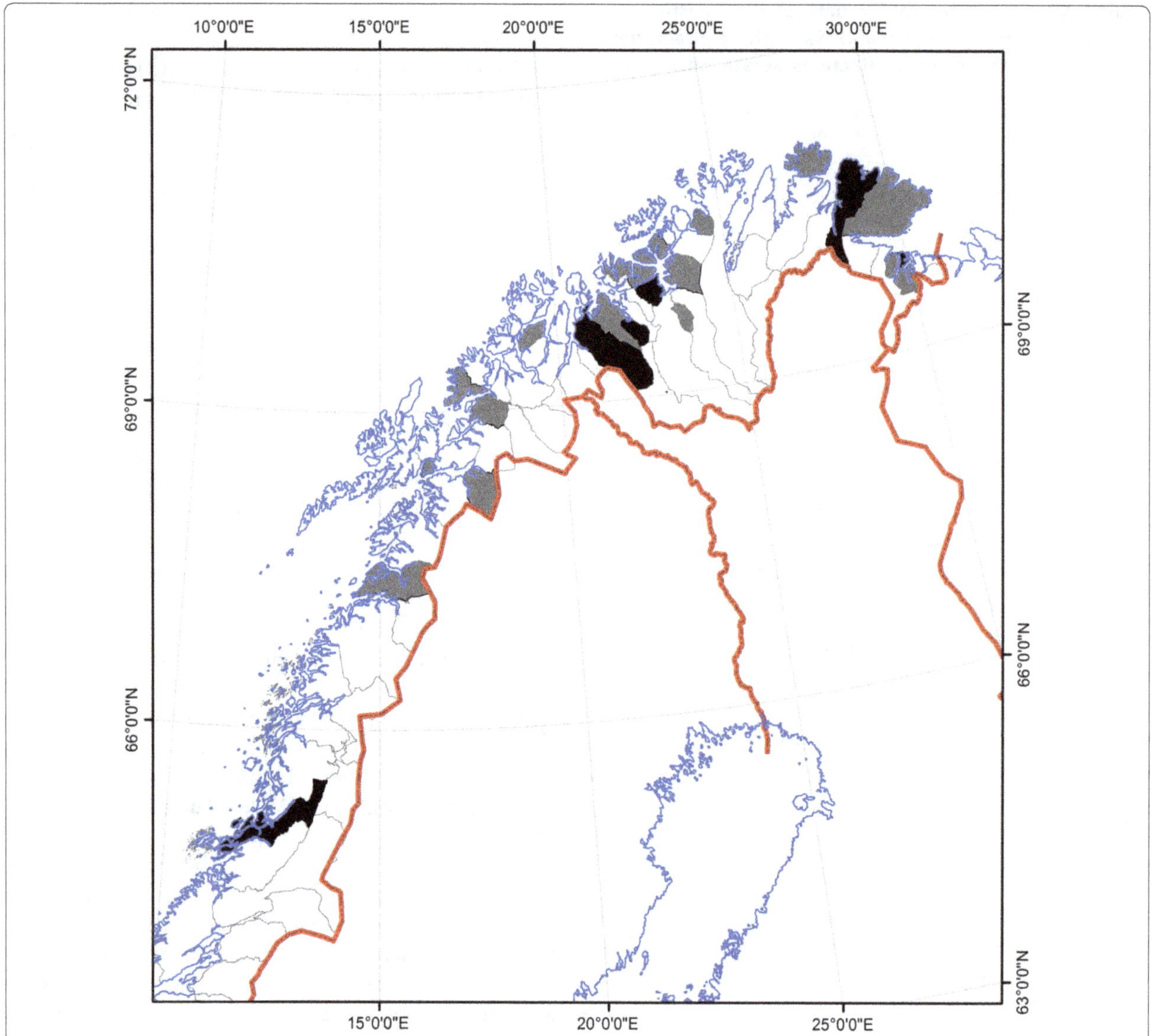

Fig. 2 Map of Northern Norway, indicating the reindeer herding districts represented by reindeer herders responding to which district they represented (n = 37; no such information were given by the Swedish herders). *Grey* = 1 herder, *black* = 2 herders

Herding and feeding

Most owners (23 %) used 1–2 weeks to translocate their animals from summer to winter pasture, whereas 19 % said that they used 1–5 h, and 12 % that they used more than 6 weeks. Most animals were herded by motorized vehicles, such as quad bikes in the summer (51 %) and snowmobiles in the winter (88 %), but 25 % of the herders said they also herded their animals on foot. On winter pasture, 21 % fed their animals regularly, whereas 64 % fed them only occasionally. The most prevalent feeds used were dry hay (32 %) and pellets (28 %), usually pelleted feed produced for reindeer. Combinations of different feeds were also used during the winter, with pellets and lichens being the most frequent (27 %).

Predators

Of all the respondents, 49 (82 %) regarded predators as the most important factor related to loss of animals, with wolverine (*Gulo gulo*; 32 %) and lynx (*Lynx lynx*; 25 %) being the two most important species, followed by eagle (species not specified but assumed to be Golden eagle, *Aquila chrysaetos*; 20 %) and brown bear (*Ursus arctos*; 16.6 %), as well as red fox (*Vulpes vulpes*), wolf (*Canis lupus*) and dog (*Canis familiaris*) (each of them 2.4 %).

Other diseases than IKC

When asked about the occurrence of diseases in general, 17 % of the respondents answered that they considered infestation of the reindeer warble fly larvae (*Hypoderma*

Table 2 Answers about the appearance of infectious keratoconjunctivitis in reindeer based on 63 reindeer herder respondents, 48 in Norway and 14 in Sweden

Question	Category	Number	Percentage[a]
When did you observe eye disease as illustrated?[b]	Never observed	11	18
	Last year	26	43
	2 years ago	8	13
	3 years ago	5	8
	4 years ago or more	10	17
If this eye disease was observed last year (2010), how many animals were affected?	1–5	31	67
	6–10	7	15
	11–15	1	2
	16–20	3	7
	21–30	1	2
	>30	3	7
How does the disease normally look like in your herd?	A	23	47
	B	22	45
	C	1	2
	D	0	0
	All types occur	3	6

[a] Since decimals are omitted, the sum (percentage) is not always 100 for each question

[b] Refers to illustrations given in (Fig. 1a–d)

tarandi) and reindeer throat bot fly larvae (*Cephenemyia trompe*) as the most common diseases. Sixty percent of the owners conducted annual anti-parasitic treatment, whereas 19 % did not give any parasitic treatment. The treatment was usually done in September–November, and most animals in the herd were treated (both sexes, all ages). Lameness and other problems with the legs is given as the second most important cause of disease (8 %), whereas other diseases mentioned specifically in the questionnaire, such as abortion, emaciation, other parasite infestations or trauma, were not, from the herders point of view, regarded as common disease conditions.

Among the herders that had no or only restricted access to a veterinarian, 31 % responded that the parasite burden represented the most frequent disease condition, whereas those who had access to veterinary services did not to the same extent experience the parasite burden as important ($P = 0.003$).

Discussion

This survey aimed at gathering traditional knowledge and experience from reindeer herders regarding IKC in reindeer, to identify herding conditions and management

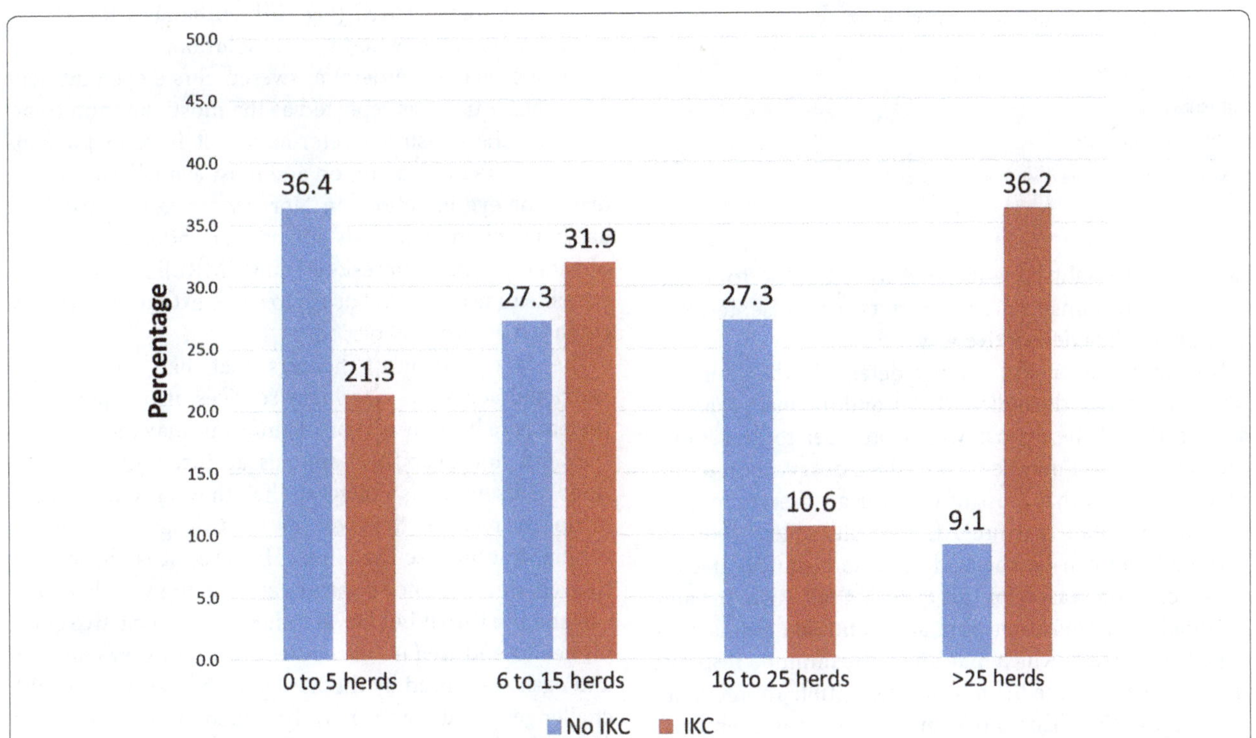

Fig. 3 The association between the occurrence of infectious keratoconjunctivitis among reindeer in a herd and the number of contact herds for that particular herd, i.e. sharing pastures, corrals, transport vehicles etc. during the year

Table 3 Management actions taken by the herder when the disease infectious keratoconjunctivitis occurred in semi-domesticated reindeer (*Rangifer t. tarandus*). *Question* what do you do when this disease occurs in a single/a few animals in the herd?

Management action taken by the herder	Percentage of responders (n = 57)
No measures taken	23
Separate the affected animal from the herd	0
Initiate a treatment (by the owner)	12
Slaughter/euthanize the animal	56
Consult a veterinarian	7
Other action (not specified)	2

Table 4 Management (by the veterinarian, according to the herder) of infectious keratoconjunctivitis in semi-domesticated reindeer (*Rangifer t. tarandus*). *Question* if a veterinarian is initiating measures—what measures are most common?

Measures by the veterinarian	Percentage of responders (n = 34)[a]
Ophthalmic ointment containing antibiotics	41
Systemic treatment with antibiotics	3
Both systemic and local (ointment) antibiotic treatment	6
Slaughter the animal (consumption)	56
Euthanasia	12
Other action (not specified)	38

[a] Multiple answers were given by some responders

factors that might be associated to IKC. Due to a relatively low response rate, the results are presented predominantly in a descriptive way.

IKC in reindeer was mainly detected when animals were gathered and handled (89 %), and the main seasonal appearance of the disease was September to November. This information may be biased, since observation of disease in animals that most of the year are free-ranging in remote mountain pastures, is difficult, unless they are gathered and can be checked at close distance, and the most common season for this is during fall. Also, through herding, gathering, transport and handling, animals are exposed to stress, which may affect the immune response negatively and make them more susceptible to infections and disease [21]. This is relevant, since it has been demonstrated that experimentally immune-compromised reindeer have reactivated latent herpesvirus (CvHV2) infections [22], which has been identified as the cause of an IKC outbreak [10]. Thus, the fact that most IKC cases are reported to appear in September to November may reflect that this is when most of the animals are inspected at close range. However, it may also be a result of the disease being initiated during this period, due to the handling and the stress they experience, or a combination of the two.

Another interesting finding was that some herders claimed they had no access to a veterinarian, and that only four of 57 respondents (7 %) were considering consulting a veterinarian should disease symptoms of IKC occur. This may reflect scarce availability of a veterinarian in that area. It may also indicate a restricted willingness to spend resources on disease treatment or limited trust in the probability that veterinary advice and treatment will change the course and outcome of the disease, since most of the herders responded to IKC by slaughtering the animal. Since IKC is a transmissible disease, sometimes affecting tens or hundreds of animals, it was somewhat surprising that none of the respondents mentioned separation of the diseased animals from the healthy as a measure to restrict disease spreading.

The treatment of IKC in a reindeer herd will depend on a range of factors, such as the severity of the disease, the number of affected individuals and the herder´s ability and willingness to invest time and money on treatment and care. For some animals, displaying severe and late stage symptoms of IKC (Fig. 1d), euthanasia for animal welfare reasons may be the best solution, which 12 % of the respondents (herders) answered. Since eye ointment with antibiotics was reported as the most common treatment by the consulted veterinarian, it is of major concern that the most common and most available antibiotic drugs for eye infections in Norway are not licensed for use in production animals, including reindeer, due to lack of data on maximum residue limits (MRL). It is, however, possible to use off-label drugs to some extent, but with an extended withdrawal period.

The fact that most herders that had no or only restricted access to veterinary services also experienced the parasite burden as more significant, may indicate that they did not treat their animals against parasite infections. This may also suggest that they lack knowledge or do not receive advice on the right drugs, dose and/or timing, to optimize the effect. However, it is challenging to evaluate this, since parasites such as the warble fly larvae and the throat bot larvae, which have a negative effect on health and welfare of reindeer [23], are very common and easily recorded by the herders, whereas other health challenges or diseases may be much more difficult to identify.

Almost all the respondents in both Norway and Sweden claimed that their summer and winter pastures during 2010, the year before the survey, were of good or very

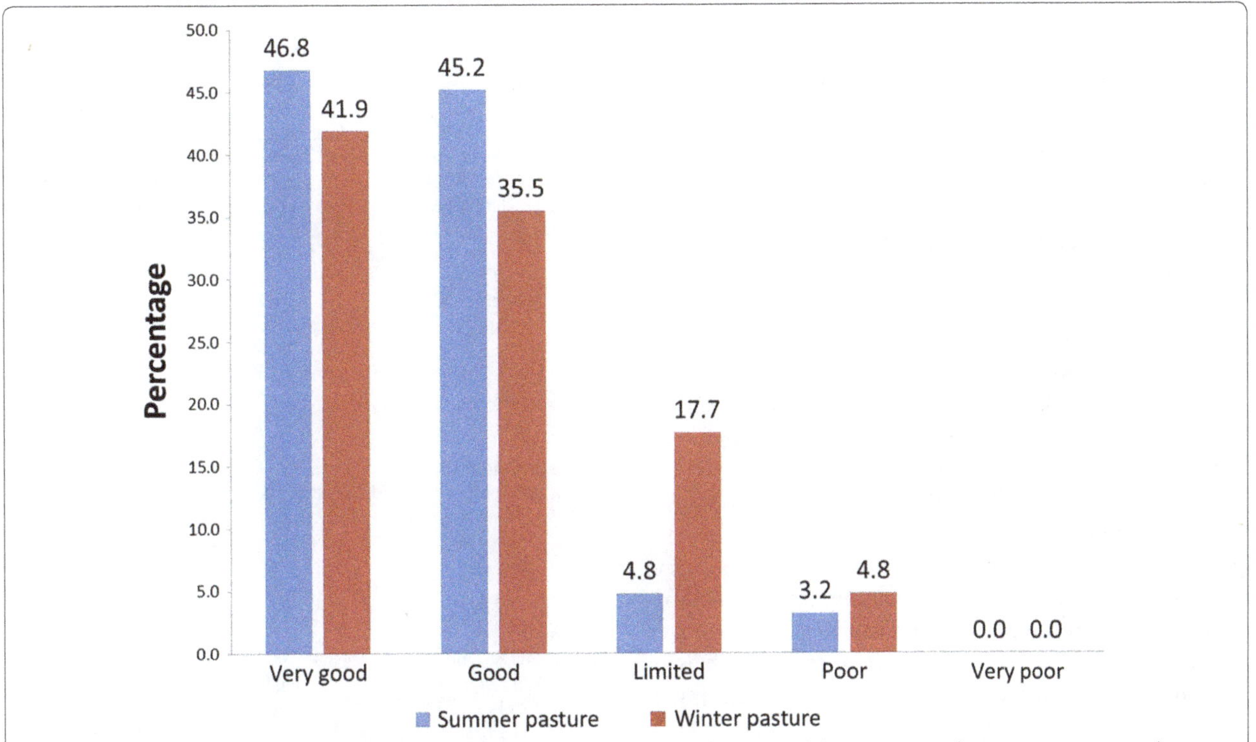

Fig. 4 Most of the reindeer herders (percentages given) responding to the survey characterized their summer and winter pastures as good or very good in 2010, whereas 8 and 23 % of the herders evaluated their pastures as poor or limited during summer and winter, respectively

good quality. Although some supplementary feeding was conducted, this indicates that among these herders, of whom 43 % observed IKC in 2010, starvation and poor pasture quality did not stand out as the main characteristic determinant for this disease. It is also important to note that herd size alone was not significantly associated to the occurrence of IKC. Most herders regarded precipitation as rain as having a negative impact on reindeer herding, during both summer and winter. This is relevant, since the effects of climatic changes in arctic and sub-arctic regions is predicted to consist of increased precipitation in the form of rain, especially associated to an increased frequency of freeze–thaw cycles during winter [18], which may hinder the animals to find their necessary food resources.

The questionnaire revealed that 21 % of the herders fed their animals regularly during the winter, whereas 64 % fed them only occasionally. Supplementary feeding has been described by herders as an emergency solution only, which may be necessary during the winter due to challenging winter pasture conditions [24]. Supplementary feeding of reindeer is costly and results in a heavier workload with more herd supervision and feed management, compared to free grazing. It may also induce a different fat composition in the meat and a taste different from the characteristic flavours of reindeer meat [24]. Further, corralling and supplementary feeding may facilitate the transmission of infectious agents among the animals [20] and also lead to feeding related disorders like diarrhoea and ruminal acidosis [25]. However, Josefsen and colleagues have found, by conducting routine reindeer necropsies over a period of time (1998–2011) in Norway, that lack of feed, hunger and emaciation was a more common cause of mortality compared to feeding related disorders [26]. Supplementary feeding may also affect the behaviour of the animals and their use of pasture, making the reindeer more dependent on human care [27]. However, it has been shown that supplementary feeding generally increases body weight and reproduction success of the females and contributes to a decrease in calf mortality [28, 29].

Somewhat surprisingly, almost 30 % of the herds represented in the survey were in contact with as many as 25 other herds or more during a year of herding (summer and winter pastures). This contact also includes exposure to circulating and enzootic infectious agents of other herds. This is in line with serological studies covering many different herding districts and regions, showing that the prevalence of some virus infections, such as pestivirus and alphaherpesvirus, has been quite stable over time [16, 30, 31]. It also suggests that managing infectious diseases should be considered a communal responsibility among herders within a district. Even if no significant association was found between the occurrence of IKC and the number of contact herds for each particular herd, the herds where IKC was reported did have a larger number of contact herds (>25). This is in line with the fact that IKC is infectious and spreads between animals and herds, although it also might reflect that the chance of having an animal with IKC probably increases with the number of animals.

In our data, we found no association between the appearance of IKC and the different methods of herding and translocation of animals between pastures, such as walking with the animals, the use of motorized vehicles on the ground, transporting them by trucks, or use of helicopter in the field, although these methods may represent different stress exposure to the animals. Also predators represent stress for free ranging animals, but in our data we did not find an association between appearance of IKC and the presence and types of predators of importance. This may reflect that there are no such associations, or that our study, due to the restricted number of respondents, lacked the power to reveal them.

Conclusions

From this survey, it can be concluded that IKC is to be considered a common disease in reindeer (55 % of the herds in 2010), typically affecting 1–5 animals at a time, and appearing most often during September to November. The chance of having registered the disease in a herd was higher for herds having >25 contact herds. In spite of the contagious nature of IKC, none of the herders responded that they isolated affected animals from healthy, and the majority of the herders usually slaughtered affected animals rather than consulting a veterinarian for medical treatment. The herder´s experience, that precipitation as rain had a negative impact on reindeer herding, is of relevance when investigating possible effects of climatic changes in arctic and sub-arctic regions. We recommend herders to be aware of this disease, recognize the initial symptoms, isolate affected animals from healthy, and to make use of local veterinary expertise in order to safeguard animal welfare and limit the spread and economical loss due to having a disease outbreak in the herd.

Authors' contributions

MT and EÅ secured funding. MT, SMS, EÅ and CK planned the study and the questionnaire. MT, SMS and CK distributed the questionnaire in Norway, EÅ in Sweden. CK organized the data and conducted statistics. BJ organized the herding districts and produced Fig. 2 (map). MT wrote first draft of the manuscript, SMS, CK, EÅ and BJ contributed and all authors read and approved the final manuscript.

Author details

[1] Arctic Infection Biology, Department of Arctic and Marine Biology, UiT-Arctic University of Norway, Stakkevollveien 23, 9010 Tromsø, Norway. [2] Department of Health Surveillance, Section for Disease Prevention and Animal Welfare, Norwegian Veterinary Institute, P.O. Box 750, Sentrum, 0106 Oslo, Norway. [3] Department of Pathology and Wildlife Diseases, National Veterinary Institute, 751 89 Uppsala, Sweden. [4] Northern Research Institute-Tromsø, Tromsø Science Park, 9294 Tromsø, Norway. [5] Department of Production Animal Clinical Sciences, Faculty of Veterinary Medicine and Biosciences, Norwegian University of Life Sciences, Ullevålsveien 72, 0454 Oslo, Norway.

Acknowledgements

Thanks to veterinarian Sire Fors Grønmo for translation of the questionnaire to the Sami language. Thanks to the Reindeer Development Fund (Reindriftens utviklingsfond; RUF, Norway) and Nordic Council of Ministers (Nordisk Råd) for funding the study.

Competing interests

The authors declare that they have no competing interests in the manuscript. MT is deputy editor of Acta Veterinaria Scandinavica, but has not in any way been involved in or interacted with the review process or editorial decision-making.

References

1. Postma GC, Carfagnini JC, Minatel L. *Moraxella bovis* pathogenicity: and update. Comp Immunol Microbiol Infect Dis. 2008;31:449–58.
2. Motha MX, Frey J, Hansen MF, Jamaludin R, Tham KM. Detection of *Mycoplasma conjunctiva* in sheep affected with conjunctivitis and infectious keratoconjunctivitis. N Z Vet J. 2003;51:186–90.
3. Giacometti M, Janovsky M, Belloy L, Frey J. Infectious keratoconjunctivitis of ibex, chamois and other caprinae. Rev Sci Tech. 2002;21:335–45.
4. Dubay SA, Williams ES, Mills K, Boerger-Fields AM. Association of *Moraxella ovis* with keratokonjunctivitis in mule deer and moose in Wyoming. J Wildl Dis. 2000;36:241–7.
5. Gortázar C, Fernández-de-Luco D, Frölich K. Keratoconjunctivitis in a free-ranging red deer (*Cervus elaphus*) population in Spain. Z Jagdwiss. 1998;44:257–61.
6. Angelos JA. *Moraxella bovoculi* and infectious bovine keratoconjunctivitis: cause or coincidence? Vet Clin North Am Food Anim Pract. 2010;26:73–8. doi:10.1016/j.cvfa.2009.10.002.
7. Bergman A. Contagious keratitis in reindeer. Scand Vet J. 1912;2:145–77.
8. Skjenneberg S, Slagsvold L. Reindeer husbandry and its ecological principles [In Norwegian]. Oslo: Universitetsforlaget; 1968.
9. Rehbinder C, Nilsson A. An outbreak of kerato-conjunctivitis among corralled, supplementary fed, semi-domesticated reindeer calves. Rangifer. 1995;15:9–14.
10. Tryland M, Das Neves CG, Sunde M, Mørk T. Cervid herpesvirus 2, the primary agent in an outbreak of infectious keratoconjunctivitis in semi-domesticated reindeer. J Clin Microbiol. 2009;47:3707–13.
11. Kummeneje K. Isolation of *Neisseria ovis* and a *Colesiota conjunctivae*-like organism from cases of kerato-conjunctivitis in reindeer in northern Norway. Acta Vet Scand. 1976;17:107–8.
12. Rehbinder C. Keratitis in reindeer. Investigations of mycoplasma, rickettsia, rickettsia-like organisms and virus. Acta Vet Scand. 1977;18:65–74.
13. Rehbinder C, Glatthard V. Keratitis in reindeer. Relation to bacterial infections. Acta Vet Scand. 1977;18:54–64.
14. Oksanen A, Laaksonen S, Hirvelä-Koski V. Pink-eye in a winter-corralled reindeer herd [In Finnish]. Suomen Eläinlääkärilehti. 1996;102:138–41.
15. Aschfalk A, Josefsen TD, Steingass H, Müller W, Goethe R. Crowding and winter emergency feeding as predisposing factors for kerato-conjunctivitis in semi-domesticated reindeer in Norway. Dtsch Tierarztl Wochenschr. 2003;110:295–8.
16. Das Neves CG, Roth S, Rimstad E, Thiry E, Tryland M. Cervid herpesvirus 2 infection in reindeer: a review. Vet Microbiol. 2010;143:70–80.
17. Moen J. Climate change: effects on the ecological basis for reindeer husbandry in Sweden. Ambio. 2008;37:304–11.
18. Pachauri RK, Meyer LA, IPCC. Climate change 2014: synthesis Report. Contribution of working groups I, II and III to the fifth assessment report

of the intergovernmental panel on climate change. Geneva: IPCC; 2014. p. 151.

19. Tryland M, Josefsen TD, Oksanen A, Aschfalk A. Contagious ecthyma in Norwegian semidomesticated reindeer (*Rangifer tarandus tarandus*). Vet Rec. 2001;149:394–5.
20. Tryland M. Are we facing new health challenges and diseases in reindeer in Fennoscandia? Rangifer. 2012;32:35–48.
21. Stubsjøen SM, Moe RO. Stress and animal welfare for reindeer: a review [In Norwegian]. Norsk Vet. 2014;126:116–20.
22. Das Neves CG, Mørk T, Thiry J, Godfroid J, Rimstad E, Thiry E, et al. Cervid herpesvirus 2 experimentally reactivated in reindeer can produce generalized viremia and abortion. Virus Res. 2009;145:321–8.
23. Ballesteros M, Baardsen BJ, Langeland K, Fauchald P, Stien A, Tveraa T. The effect of warble flies on reindeer fitness: a parasite removal experiment. J Zool. 2012;287:34–40.
24. Furberg M, Evengård B, Nilsson M. Facing the limit of resilience: perceptions of climate change among reindeer herding Sami in Sweden. Global Health Action. 2011;4:148.
25. Josefsen TD, Sundset MA. Feeding and feeding related disorders in reindeer [In Norwegian]. Norsk Vet. 2014;126:160–9.
26. Josefsen TD, Mørk T, Sørensen KK, Knudsen SK, Hasvold HJ, Olsen L. Necropsies and organ investigations of reindeer 1998–2011 [In Norwegian]. Norsk Vet. 2014;126:172–81.
27. Magga OH, Oskal N, Sara MN. Animal welfare in the Sami culture [In Norwegian]. Sàmi University College 2001. Attachement to White Paper 12 (2002–2003); summary printed as 4.1.3. p. 21.
28. Tveraa T, Ballesteros M, Bårdsen B-J, Fauchald P, Lagergren M, Langeland K, et al. Predators and reindeer herding. Status of knowledge for Finnmark [In Norwegian]. Norwegian Institute of Nature Research. Report 2012; 821. http://www.nina.no/archive/nina/PppBasePdf/rapport/2012/821.pdf.
29. Ballesteros M, Bårdsen B, Fauchald P. Combined effects of long-term feeding, population density and vegetation green-up on reindeer demography. Ecosphere. 2013;4:1–13.
30. Stuen S, Krogsrud J, Hyllseth B, Tyler NJC. Serosurvey of three virus infections in reindeer in northern Norway and Svalbard. Rangifer. 1993;13:215–9.
31. Tryland M, Mørk T, Ryeng KA, Sørensen KK. Evidence of parapox-, alphaherpes- and pestivirus infections in carcasses of semi-domesticated reindeer (*Rangifer tarandus tarandus*) from Finnmark, Norway.

Diagnostic accuracy of blood sucrose as a screening test for equine gastric ulcer syndrome (EGUS) in adult horses

Michael Hewetson[1,4*], Ben William Sykes[2], Gayle Davina Hallowell[3] and Riitta-Mari Tulamo[1]

Abstract

Background: Equine gastric ulcer syndrome (EGUS) is common in adult horses, particularly those involved in performance disciplines. Currently, detection of EGUS by gastroscopy is the only reliable ante mortem method for definitive diagnosis; however it is unsuitable as a screening test because it is expensive, time consuming, and is not readily available to most veterinarians. Sucrose permeability testing represents a simple, economical alternative to gastroscopy for screening purposes, and the feasibility of this approach in the horse has been previously reported. The aim of this study was to determine the diagnostic accuracy of blood sucrose as a screening test for EGUS in a large group of adult horses with and without naturally occurring gastric disease.

Results: One hundred and one adult horses with or without naturally occurring gastric ulceration were studied. The diagnostic accuracy of blood sucrose for diagnosis of gastric lesions (GL), glandular lesions (GDL), squamous lesions (SQL), and clinically significant lesions (CSL) at 45 and 90 min after administration of 1 g/kg of sucrose via nasogastric intubation was assessed using receiver operator characteristics (ROC) curves and calculating the area under the curve (AUC). For each lesion type, sucrose concentration in blood was compared to gastroscopy, as the gold standard, and sensitivities (Se) and specificities (Sp) were calculated across a range of sucrose concentrations. Ulcer grading was performed blindly by one observer; and the results were validated by comparing them with that of two other observers, and calculating the level of agreement. Cut-off values were selected manually to optimize Se. The prevalence of GL, GDL, SQL, and CSL was 83, 70, 53 and 58% respectively. At the selected cut-offs, Se ranged from 51 to 79% and Sp ranged from 43 to 72%, depending upon the lesion type and time of sampling.

Conclusions: Blood sucrose is neither a sensitive or specific test for detecting EGUS in this population of adult horses with naturally occurring gastric ulceration. Further studies aimed at evaluating the performance characteristics of the test in different study populations are warranted. Given the limitations of endoscopy, due consideration should also be given to alternative methods for comparison of blood sucrose with a gold standard.

Keywords: Sucrose, Equine, Ulcer, Glandular, Squamous, EGUS, EGGD, ESGD, Permeability, Sensitivity, Specificity

Background

Equine gastric ulcer syndrome (EGUS) is a term used to describe erosive and ulcerative diseases of the equine stomach; and can be further classified into equine squamous gastric disease (ESGD) and equine glandular gastric disease (EGGD) based on the anatomical region affected [1]. EGUS is common in horses and although the clinical ramifications of this disease have as yet, not been completely elucidated, it remains an important disease in the equine industry. Performance horses are particularly susceptible, with 47–100% of Thoroughbred racehorses [2–5], 44–87% of Standardbred racehorses [6–8], 33–93% of endurance horses [9, 10] and 58–64% of show and sport horses [11, 12] found to have gastric lesions on gastroscopy. Non-performance horses are also susceptible to EGUS, with ulcers found in the gastric mucosa of

*Correspondence: michael.hewetson@up.ac.za
[4] Department of Companion Animal Clinical Studies, Faculty of Veterinary Science, University of Pretoria, Onderstepoort, South Africa

11–67% of sedentary horses and horses that partake in less strenuous activities [13–15].

Currently, detection of EGUS by gastroscopy is the only reliable ante mortem method for definitive diagnosis in horses [16] and is considered the gold standard against which all other diagnostic tests are compared [1]. Disadvantages of gastroscopy are that it's not readily available to most veterinarians, it is an inefficient expenditure of time, and it requires a minimum level of expertise to perform and interpret. Furthermore, gastroscopy is costly to the client and with an increase in public awareness of EGUS and its popularity as a 'catch-all' diagnosis for poor performance in sport horses, many owners are electing to treat their horses on an empirical basis without the benefit of a definite diagnosis. Given the current economic climate and the rising costs of omeprazole, it is easy then to imagine that owners and veterinarians would be interested in using an economical screening test to rule out gastric ulcers. Such a screening test should ideally have a high sensitivity as it will correctly identify most horses with gastric ulcers, remembering that many horses with EGUS will not demonstrate clinical signs, and are considered to have 'silent' or non-clinical gastric ulceration [14, 17–20].

Sucrose permeability testing represents a simple, economical alternative to gastroscopy for screening purposes, and the feasibility of this approach in the horse has been previously reported [21–23]. Because of its large molecular size (342 Da), sucrose is not able to permeate across healthy gastrointestinal mucosa, but it has been reported to cross the mucosa in the presence of gastrointestinal disease, presumably due to an changes in intestinal tight junction permeability or directly through gaps in the epithelium caused by erosion or ulceration [24–26]. The efficiency of the mucosal disaccharidases and the monosaccharide transport systems in the equine small intestine has been established by a series of oral disaccharide and monosaccharide tolerance tests, and it has been demonstrated that adult horses are fully capable of rapidly hydrolyzing sucrose [27, 28]. Furthermore, sucrase has the highest activity in the duodenum of the horse, with concentrations similar to those reported in the intestine of other non-ruminant species [29]. If present in blood, sucrose is cleared via the urine; it is not metabolized and the body does not produce it [30, 31]. Therefore, increased amounts of sucrose in blood after an oral dose is site specific for increased gastric permeability, and can be used to predict the presence of gastric disease [32–38].

The objective of this study was to determine the diagnostic accuracy of blood sucrose as a potential screening test for EGUS in adult horses by comparing it to gastroscopy as the gold standard.

Methods

Study design

The study was conducted as a blind comparison to a gold standard.

Study population

One hundred and one adult horses were eligible for inclusion in the study and were recruited from horses that had been referred to the University of Helsinki Equine Teaching Hospital, Finland for gastroscopy and from a local riding center. The horses were used for a wide range of equestrian activities, ranging from dressage to racing, and were recruited on the assumption that up to 53% of them would be affected by naturally occurring gastric ulceration of EGUS severity score ≥ 2 [14, 16]. Horses were excluded from the study if they had received non-steroidal anti-inflammatory drugs or omeprazole within 7 days prior to testing. This was done to avoid confounding changes in gastric permeability secondary to administration of these drugs [23, 39, 40].

Gastroscopy

Owners were asked to withhold food from their horses for 16 h and water for 6 h prior to sucrose testing. Following completion of fasting, blood samples (10 ml) were collected in vacuumed clot tubes from the jugular vein; horses were sedated with a combination of intravenous detomidine hydrochloride (10 μg/kg body weight (BW))[1] and butorphanol (0.025 mg/kg BW)[2]; and gastroscopy was performed using a previously described technique [21].

All endoscopic examinations were recorded and archived. For each horse, video recordings and still-frame images were taken of the stomach from the right side of the stomach along the margo plicatus, the dorsal part of the fundus, the greater curvature along the margo plicatus, the lesser curvature along the margo plicatus, the glandular mucosa in the region of the pylorus and the proximal duodenum [41].

Administration of sucrose and collection of samples

Immediately following gastroscopy, 1 g/kg BW of sucrose[3] was administered as a 10% solution via nasogastric tube to each horse. Blood samples (10 ml) were then collected in vacuumed clot tubes from the jugular vein at 45 and 90 min after administration of sucrose. These time points were chosen based upon data from a previous study which indicated that peak sucrose concentrations occur approximately between 45 and 90 min after sucrose

---

[1] Domosedan, Elanco Animal Health, UK.

[2] Butador, Chanelle Vet animal health, UK.

[3] Kidesokeri 530, Sucros Oy, Finland.

administration [21]. Horses were not given access to food until the final blood sample had been collected to prevent ingestion of sucrose that may have been present in the food. Following blood collection, the serum was separated by centrifugation (10 min at 2000×*g*) and then stored in a freezer at −80 °C until analysis.

Lesion assessment

Following completion of data collection, video recordings and still-frame images from each horse were reviewed independently by a board-certified internist (BS) who was blinded to the results of the sucrose assay. For each set of videos/images, the observer was asked to answer a set of dichotomous (yes or no) questions: does the horse have (1) gastric lesions? (2) glandular lesions? (3) squamous lesions? and (4) are the gastric lesions clinically significant? The term "gastric lesion" was used to describe lesions throughout the gastric mucosa and is synonymous with the term EGUS. In contrast, the terms "glandular lesion" and "squamous lesion" were used to differentiate the two different anatomical regions of the equine stomach and are synonymous with the term EGGD and ESGD respectively [1]. Clinically significant gastric lesions were used as a proxy indicator of ulcer severity and were defined as lesions that the observer would consider severe enough to warrant treatment. The term 'lesion' rather than 'ulceration' was used to enable the observer to report on the presence of other types of lesions (e.g. erosions) in addition to ulceration, as any damage to the mucosa of the stomach has the theoretical potential to increase permeability to sucrose [24–26].

Inter-observer agreement

In order to assess the validity of the gastroscopy assessment, the observations for each horse were compared with observations made by two other board certified internists on the same set of video recordings and still-frame images (GH, MH), and the level of agreement was calculated.

Sample processing and analyses

Serum was analyzed for sucrose using a previously validated gas chromatography-flame ionization detection (GC-FID) assay for quantifying sucrose in equine serum [42].

Statistical analysis

The overall diagnostic accuracy of blood sucrose for diagnosis of GL, GDL, SQL and CSL was assessed using receiver operator characteristics (ROC) curves and calculating the area under the curve (AUC). For each diagnostic criterion, sucrose concentration in blood at 45 and 90 min was compared with gastroscopy as the gold standard; and sensitivities (Se), specificities (Sp), positive predictive values (PPV) and negative predictive values (NPV) were calculated across a range of sucrose concentrations. Optimal cut-off values were then selected manually to optimize sensitivity and provide a practical threshold for practitioners in the field when screening horses for EGUS. Confidence intervals were set at 95% (95% CI).

Inter-observer agreement was summarized as the percentage of perfect (100%) agreements between observers for each diagnostic criterion, and a kappa coefficient (K) was calculated.

Statistical analyses were performed with R for Windows® version 3.0.2[4].

Results

Horses

One hundred and one adult horses were accepted into the study; 59 mares, 4 stallions, and 38 geldings. Horses ranged from two to 22 years of age (median, 9.9 years). Body weight ranged from 400 to 683 kg (median, 518 kg). Breeds included 37/101 Warmbloods, 25/101 Finnhorses, 34/101 Standardbreds, 3/101 Welsh Ponies, 1/101 Trakhener, and 1/101 Arab. Horses were used for a variety of purposes, including eventing, show jumping, dressage, trotting and general riding purposes. Fifty-three horses were demonstrating clinical signs suggestive of EGUS at the time of gastroscopy.

Gastroscopy

The overall prevalence of gastric lesions (ulcers or erosions) was 83%. Lesions were most common in the glandular mucosae (70%), followed by the squamous mucosae (53%). Fifty eight percent of the horses had gastric lesions that were severe enough to be considered clinically significant i.e. requiring treatment. Squamous lesions were most frequently observed in the region of the cardia and along the lesser curvature of the stomach adjacent to the margo plicatus; and consisted primarily of small single ulcers characteristic of EGUS severity score ≤ 2. Glandular lesions were exclusively observed around the pylorus and consisted primarily of focal raised hemorrhagic or fibrinous lesions.

Sucrose permeability

All horses tolerated sucrose permeability testing and no adverse effects were noted following administration of the sucrose solution. On analysis of the serum samples, all horses demonstrated an increase in serum sucrose concentration over time, with peak serum sucrose concentrations occurring 90 min after administration of the sucrose solution.

---
[4] R Foundation for Statistical Computing, Vienna, Austria.

The mean ± SD serum sucrose concentration at 45 min was 6.85 ± 4.90 μmol/l for normal horses (n = 17); 9.66 ± 9.16 μmol/l for horses with GL (n = 84); 9.44 ± 9.27 μmol/l for horses with GDL (n = 71); 10.56 ± 8.66 μmol/l for horses with SQL (n = 54); and 10.43 ± 9.22 μmol/l for horses with CSL (n = 59). The mean ± SD serum sucrose concentration at 90 min was 7.22 ± 4.65 μmol/l for normal horses (n = 17); 10.29 ± 8.12 μmol/l for horses with GL (n = 84); 9.86 ± 7.54 μmol/l for horses with GDL (n = 71); 11.53 ± 8.17 μmol/l for horses with SQL (n = 54); and 11.24 ± 8.55 μmol/l for horses with CSL (n = 59).

Diagnostic accuracy of blood sucrose for diagnosis of EGUS

ROC curves for each diagnostic criterion at 45 and 90 min after sucrose administration are illustrated in Figs. 1 and 2.

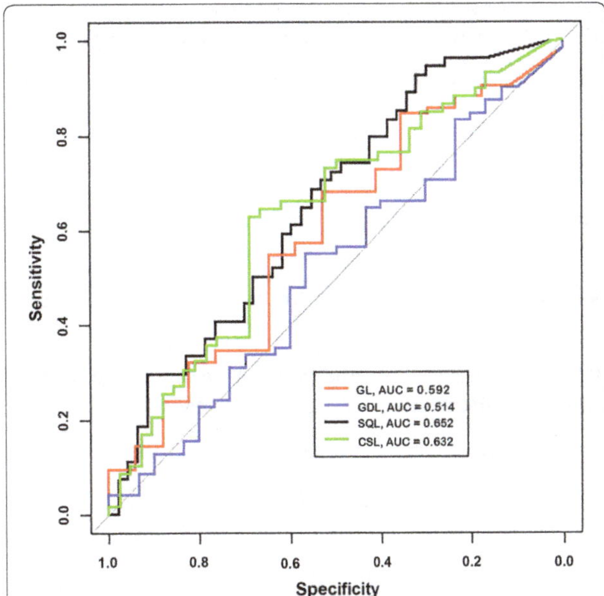

Fig. 1 ROC curves for blood sucrose concentration when used to distinguish between normal horses and horses with GL, GDL, SQL and CSL at 45 min after administration of 1 g/kg of sucrose via nasogastric intubation. *AUC* area under the curve

Gastric lesions

The AUC ± 95% CI for blood sucrose concentration when used to distinguish between normal horses and horses with GL at 45 and 90 min was 0.59 (0.44–0.74) and 0.62 (0.47–0.76) respectively. Sucrose concentrations of 4.61 μmol/l at 45 min and 4.57 μmol/l at 90 min were selected as the optimal cut-offs for discriminating between normal horses and horses with GL. The Se, Sp, PPV and NPV of blood sucrose at 45 and 90 min for diagnosis of GL using the selected cut-off values are depicted in Table 1.

Glandular lesions

The AUC ± 95% CI for blood sucrose concentration when used to distinguish between normal horses and horses with GDL at 45 and 90 min was 0.51 (0.39–0.64) and 0.53 (0.40–0.66) respectively. Sucrose concentrations of 5.80 μmol/l at 45 min and 6.05 μmol/l at 90 min were selected as the optimal cut-offs for discriminating between normal horses and horses with GDL. The Se, Sp, PPV and NPV of blood sucrose at 45 and 90 min for diagnosis of GDL using the selected cut-off values are depicted in Table 2.

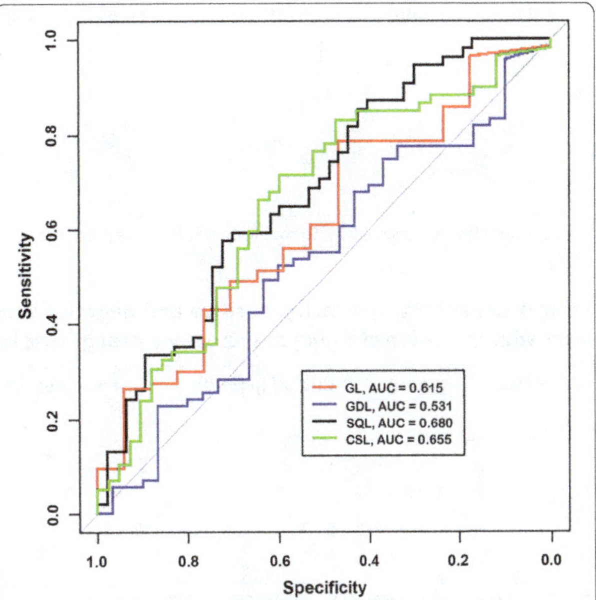

Fig. 2 ROC curves for blood sucrose concentration when used to distinguish between normal horses and horses with GL, GDL, SQL and CSL at 90 min after administration of 1 g/kg of sucrose via nasogastric intubation. *AUC* area under the curve

Squamous lesions

The AUC for blood sucrose concentration when used to distinguish between normal horses and horses with SQL at 45 and 90 min was 0.65 (0.55–0.76) and 0.68 (0.58–0.79) respectively. Sucrose concentrations of 7.86 μmol/l at 45 min and 8.24 μmol/l at 90 min were selected as the optimal cut-offs for discriminating between normal horses and horses with SQL. The Se, Sp, PPV and NPV of blood sucrose at 45 and 90 min for diagnosis of SQL using the selected cut-off values are depicted in Table 3.

Clinically significant gastric lesions

The AUC for blood sucrose concentration when used to distinguish between normal horses and horses with CSL

Table 1 Sensitivity, specificity, positive and negative predictive values of blood sucrose for diagnosis of GL in horses after administration of 1 g/kg of sucrose via nasogastric intubation

Time of sampling (min)	Cut-off (µmol/l)	Disease present	Disease absent	Sp (%) 95% CI	Se (%) 95% CI	NPV (%) 95% CI	PPV (%) 95% CI
45	4.61	84	17	52.9	67.9	25.0	87.7
				28–77	57–78	12–42	77–95
90	4.57	84	17	47.1	78.6	30.8	88.0
				23–72	68–87	14–52	78–94

GL gastric lesions, *Se* sensitivity, *Sp* specificity, *NPV* negative predictive value, *PPV* positive predictive value, *95% CI* 95% confidence intervals

Table 2 Sensitivity, specificity, positive and negative predictive values of blood sucrose for diagnosis of GDL in horses after administration of 1 g/kg of sucrose via nasogastric intubation

Time of sampling (min)	Cut-off (µmol/l)	Disease present	Disease absent	Sp (%) 95% CI	Se (%) 95% CI	NPV (%) 95% CI	PPV (%) 95% CI
45	5.80	71	31	48.1	50.7	30.0	69.2
				30–67	39–63	18–45	55–81
90	6.05	71	31	43.3	66.2	35.1	73.4
				26–63	54–77	20–53	61–84

GL gastric lesions, *Se* sensitivity, *Sp* specificity, *NPV* negative predictive value, *PPV* positive predictive value, *95% CI* 95% confidence intervals

Table 3 Sensitivity, specificity, positive and negative predictive values of blood sucrose for diagnosis of SQL in horses after administration of 1 g/kg of sucrose via nasogastric intubation

Time of sampling (min)	Cut-off (µmol/l)	Disease present	Disease absent	Sp (%) 95% CI	Se (%) 95% CI	NPV (%) 95% CI	PPV (%) 95% CI
45	7.86	54	47	68.1	50.0	54.2	64.3
				53–81	36–64	41–67	48–79
90	8.24	54	47	72.3	57.4	59.7	70.5
				57–84	43–71	46–72	55–83

SQL squamous lesions, *Se* sensitivity, *Sp* specificity, *NPV* negative predictive value, *PPV* positive predictive value, *95% CI* 95% confidence intervals

Table 4 Sensitivity, specificity, positive and negative predictive values of blood sucrose for diagnosis of CSL in horses after administration of 1 g/kg of sucrose via nasogastric intubation

Time of sampling (min)	Cut-off (µmol/l)	Disease present	Disease absent	Sp (%) 95% CI	Se (%) 95% CI	NPV (%) 95% CI	PPV (%) 95% CI
45	4.61	59	42	50.0	74.6	58.3	67.7
				34–66	62–85	41–75	55–79
90	5.87	59	42	52.4	76.3	61.1	69.2
				36–68	63–86	44–77	57–80

CSL clinically significant lesions, *Se* sensitivity, *Sp* specificity, *NPV* negative predictive value, *PPV* positive predictive value, *95% CI* 95% confidence intervals

at 45 and 90 min was 0.63 (0.52–0.74) and 0.66 (0.55–0.77) respectively. Sucrose concentrations of 4.61 µmol/l at 45 min and 5.87 µmol/l at 90 min were selected as the optimal cut-offs for discriminating between normal horses and horses with clinically significant lesions. The Se, Sp, PPV and NPV of blood sucrose at 45 and 90 min for diagnosis of CSL using the selected cut-off values are depicted in Table 4.

Inter-observer agreement

When asked to answer if each horse has (1) gastric lesions; (2) glandular lesions; (3) squamous lesions; and

(4) clinically significant gastric lesions, perfect agreement between-observers within the 101 sets of observations was achieved on average, in 83% (K = 0.50; $P < 0.0001$; 95% CI 0.24–0.76); 78% (K = 0.57; $P < 0.0001$; 95% CI 0.39–0.75); 74% (K = 0.65; $P < 0.0001$; 95% CI 0.53–0.77); and 75% (K = 0.62; $P < 0.0001$; 95% CI 0.48–0.75) of the cases respectively.

Discussion

The objective of this study was to validate the sucrose blood test as a screening test for EGUS in adult horses by determining its performance characteristics in a large group of horses with and without naturally occurring gastric disease. ROC curve analysis was used to visually demonstrate the cut-off dependency of the test across a range of sucrose concentrations and to provide an estimate of the overall diagnostic accuracy of the test that is independent of specific cut-off values or prevalence of gastric lesions in the study population. For this study, ROC curves of true positive rates (Se) against false positive rates (1-Sp) were plotted using blood sucrose concentrations from normal horses, and horses with GL, GDL, SQL and CSL at 45 and 90 min after administration of sucrose (Figs. 1, 2). The AUC's in each plot represents a summary of the overall diagnostic accuracy of the test by combining accuracy over a range of cut-offs, with a value approaching 1.0 indicating perfect discrimination and 0.5 representing zero discrimination. Using an arbitrary guideline, the AUC can be used to distinguish between a non-informative (AUC = 0.5); less accurate (0.5 < AUC $\leq$ 0.7); moderately accurate (0.7 < AUC $\leq$ 0.9); highly accurate (0.9 < AUC < 1); and perfect test (AUC = 1) [43]. Depending upon the lesion type and time of sampling, the AUC for the blood sucrose test ranged from 0.51 to 0.68, indicating that blood sucrose concentration is poor at discriminating between normal horses and horses with EGUS and is therefore not considered to be a very accurate test.

Because the AUC summarizes the ROC curve as a whole, and therefore attributes the same weighting to both relevant and irrelevant parts of the curve [44], cut-off values were inserted on the continuous scale of test results that allowed calculation of Se and Sp for horses with GL, GDL, SQL and CSL at each time point. Using the selected cut-offs, the Se and Sp of the blood sucrose test for detecting the presence or absence of EGUS was low (Tables 1, 2, 3, 4), confirming the poor diagnostic accuracy of the test in this study population.

It is not immediately evident why the sucrose blood test has a poor diagnostic accuracy in adult horses despite previous literature to suggest otherwise [21–23]. In this study, there was a predominance of glandular lesions (70%) whereas in previous studies, sucrose permeability was assessed primarily on horses with squamous lesions; and it may be that there are fundamental differences in the permeability of the sucrose molecule between the glandular and squamous epithelium. It has been found that gap junctional intercellular communication (GJIC) plays an important role in the gastric mucosal defense system, and loss of GJIC is associated with ulcer formation. A recent study demonstrated the presence of specific gap junctions in the glandular mucosa of the equine stomach, however these gap junctions were absent in the squamous mucosa of the stomach [45]. This suggests that there are significant differences in the permeation pathway of the glandular vs. the squamous epithelium which may explain (in part) why in this study population, with a predominace of glandular ulcers, the sucrose blood test had a poorer diagnostic accuracy than expected. Furthermore, glandular lesions are often smaller in cross-sectional area and are usually not ulcerative per se, but rather erosive or may even consist of intact mucosa with hyperemia [1]. In such cases, it is possible that sucrose is less likely to permeate in quantities large enough to appreciate differences between affected and unaffected horses, although this has yet to be substantiated.

The authors do recognize however, that the sensitivity and specificity for squamous lesions was also poor, albeit less so than for glandular ulcers. Another factor to consider therefore, is the fact that in this particular study, very few of the squamous lesions were extensive or demonstrated areas of apparent deep ulceration characteristic of EGUS severity score $\geq$3 [1]. It is therefore possible that in such cases, the total surface area for sucrose permeation was too small to differentiate between affected and unaffected horses. Based on this premise, re-analysis of the data using a scoring system that takes into account not only the severity of the lesion, but also the number of lesions should be considered [46].

Alternatively, the validity of the gold standard itself can be questioned. It may be that the sucrose test is too sensitive and may detect slight and clinically insignificant mucosal damage that cannot be seen on endoscopy, thus limiting its use in clinical decision-making regarding gastric ulceration [33]. We postulate that sucrose permeability is in fact an accurate representation of the true mucosal integrity of the stomach based on a number of previous publications documenting its effectiveness in both humans and other species [35, 36, 38, 47]; and that assessment via endoscopy is under- or overestimating the severity or depth of gastric lesions. This is based on the fact that assessment of lesion severity (and even the presence or absence of lesions) using gastroscopy is subjective, and agreement between observers for endoscopic diagnosis is notoriously poor, particularly if they are inexperienced [48,

49]. Furthermore, it has been demonstrated that there is a poor correlation between endoscopic assessment of gastric ulcers ante mortem and histological appearance at necropsy [46, 50]. Because of these limitations, an attempt was made in this study to determine if the gold standard was reproducible between-observers. All assessments made by the observer were compared with assessments made by two other board certified internists that have experience with gastroscopy, and the level of agreement for each outcome was determined. Agreement was moderate [51], but still unacceptably low, and it is possible that in the hands of different observers, the diagnostic accuracy of the test will vary. Considering these limitations, it is the authors' opinion that histopathology rather than endoscopy should be utilized as a gold standard for comparison in future gastric permeability studies. Alternatively, Bayesian statistical approaches that are used for evaluation of diagnostic tests in the absence of a gold standard test should be considered [52].

The choice to include the severity of gastric ulceration in the study was based on the premise that the sucrose blood test would be able to differentiate between severe and less severe lesions, enabling practitioners to select cases for treatment based upon the outcome of the test. Unfortunately there are no grading systems that can be used interchangeably for horses with both ESGD and EGGD [53], and so the authors elected to use the concept of a 'clinically significant gastric lesion' as a proxy indicator of ulcer severity, where clinically significant lesions were defined as lesions that the observer would consider severe enough to warrant treatment if seen in a clinical case. While the authors recognize that this is not a perfect solution, as clinicians will usually use both gastroscopic appearance of lesions in combination with the clinical history to determine clinically significance, the authors believe that this proxy is the best possible compromise. While a scoring system (e.g. EGUS 0-4) would have been more objective, the fact that it cannot be used for EGGD makes it impossible to be used in this study. In future, assessment of both clinical and endoscopic outcomes when determining the diagnostic accuracy of the sucrose test is recommended.

When conducting a validation study to determine the diagnostic accuracy of a test, it is essential that the study include an appropriate spectrum of subjects which is representative of the population for which the test is intended. We aimed to determine the diagnostic accuracy of the sucrose blood test as a screening test for EGUS in adult horses and therefore we selected horses used for a wide spectrum of activities, ranging from dressage to racing. Eighty four percent of the horses in the study population had gastric lesions, which is similar to previously reported prevalence data for this geographical region [14]. Unfortunately, there was a limited spectrum of disease in the study population, with a predominance of small single lesions and a noticeable absence of extensive lesions with areas of apparent deep ulceration. As discussed earlier, this has the potential to skew the results by virtue of the fact that permeability of sucrose is directly proportional to the surface area of the damaged gastric mucosa available for permeation. An additional limitation of the study was the fact that that a proportion of the horses in this study (58/101) showed no clinical signs of gastric ulceration at the time of sucrose testing. There is currently little evidence to suggest a direct cause-and-effect relationship between clinical signs of EGUS and the presence, severity or location of gastric ulcers in adult horses [1] and, therefore, it is possible that the diagnostic accuracy of the sucrose test would be improved when testing a population of horses that were all demonstrating clinical signs at the time of gastroscopy.

Conclusions

Blood sucrose was neither a sensitive nor specific test for detecting EGUS in this population of adult horses with naturally occurring disease. This study included both horses with and without clinical signs of gastric ulceration. Further studies aimed at evaluating the performance characteristics of the test in a selected population of horses demonstrating clinical signs consistent with EGUS may be warranted. Given the limitations of endoscopy, due consideration should also be given to alternative methods for comparison of blood sucrose with a gold standard (Additional file 1).

Abbreviations

BW: body weight; EGUS: equine gastric ulcer syndrome; GL: gastric lesion; GDL: glandular lesions; SQL: squamous lesion; CSL: clinically significant lesion; GC-FID: gas chromatography-flame ionization detection; ROC: receiver operator characteristic; AUC: area under the curve; Se: sensitivity; Sp: specificity; PPV: positive predictive value; NPV: negative predictive value; 95% CI: 95% confidence intervals; SD: standard deviation.

Authors' contributions

MH participated in the hypothesis generation, study design, organizing and acquisition of data, interpreting and analyzing the results, and drafting the manuscript. BS and GH participated in the acquisition of data, interpreting and analyzing the results, and critical revision of the manuscript. RMT participated in the study design, interpreting the results, and critical revision of the manuscript. All authors read and approved the final manuscript.

Author details

[1] Department of Equine and Small Animal Medicine, Faculty of Veterinary Medicine, University of Helsinki, Helsinki, Finland. [2] School of Veterinary Sciences, University of Queensland, Brisbane, Australia. [3] School of Veterinary Medicine and Science, University of Nottingham, Nottingham, UK. [4] Department of Companion Animal Clinical Studies, Faculty of Veterinary Science, University of Pretoria, Onderstepoort, South Africa.

Acknowledgements
The authors would like to thank professors Allen Rousell, Sandy Love, Satu Sankari, Noah Cohen and Anna-Maija Virtala for their support, guidance and vision; Kaisa Aaltonen and Anne Sjöhölm for their technical assistance; and Jouni Junnila and Geoffry Fosgate for their assistance with the statistical analysis.

Competing interests
The authors declare that they have no competing interests.

References
1. Sykes BW, Hewetson M, Hepburn RJ, Luthersson N, Tamzali Y. European College of Equine Internal Medicine Consensus Statement—equine gastric ulcer syndrome in adult horses. J Vet Intern Med. 2015;29:1288–99.
2. Murray MJ, Schusser GF, Pipers FS, Gross SJ. Factors associated with gastric lesions in thoroughbred racehorses. Equine Vet J. 1996;28:368–74.
3. Begg LM, O'Sullivan CB. The prevalence and distribution of gastric ulceration in 345 racehorses. Aust Vet J. 2003;81:199–201.
4. Vatistas NJ, Snyder JR, Carlson G, Johnson B, Arthur RM, Thurmond M, et al. Cross-sectional study of gastric ulcers of the squamous mucosa in thoroughbred racehorses. Equine Vet J. 1999;29:34–9.
5. Sykes BW, Sykes KM, Hallowell GD. A comparison of three doses of omeprazole in the treatment of equine gastric ulcer syndrome: a blinded, randomised, dose-response clinical trial. Equine Vet J. 2015;47:285–90.
6. Rabuffo TS, Orsini JA, Sullivan E, Engiles J, Norman T, Boston R. Associations between age or sex and prevalence of gastric ulceration in Standardbred racehorses in training. J Am Vet Med Assoc. 2002;221:1156–9.
7. Dionne RM, Vrins A, Doucet MY, Pare J. Gastric ulcers in standardbred racehorses: prevalence, lesion description, and risk factors. J Vet Intern Med. 2003;17:218–22.
8. Jonsson H, Egenvall A. Prevalence of gastric ulceration in Swedish Standardbreds in race training. Equine Vet J. 2006;38:209–13.
9. Nieto JE, Snyder JR, Beldomenico P, Aleman M, Kerr JW, Spier SJ. Prevalence of gastric ulcers in endurance horses-a preliminary report. Vet J. 2004;167:33–7.
10. Tamzali Y, Marguet C, Priymenko N, Lyazrhi F. Prevalence of gastric ulcer syndrome in high-level endurance horses. Equine Vet J. 2011;43:141–4.
11. McClure SR, Glickman LT, Glickman NW. Prevalence of gastric ulcers in show horses. J Am Vet Med Assoc. 1999;215:1130–3.
12. Hartmann AM, Frankeny RL. A preliminary investigation into the association between competition and gastric ulcer formation in non-racing performance horses. J Equine Vet Sci. 2003;23:560–1.
13. le Jeune SS, Nieto JE, Dechant JE, Snyder JR. Prevalence of gastric ulcers in Thoroughbred broodmares in pasture: a preliminary report. Vet J. 2009;181:251–5.
14. Luthersson N, Nielsen KH, Harris P, Parkin TD. The prevalence and anatomical distribution of equine gastric ulceration syndrome (EGUS) in 201 horses in Denmark. Equine Vet J. 2009;41:619–24.
15. Chameroy KA, Nadeau JA, Bushmich SL, Dinger JE, Hoagland TA, Saxton AM. Prevalence of non-glandular gastric ulcers in horses involved in a university riding program. J Equine Vet Sci. 2006;26:207–11.
16. Andrews FM, Bernard WV, Byars TD, Cohen ND, Divers TJ, MacAllister CG, et al. Recommendations for the diagnosis and treatment of equine gastric ulcer syndrome (EGUS). Equine Vet Educ. 1999;1:122–34.
17. Bell RJW, Kingston JK, Mogg TD, Perkins NR. The prevalence of gastric ulceration in racehorses in New Zealand. N Z Vet J. 2007;55:13–8.
18. Andrews FM, Nadeau JA. Clinical syndromes of gastric ulceration in foals and mature horses. Equine Vet J. 1999;31:30–3.
19. Murray MJ, Grodinsky C, Anderson CW, Radue PF, Schmidt GR. Gastric ulcers in horses: a comparison of endoscopic findings in horses with and without clinical signs. Equine Vet J. 1989;7:68–72.
20. Murray MJ, Murray CM, Sweeney HJ, Weld J, Digby NJ, Stoneham SJ. Prevalence of gastric lesions in foals without signs of gastric disease: an endoscopic survey. Equine Vet J. 1990;22:6–8.
21. Hewetson M, Cohen ND, Love S, Buddington RK, Holmes W, Innocent GT, et al. Sucrose concentration in blood: a new method for assessment of gastric permeability in horses with gastric ulceration. J Vet Intern Med. 2006;20:388–94.
22. O'Conner MS, Steiner JM, Roussel AJ, Williams DA, Meddings JB, Pipers F, et al. Evaluation of urine sucrose concentration for detection of gastric ulcers in horses. Am J Vet Res. 2004;65:31–9.
23. D'Arcy-Moskwa E, Noble GK, Weston LA, Boston R, Raidal SL. Effects of meloxicam and phenylbutazone on equine gastric mucosal permeability. J Vet Intern Med. 2012;26:1494–9.
24. Pantzar N, Westrom BR, Luts A, Lundin S. Regional small-intestinal permeability in vitro to different-sized dextrans and proteins in the rat. Scand J Gastroenterol. 1993;28:205–11.
25. Gryboski JD, Thayer WR Jr, Gabrielson IW, Spiro HM. Disacchariduria in gastrointestinal disease. Gastroenterology. 1963;45:633–7.
26. Lindemann B, Solomon AK. Permeability of luminal surface of intestinal mucosal cells. J Gen Physiol. 1962;45:801–10.
27. Roberts MC. Carbohydrate digestion and absorption studies in the horse. Res Vet Sci. 1975;18:64–9.
28. Roberts MC. Carbohydrate digestion and absorption in the equine small intestine. J S Afr Vet Assoc. 1975;46:19–27.
29. Dyer J, Fernandez-Castano Merediz E, Salmon KS, Proudman CJ, Edwards GB, Shirazi-Beechey SP. Molecular characterisation of carbohydrate digestion and absorption in equine small intestine. Equine Vet J. 2002;34:349–58.
30. Vettorazzi G, MacDonald I. Sucrose: nutritional and safety aspects. New York: Springer; 1988. p. 35–8.
31. Keith NM, Power MH. The urinary excretion of sucrose and its distribution in the blood after intravenous injection into normal men. Am J Physiol. 1937;120:203–11.
32. Davies NM, Corrigan BW, Jamali F. Sucrose urinary excretion in the rat measured using a simple assay: a model of gastroduodenal permeability. Pharm Res. 1995;12:1733–6.
33. Erlacher L, Wyatt J, Pflugbeil S, Koller M, Ullrich R, Vogelsang H, et al. Sucrose permeability as a marker for NSAID-induced gastroduodenal injury. Clin Exp Rheumatol. 1998;16:69–71.
34. Goodgame RW, Malaty HM, el-Zimaity HM, Graham DY. Decrease in gastric permeability to sucrose following cure of *Helicobacter pylori* infection. Helicobacter. 1997;2:44–7.
35. Meddings JB, Kirk D, Olson ME. Noninvasive detection of nonsteroidal anti-inflammatory drug-induced gastropathy in dogs. Am J Vet Res. 1995;56:977–81.
36. Meddings JB, Sutherland LR, Byles NI, Wallace JL. Sucrose: a novel permeability marker for gastroduodenal disease. Gastroenterology. 1993;104:1619–26.
37. Meddings JB, Wallace JL, Sutherland LR. Sucrose permeability: a novel means of detecting gastroduodenal damage noninvasively. Am J Ther. 1995;2:843–9.
38. Sutherland LR, Verhoef M, Wallace JL, Van Rosendaal G, Crutcher R, Meddings JB. A simple, non-invasive marker of gastric damage: sucrose permeability. Lancet. 1994;343:998–1000.
39. Hopkins AM, McDonnell C, Breslin NP, O'Morain CA, Baird AW. Omeprazole increases permeability across isolated rat gastric mucosa pre-treated with an acid secretagogue. J Pharm Pharmacol. 2002;54:341–7.
40. Jenkins AP, Trew DR, Crump BJ, Nukajam WS, Foley JA, Menzies IS, et al. Do non-steroidal anti-inflammatory drugs increase colonic permeability? Gut. 1991;32:66–9.
41. Murray MJ, Eichorn ES. Effects of intermittent feed deprivation, intermittent feed deprivation with ranitidine administration, and stall confinement with ad libitum access to hay on gastric ulceration in horses. Am J Vet Res. 1996;57:1599–603.
42. Hewetson M, Aaltonen K, Tulamo RM, Sankari S. Development and validation of a gas chromatography-flame ionization detection method for quantifying sucrose in equine serum. J Vet Diagn Invest. 2014;26:232–9.
43. Swets JA. Measuring the accuracy of diagnostic systems. Science. 1988;240:1285–93.
44. Greiner M, Pfeiffer D, Smith RD. Principles and practical application of the receiver-operating characteristic analysis for diagnostic tests. Prev Vet Med. 2000;45:23–41.
45. Fink C, Hembes T, Brehm R, Weigel R, Heeb C, Pfarrer C, et al. Specific localisation of gap junction protein connexin 32 in the gastric mucosa of horses. Histochem Cell Biol. 2006;125:307–13.
46. Andrews FM, Reinemeyer CR, McCracken MD, Blackford JT, Nadeau JA, Saabye L, et al. Comparison of endoscopic, necropsy and histology scoring of equine gastric ulcers. Equine Vet J. 2002;34:475–8.

47. Craven M, Chandler ML, Steiner JM, Farhadi A, Welsh E, Pratschke K, et al. Acute effects of carprofen and meloxicam on canine gastrointestinal permeability and mucosal absorptive capacity. J Vet Intern Med. 2007;21:917–23.
48. Amano Y, Ishimura N, Furuta K, Okita K, Masaharu M, Azumi T, et al. Interobserver agreement on classifying endoscopic diagnoses of nonerosive esophagitis. Endoscopy. 2006;38:1032–5.
49. Hyun YS, Han DS, Bae JH, Park HS, Eun CS. Interobserver variability and accuracy of high-definition endoscopic diagnosis for gastric intestinal metaplasia among experienced and inexperienced endoscopists. J Korean Med Sci. 2013;28:744–9.
50. Pietra M, Morini M, Perfetti G, Spadari A, Vigo P, Peli A. Comparison of endoscopy, histology, and cytokine mRNA of the equine gastric mucosa. Vet Res Commun. 2010;34(Suppl 1):S121–4.
51. Viera AJ, Garrett JM. Understanding interobserver agreement: the kappa statistic. Fam Med. 2005;37:360–3.
52. Toft N, Jorgensen E, Hojsgaard S. Diagnosing diagnostic tests: evaluating the assumptions underlying the estimation of sensitivity and specificity in the absence of a gold standard. Prev Vet Med. 2005;68:19–33.
53. Sykes BW, Jokisalo J, Hallowell GD. Evaluation of a commercial faecal blood test for the diagnosis 636 of gastric ulceration in Thoroughbred racehorses: a preliminary report. BMC Vet Res. 2014;9:10.

16

Exceptional longevity and potential determinants of successful ageing in a cohort of 39 Labrador retrievers

Vicki Jean Adams[1*], Penny Watson[2], Stuart Carmichael[3], Stephen Gerry[4], Johanna Penell[5] and David Mark Morgan[6]

Abstract

Background: The aim of this study was to describe the longevity and causes of mortality in 39 (12 males, 27 females) pedigree adult neutered Labrador retrievers with a median age of 6.5 years at the start of the study and kept under similar housing and management conditions. Body condition score was maintained between two and four on a 5-point scale by varying food allowances quarterly. The impact of change in body weight (BW) and body composition on longevity was analysed using linear mixed models with random slopes and intercepts.

Results: On 31 July 2014, 10 years after study start, dogs were classified into three lifespan groups: 13 (33 %) Expected (≥9 to ≤12.9 years), 15 (39 %) Long (≥13 to ≤15.5 years) and 11 (28 %) Exceptional (≥15.6 years) with five still alive. Gender and age at neutering were not associated with longevity ($P \geq 0.06$). BW increased similarly for all lifespan groups up to age 9, thereafter, from 9 to 13 years, Exceptional dogs gained and Long-lifespan dogs lost weight ($P = 0.007$). Dual-energy x-ray absorptiometer scans revealed that absolute fat mass increase was slower to age 13 for Long compared with Expected lifespan dogs ($P = 0.003$) whilst all groups lost a similar amount of absolute lean mass ($P > 0.05$). Percent fat increase and percent lean loss were slower, whilst the change in fat:lean was smaller, in both the Exceptional and Long lifespan compared with Expected dogs to age 13 ($P \leq 0.02$). Total bone mineral density was significantly lower for Expected compared to Exceptional and Long lifespan dogs ($P < 0.04$).

Conclusions: This study shows that life-long maintenance of lean body mass and attenuated accumulation of body fat were key factors in achieving a longer lifespan. The results suggest that a combination of a high quality plane of nutrition with appropriate husbandry and healthcare are important in obtaining a greater than expected proportion of Labrador retrievers living well beyond that of the expected breed lifespan: 89.7 % (95 % CI 74.8–96.7 %) dogs were alive at 12 years of age and 28.2 % (95 % CI 15.6–45.1 %) reaching an exceptional lifespan of ≥15.6 years.

Keywords: Ageing, Exceptional longevity, Healthspan, Body weight, Sarcopenia, Lean body mass, Body fat mass, Nutrition, Husbandry, Healthcare

Background

For the domesticated dog (*Canis lupus familiaris*), changes observed through ageing can be seen as good (e.g. improved obedience), bad (e.g. dental disease) or inconsequential (e.g. greying of the muzzle) with respect to their viability and survival. Physiological changes that may be important biomarkers of ageing in dogs include increasing body fat, reducing lean body mass (of which lean muscle mass is an important component), periodontal disease, osteoarthritis, reduced renal or cardiac function, changes to the endocrine system (including

*Correspondence: vjadams12@gmail.com
[1] Vet Epi, White Cottage, Dickleburgh, Norfolk IP21 4NT, UK

insulin and glycaemic control), cognitive and behavioural changes and the development of neoplastic disease [1–4].

The goal for today's biogerontologists is to extend human healthspan, defined as the years in which an individual is generally healthy and free from serious disease, alongside increasing longevity; this goal can also be applied to our companion animals [5]. In the domestic dog, reported average longevity estimates for all breeds combined have varied between 10.0 and 12.0 years, depending on the population studied [6–8]. As part of the current project, an external panel of veterinary and academic experts was convened to independently and objectively define an average lifespan for Labrador retrievers based on median/mean age at death reported in published research and from a proprietary service dog database as well as their professional knowledge and/or personal experience. Upon review of the body of evidence available from 1999 to 2013, a consensus was reached that the typical lifespan of Labrador retrievers was 12 years of age (Table 1). The domesticated dog represents an exceptional range of phenotypic morphology with breeds varying in weight by two-orders of magnitude [9]. Canine life expectancy and body mass are inversely correlated with size explaining 40–44 % of the variance in age at death [8, 9]; small breeds typically live much longer than large breeds [8, 10–12]. It is not clear what effect neutering has on longevity as one study reported that neutering was associated with increased longevity for females but not males in the UK [6], whilst neutered males outlived entire males among US military dogs [13]. Another study has shown that neutering was strongly associated with an increase in lifespan as well as a decreased risk of death from some causes, such as infectious disease, but an increased risk of death from others, such as cancer [14]. The discrepancies might be related to the age of neutering, however, there is a lack of information on this.

Table 1 Evidence used in consensus for 'Typical' Labrador retriever lifespan based on reported ages at death with reference numbers in square brackets

Reference material	Country	#Dogs	Median lifespan, years
Assistance dog database[a]	US	498	12.0
Lawler et al. [2]	US	48	'Restricted' group: 13.0
Kealy et al. [19]			'Control' group: 11.2
Adams et al. [8]	UK	574	12.25
O'Neill et al. [12]	UK	418	12.5
Michell [6]	UK	328	12.6
Proschowsky et al. [7]	Denmark	199	10.5
Typical lifespan of Labrador retrievers[b]			12.0

[a] Canine companions for independence (Santa Rosa, CA, USA)

[b] Consensus age provided by Jan Bellows, DVM, DAVDC, DABVP, FAVD; Carmen M. H. Colitz, DVM, Ph.D., DACVO, Donald Ingram, Ph.D.; Stanley L. Marks, BVSc, Ph.D., DACVIM, DACVN; Sherry L. Sanderson, DVM, Ph.D., DACVIM, DACVN; Julia Tomlinson, BVSc, Ph.D., DACVS, CCRP, CVSM

With the large disparity in longevity of individual dog breeds, the challenge is to understand the biological mechanisms that underlie these apparent differences [15]. The term 'exceptional longevity' has be used to describe both groups of, and individual, dogs that live 30 % longer than is expected for their breed's typical or average lifespan [16]. Dogs that live for a longer period than their anticipated lifespan appear to demonstrate an ability to delay the onset of life-threatening diseases [16–18]. A previous study of 24 pairs of Labrador retriever littermates from 7 litters showed that lifetime calorie restriction resulted in a 1.8 year longer median lifespan in the 'Restricted' group fed 25 % less than the 'Control' group ($P = 0.004$) [19].

The longitudinal study reported here is a continuation of efforts to understand the biology of ageing and its valuable application to companion dogs. The aim of this study was to describe the longevity and causes of mortality in a cohort of purebred Labrador retrievers kept under similar housing and management conditions. Additionally, we wished to evaluate the impact of gender, age at neutering, and changes in body weight and body composition on longevity.

Methods

Background and animal selection

The original study was designed as a clinical trial to test a novel energy restriction mimetic in the form of the dietary supplement mannoheptulose (MH). MH is a seven-carbon sugar derived from avocado that acts to reduce glycolysis via hexokinase inhibition and has been proposed as a calorie restriction mimetic that delivers anti-ageing and health promoting benefits of calorie restriction without reducing food intake [20, 21]. Initially, three groups of dogs were formed from a cohort of 59 Labrador retrievers after a 15-month acclimatisation period from May 2003 to 15 July 2004 (Fig. 1). During the acclimatisation period, fasting blood glucose and insulin were measured and the dogs were allocated to treatment groups using stratified randomisation based on these levels. The study design was approved by the Institutional Animal Care and Use Committee (IACUC) of Procter and Gamble (P&G) Pet Care (Mason, OH, USA).[1] The accommodation facility where the dogs were housed, the P&G Pet Care Pet Health and Nutrition Center in Lewisburg, OH, USA, was accredited by the Association for Assessment and Accreditation of Laboratory Animal

[1] The IACUC board had both internal and external board members. The external members were represented by a local High School teacher, and a local veterinarian from Dayton (OH, USA) with research experience but with no affiliation with any type of research institute.

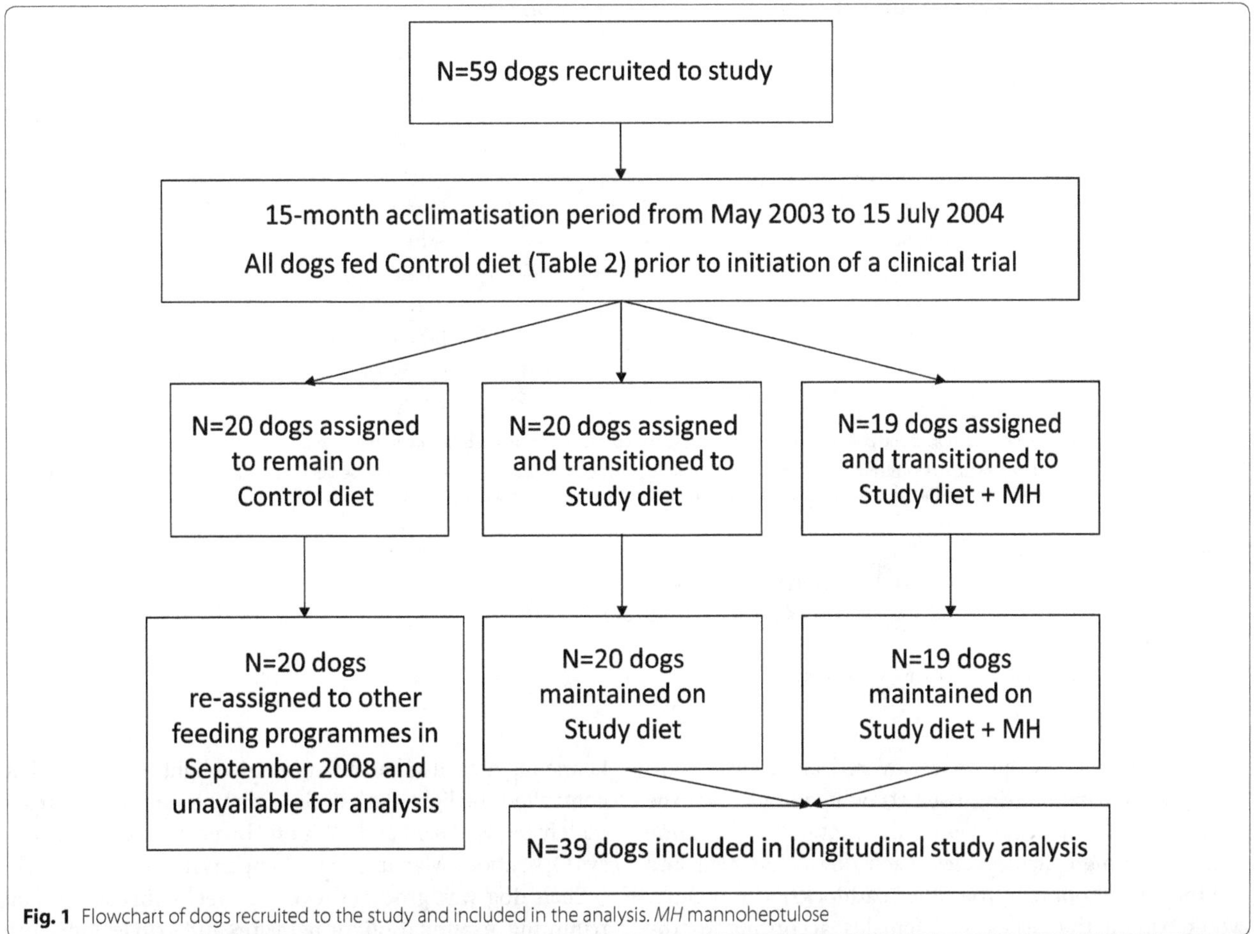

Fig. 1 Flowchart of dogs recruited to the study and included in the analysis. *MH* mannoheptulose

Care. After the initiation of the clinical trial an independent International Animal Welfare Advisory Board also had input and recommendations principally on the dogs' behaviour and enrichment interventions. This board made unannounced visits to the centre and their reports were made publically available.[2]

At the start of the original clinical trial (16 July 2004) one group was fed a control diet (n = 20, Table 2), one group was fed a study diet matrix (n = 20, Table 2) and the third group was fed the same study diet matrix with the inclusion of avocado juice extract with a concentration of <0.10 % as a source of biologically available mannoheptulose (MH) (n = 19) [22]. As a result of an internal business decision, the group of dogs that had been fed the control diet were released from the clinical trial and entered other feeding programmes in September 2008. The feeding of the two other groups continued as before with the same allocated study diet with or without MH (Fig. 1). Statistical analysis in June 2013 showed no significant effect of the diet on longevity detected between the 19 dogs that received the study diet and MH and the 20 dogs that were just fed the study diet; therefore, the data for these dogs were combined for the longevity analysis in this study (Fig. 1). For the remainder of this paper we report only on these 39 dogs.

A total of 39 adult, neutered Labrador retrievers consisting of 12 males and 27 females recruited in early to mid-adulthood, between the ages of 5.3 and 8.5 years (mean age 6.7 years, median 6.5), were included in the current longitudinal study. All dogs were acquired from private breeders or United States Department of Agriculture-inspected provider. One breeder provided 33 (85 %) Labrador retrievers from breeding a total of 12 sires and 19 dams. For these 33 dogs, the husbandry (feeding and kennelling) and medical care (worming and vaccinations) was kept consistent for all the dogs from birth and through early adulthood prior to them being recruited for the study. Furthermore, these dogs were housed in groups of three (one male and two female) in large open paddocks that were 15 metres wide by 45 m long covered

[2] International Animal Welfare Advisory Board annual report 2013 is available at https://www.iams.com/iams-truth/international-advisory-board-activities.

Table 2 General ingredient and nutrient composition of the control and study diets

Ingredient composition			Analysis %		
Control diet[a]	**Study diet[b]**		**Nutrient[f]**	**Control**	**Study**
Maize	Chicken meal	Egg product	Protein (%)	25.1	24.7
Chicken by-product meal	Chicken by-product meal	Brewer's yeast	Fat (%)	13.8	15.0
Maize gluten meal	Maize	FOS[c]	Fibre (%)	2.1	2.1
Soybean meal	Sorghum	sHMP[d]	Ash (%)	5.3	7.0
Animal fat	Barley	Linseed	Moisture (%)	7.8	7.5
Palatant	Chicken fat	L-carnitine	Vitamin E (IU/kg)	163	328
Minerals	Fishmeal	Minerals	β-carotene (ppm)	2.9	39
Vitamins	Palatant	Vitamins	GE[g] (kcal/kg)	4716	4695
	Beet pulp	Other[e]	6:3 fatty acids[h]	19:1	9:1

[a] The control diet was nutritionally complete and balanced and formulated to be representative of a mid-tier adult dog food product

[b] Study diet was formulated to contain the same nutritional technologies found in the Eukanuba nutritional matrix for senior dogs (Eukanuba® Senior Maintenance Dog Food. For the study period reported this product was owned and manufactured by Procter & Gamble, Cincinnati, Ohio, USA)

[c] Fructo-oligosaccharide

[d] Sodium hexametaphosphate

[e] Avocado juice concentrate (<0.10 %) was included in the diet matrix for 19 dogs

[f] Nutrient composition is actual laboratory analytical results expressed on as-fed basis

[g] Gross energy

[h] Ratio of dietary omega-6 fatty acids and omega-3 fatty acids

with gravel on a concrete base. Covered shelter was available (the internal housing used straw bedding) from the heat/cold and the dogs were all exposed to the same natural day/night light cycles. Each dog could hear and see their neighbours in the other paddocks. The breeder would rotate the males and females according to the breeding programme. After recruitment, 38 entire dogs were surgically neutered by the supervising veterinarian in 2003 prior to the start of the study period in July 2004 with only one dog, a male, that had been neutered at 4.4 years of age just prior to being recruited into the study in 2003. The mean and median age at neutering was 5.5 years (range 4.3–7.5 years).

Animal husbandry and veterinary care

Dogs were housed in a kennel system that include indoor kennels and outdoor runs. Both the indoor kennels and outdoor runs were cleaned and disinfected on a regular basis, and all had size-appropriate dog toys that were cleaned and interchanged regularly to provide environmental enrichment. The temperature of the indoor kennel was kept at approximately 22 °C (range 18–25 °C) with a relative humidity of 50 % (range 40–70 %). Air flow through the kenneling facility was maintained with approximately 15 fresh air changes per hour (range 10–30). Natural light was provided by large rectangular windows that were positioned above each of the individual indoor kennels and ran on both sides of an open corridor and for the entire length of the facility. The indoor kenneling area also had an automated lighting system that controlled the light/dark cycle with 12 h on from approximately 06.00–18.00 and 12 h off (Invensys system, Invensys Operations Management Company, Plano, TX, USA).

Each dog was groomed every 2 weeks (brushing, nail trimming, examination for parasites and skin lesions) and bathing was done quarterly. Daily socialisation of all dogs took place (20 min) with a qualified animal welfare specialist and additionally social groups of three to six dogs were exercised outdoors daily (30 min minimum) in a large gravel lined or grass exercise area. Furthermore, compatible groups of dogs had 24-h access to each other through their partially covered run that interconnected neighbouring kennels.[3] Equipment designed to provide environmental enrichment (e.g. agility course apparatus, wading pools, a variety of dog toys and shaded areas) was provided in the large areas.

The preventative healthcare plan for each dog included faecal examinations annually for endoparasites alongside blood testing for heartworm. Heartworm prevention was given monthly (Interceptor®, Novartis Animal Health,

[3] Dogs were housed in indoor kennels either on their own or in pairs. The kennels were 122 × 122 cm (single) or 244 × 244 cm (double) and arranged either side of an open corridor allowing dogs to see and hear other dogs in the group. Suitable bedding (Kuranda Dog Beds, Glen Burnie, Maryland, USA) was provided for each dog. The kennels were made from welded stainless steel mesh and polycarbonate panels. The floors were epoxy and were heated. A two-way door led from each kennel to a partially covered outdoor run (365 × 243 cm) which provided additional access to natural light. All runs had concrete flooring and dogs had free access to their run throughout the day and night.

US) and flea and tick treatment was given when required (Frontline Plus®, Merial) [23]. The vaccination routine consisted of adenovirus type 2, distemper, parvovirus, parainfluenza, (± leptospira given according to a health risk assessment) and an intranasal vaccine for Bordetella administered annually according to manufacturer's recommendations (Fort Dodge Duramune Max 5/4L®; Shering-Plough Intra-Trac II ®Bordetella Vaccine). Vaccination against Rabies was given every three years (Fort Dodge RabVac® 3TF). Oral health was evaluated with dental examinations performed every 6 months; standard dental prophylaxis/treatment (e.g. extractions, descaling and polishing under anaesthesia) was performed for each dog when necessary as recommended by the attending veterinarian. Standard physical examinations were undertaken annually and blood samples collected every 6 months for routine clinical assessment. Clinical parameters measured included complete blood cell counts, serum biochemistry and thyroid function. Aside from the regular veterinary examinations, each dog was monitored daily by their animal welfare specialist and the animal husbandry staff, and any health related concerns (e.g. medical, orthopaedic, oncologic) were brought to the attention of the attending healthcare staff. At this point the healthcare staff would initiate a regular quality of life assessment to monitor the dog's health and to assess if it remained stable or declined.[4] The case was then discussed by a group that was blinded to the identity of the dog. Decisions about medications and end-of-life issues were made by the group based on whether the quality of life was declining and the dog's overall well-being was compromised (see footnote 4). The group consisted of the study director, several veterinarians within other business units of the company as well as other veterinarians from the pet care unit. The on-site attending veterinarian also was authorised to make an end-of-life decision if there was a rapid deterioration in any dog's health.

Diet and feeding

From May 2003 until the start of the study on 16 July 2004 all dogs spent 1 year on a nutritionally complete and balanced control diet which was formulated to be representative of a mid-tier adult dog food (Control diet, Table 2). This was to help acclimatise the dogs to their environment and to help adjust their body weight and body condition score so that they entered the study in 2004 with a body condition score (BCS) between two and four, based on a 5-point BCS [24]. This adaptation period also helped establish the individual food allowance required to maintain body weight with a BCS between two and four. Following this year of acclimation, the 39 dogs were transitioned onto a study diet formulated with the same nutritional technologies shown to help support the health and well-being of both adult and senior dogs (Study diet, Table 2). This dietary matrix was created to comprise the same nutritional components found in Eukanuba® Senior Maintenance[5] for large breed dogs but with a slightly lower protein (24.7 % 'as fed') and slightly higher fat (15 % 'as fed') level.

BCS was assessed by trained staff on a quarterly basis both during the adaptation year and during the study using a five-point scale. A score of 3 was considered ideal. A dog's daily food allowance was changed if the quarterly BCS was not between the 2–4 range to avoid the extremes of thinness (BCS = 1) or obesity (BCS = 5) conditions. The maximum allowable change to an individual dog's daily food allowance was ±50 g and this food amount was maintained until the next quarterly BCS assessment. The daily food allowance could also be changed by the supervising veterinarian for medical purposes.

The daily ration of food was weighed for each dog, divided into two equal portions, and offered in stainless steel food bowls inserted into rings located at the front of each indoor pen at 07:30 and 14:30 each day. Dogs were separated for feeding. Each dog was allowed 30 min to consume their food and food intake was recorded daily. Fresh water was constantly available using automatic adjustable water bowls mounted on the side of each housing unit.

Body weight and composition

Body weight was measured every 2 weeks, BCS was evaluated quarterly and whole-body composition measures were obtained prior to the start of the study and then annually using a Dual-Energy X-ray Absorptiometer (DEXA scan) (Model Delphi-A, Serial No. 70852; Bedford, MA). For the DEXA scan, dogs were fasted for a minimum of 12 h prior to being sedated using a pre-anaesthetic combination of Acepromazine (PromAce® Injectable, Fort Dodge, Fort Dodge, Iowa; 0.55 mg/kg intramuscular injection) and Atropine Sulfate (Med-Pharmex, Pomona, CA; 0.04 mg/kg subcutaneous injection). Dogs were then anaesthetised

[4] Assessments were conducted by animal welfare specialists, animal husbandry staff and healthcare staff (attending veterinarian, veterinary nurses) to assess quality of life using a 10-point Likert scale ratings to assess food/water intake (hunger/thirst), pain/discomfort, mobility, hygiene, happiness and number of "good days". When the dog was having more "bad days" than "good days" then the attending veterinarian convened a panel to discuss an end-of-life decision; original concept, Oncology Outlook, by Dr. Alice Villalobos, Quality of Life Scale Helps Make Final Call, VPN, 09/2004; scale format created for author's book, Canine and Feline Geriatric Oncology: Honouring the Human-Animal Bond, Blackwell Publishing, 2007. Revised for the International Veterinary Association of Pain Management (IVAPM) 2011 Palliative Care and Hospice Guidelines.

[5] Eukanuba® Senior Maintenance Dog Food. For the study period reported this product was owned and manufactured by Procter & Gamble, Cincinnati, Ohio, USA.

with Propofol administered via a secured intravenous catheter (Propoflo®, Abbot Labs, Chicago, IL; 7 mg/kg), intubated with an endotracheal tube and delivered 100 % oxygen. Routine anaesthetic monitoring was performed. Dogs were positioned in sternal recumbency with hind limbs extended caudally. A calibration was completed prior to each DEXA scan and measurements were taken using the whole body scanner (single-beam mode). After the scans, anaesthesia was discontinued and oxygen was continued for several minutes. Dogs were moved to a recovery cage and the endotracheal tube was removed once the swallowing reflex was regained. Whole-body measures obtained from the DEXA scans included total bone mineral density (BMD in grams), total bone mineral content (BMC in grams), total body mass (g), total fat mass (g), total lean mass (g), % body fat, % body lean and fat to lean ratio (determined as total fat mass/total lean mass).

Statistical analysis

Dogs were classified into three groups derived from tertiles of lifespan data as of 31 March 2014: Expected' when they experienced a lifespan of ≥9 to ≤12.9 years, 'Long' when they experienced a lifespan between ≥13 and ≤15.5 years and 'Exceptional' when they achieved ≥15.6 years and beyond. The value of 15.6 for the Exceptional lifespan group is 30 % longer than the 12-year typical lifespan of the breed determined by the consensus group (Table 1) [16]. Average body weights and ages among the three longevity groups at the start of the longitudinal study were compared using analysis of variance with post hoc pairwise comparisons. Cross-tabulations and Chi square or Fishers Exact tests were used to compare proportions of dogs within various groups. Survival analysis, using Kaplan–Meier (KM) and Cox proportional hazards regression (Cox) models, was performed to examine the effect of potential predictors on time to death. Monthly body weights up to December 2013 and annual body composition data up to 13 years of age were analysed using linear mixed models with random effects for slopes and intercepts and a fixed effect for the lifespan grouping variable. The models allowed an intercept and slope to be estimated for each dog with the assumption that each endpoint response for a dog had a linear trajectory across age. Body weight against age presented by longevity category in a polynomial smooth plot did not show a linear trend but a curve that follows an inverted U shape (Fig. 2); therefore, a random coefficient model was used to compare the slopes as a measure of body weight change (kg/dog/year) for three groups: up to 9 years, 9–13 years and >13 years of age. An age cut-off point of 13 years was chosen for statistical analysis because all three lifespan groups were fully represented up to age 13. Statistical analysis was

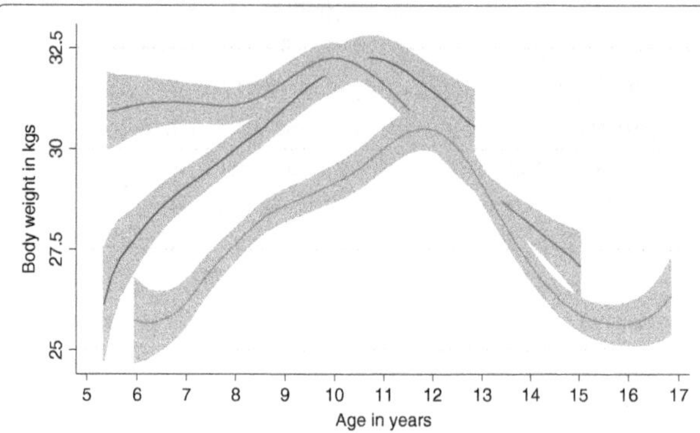

Fig. 2 Polynomial smooth *plots* of average body weight (*lines*) with 95% confidence intervals (CI, *gray shaded areas*) by age for each longevity group of dogs. The starting point for each line is the average body weight for those dogs which were in the acclimatisation period at that age on 01 July 2004 just before the study started. The end point for each line is the average body weight for those dogs which died or were censored (N = 5 in the Exceptional group) at that age at the censor date of 31 July 2014. These *plots* show that the Expected dogs (*blue line*) started at a low weight, then put on about 1 kg/year until reaching a peak at 11 years of age and this was followed by a decline of ~1.7 kg in 2 years. The Long-lived dogs (*green line*) started at a higher weight, then stayed at a rather stable weight before showing an increased weight over to reach a peak at 10 years of age and then the weight declined at ~1 kg/year. The Exceptionally long-lived dogs (*gray*) started at the lowest weight (but at an older age) and they put on weight gradually to reach a peak at 12 years of age, then slowly declined to reach a low point at 16 years before putting on some weight again

performed using commercial software.[6] The level of significance for all statistical tests was set at $P < 0.05$.

Results

Longevity and cause of death

As of July 2004, the dogs that were subsequently classified as experiencing an Exceptional lifespan were significantly older than the other dogs (P = 0.01) and there were no significant differences in body weight (P = 0.36, Table 3). The median time spent in this longitudinal study (from 16 July 2004 to death or the censor date for longevity estimation) by the 39 dogs was 7.43 years and this ranged from 2.54 to 10.04 years. As of the censor date of 31st of July 2014, the distribution of dogs based on lifespan groups was: Expected lifespan (n = 13), Long lifespan (n = 15) and Exceptional lifespan (n = 11 including 5 dogs that remained alive with a median age of 17.1 years, Table 4; Fig. 3). A total of 35 dogs (89.7, 95 % CI 75–97 %) were alive at 12 years of age and 11 dogs (28.2, 95 % CI 15.6–45.1 %) attained exceptional longevity, reaching or

[6] Statistical software: SAS version 9.3 (SAS Institute, 2011, Cary, NC, USA), Statistix version 10 (Analytical Software, 2013, Tallahassee, FL), SPSS version 22 (IBM SPSS, 2013, Chicago, IL, USA) and Stata version 13.1 (StataCorp, 2014, College Station, TX, USA).

exceeding 15.6 years of age. The five exceptionally long-lived dogs that remained alive at the censor date were considered to be 3–4 years younger than their chronological age, based on overall condition, activity level and interactive behaviour as observed by several independent veterinarians and Labrador retriever enthusiasts who interacted with these dogs in June 2014. For the 34 dogs that passed away during the study the age at death ranged from 9.7 to 16.9 years with a median age of death of 13.6 years. Each of the lifespan groups had significantly different median survival time (MST) based on KM survival analysis (Table 4; Fig. 3). A larger proportion of female dogs reached an Exceptional age (female:male ratio = 10:1) compared with the Expected (7:6) and Long (10:5) lifespan groups although this was not a statistically significant difference ($P = 0.1$). Gender was not significantly associated with survival time (KM $P = 0.06$) or risk of death (Cox $P = 0.07$) and there was no effect of the age of neutering on the risk of death for females (Cox $P = 0.2$) or males (Cox $P = 0.7$).

Cancer was the reason for euthanasia for 13 dogs (38 %) with 20 dogs (59 %) undergoing euthanasia for other reasons and one dog died overnight (enteritis, colitis and protein-losing enteropathy were found on post-mortem examination) (Table 5). Of the 13 dogs that underwent euthanasia as a result of cancer: 54 % of these dogs lived to an Expected age, 31 % were in the Long group and 15 % in the Exceptional group although these proportions were not significantly different ($P = 0.3$, Table 5).

Body weight and composition changes

From the start of the study to age 9, body weight increased for all three lifespan groups (Fig. 2) but the changes over this period were not significantly different (Table 6). In contrast, there was a significant change in body weight (kg/dog/year) during the span of 9–13 years as Exceptional dogs increased body weight while the Long lifespan dogs lost weight (+0.53 vs. −0.91 kg/dog/year respectively, $P = 0.007$). The Expected lifespan dogs also lost weight during this period (−0.15) but the loss was not significantly different from the Exceptional or Long lifespan groups. After age 13, dogs in the Exceptional and Long groups both lost a comparable amount of body weight. The polynomial plot in Fig. 2 reveals that the dogs in the Exceptional group had a lower peak in body weight and this peak occurred at a later age compared to the dogs in the Expected and Long lived groups.

The 39 dogs underwent between 3 and 10 DEXA scans during the study period with a median of seven scans per dog. Total fat mass (g/dog/year) increased in all lifespan groups to age 13 but the increase was significantly slower only for the Long lifespan dogs when compared with Expected dogs which accumulated fat at 3.1 times the rate over this time period (slopes of +320 vs. +1000, $P = 0.003$ Table 7). In contrast, all groups lost a similar amount of total lean mass (g/dog/year) through age 13 ranging from −593 (Expected), −461 (Long) to −269 (Exceptional) ($P > 0.05$). Percent body fat increased significantly more slowly to age 13 in both the Exceptional and Long-lived dogs compared with Expected dogs (1.55 and 1.25 vs. 2.69, respectively, $P = 0.02$ and $P = 0.002$). Congruently, the percentage loss of lean mass through age 13 was significantly slower for dogs of Exceptional and Long lifespans when compared with those having an Expected lifespan (−1.58 and −1.31 vs. −2.69, respectively, $P = 0.02$ and $P = 0.002$). Similarly, the change in the fat to lean ratio to age 13 was significantly greater in the Expected dogs versus both the Exceptional and Long lived dogs ($P = 0.02$ and $P = 0.002$). Total bone mineral density (BMD) was significantly lower for Expected compared to Exceptional and Long ($P < 0.04$). There were no statistically significant differences among the lifespan groups for changes in total bone mineral content (BMC) ($P = 0.2$). There were no statistically significant differences in BCS slopes over time among the three lifespan groups (data not shown).

Discussion

The results of this longitudinal study show that a greater than expected proportion of Labrador retrievers lived well beyond that of the expected breed lifespan as nearly 90 % (n = 35) of the dogs met or surpassed the consensus average life expectancy for the breed of 12 years and 28 % (n = 11) went on to achieve Exceptional longevity (≥15.6 years). In spite of being 16 and 17 years of age,

Table 3 Mean ages and body weights for the three longevity groups of dogs in July 2004

Longevity category	N	Mean body weight (kg)	SD	Min–max	Mean age (years)	SD	Min–max
Expected (≥9 to ≤12.9 years)	13	29.4	4.6	20.2–37.40	6.5*	0.6	5.3–7.6
Long (≥13 to ≤15.5 years)	15	29.4	4.3	21.1–41.4	6.4#	0.9	5.4–7.9
Exceptional (≥15.6 years)	11	26.8	3.7	19.2–33.1	7.4*#	0.8	6.0–8.5

Means among longevity groups were compared using analysis of variance with post hoc pairwise comparisons; mean body weights were not significantly different ($P = 0.36$) whilst means within the age column that share an asterisk (*) or a hash (#) were significantly different ($P = 0.01$)

N number of dogs, *SD* standard deviation, *Min–max* range from minimum to maximum values

Table 4 Number of Labrador retrievers, age at death/censor date and median survival time with 95 % CIs

Longevity category		Descriptive statistics for age in years at death/censor date[a]			MST (95 % CI) in years from Kaplan–Meier analysis
		N (%)	Mean (SD)	Median (min–max)	
Expected ≥9 to ≤12.9	Deceased	13 (33 %)	12.08* (1.04)	12.58* (9.68–12.95)	12.44* (11.70–12.80)
Long ≥13 to ≤15.5	Deceased	15 (39 %)	14.21* (0.58)	14.15* (13.18–15.19)	14.08* (13.63–14.72)
Exceptional ≥15.6	Deceased	6	15.98 (0.49)	15.80 (15.68–16.96)	
	Alive[a]	5	16.82 (0.65)	17.13 (16.04–17.50)	
	Sub-total	11 (28 %)	16.36* (0.69)	16.04* (15.68–17.50)	16.47* (15.76–NE)
Overall	Overall	39 (100 %)	14.11 (1.86)	14.01 (9.68–17.50)	14.01 (13.18–14.77)

Within each column (mean, median, MST), values which share an asterisk (*) are each significantly different from one another (P < 0.0001) by parametric and non-parametric analysis of variance for age at death/censor date and by Kaplan–Meier survival analysis; values within a column with no asterisk were not compared

CI confidence interval, *NE* not estimated using Statistix commercial software

[a] July 31, 2014

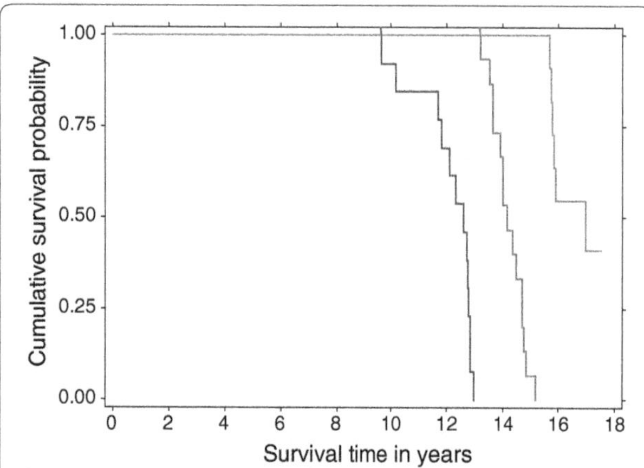

Fig. 3 Kaplan–Meier survival plot for 39 Labrador retrievers in three lifespan groups. Expected (*blue*): 13 dogs; Long (*green*): 15 dogs; and Exceptional (*gray*): six deceased and five dogs remaining alive as of the July 31, 2014 censor date

the five dogs remaining alive at the end of the study continued to be full of life, active, social and highly engaged with their animal welfare specialists and social groups according to the independent veterinarians and Labrador retriever enthusiasts who interacted with these dogs in June 2014. This supports our findings that an increase in healthspan was present in this study population. These findings are similar to those reported in an earlier longitudinal study of the effect of calorie restriction in Labrador retrievers where the 'Restricted' group experienced a median lifespan of 13.0 years with a maximum lifespan of 14.5 years compared to 11.2 and 13.2 years, respectively, for the 'Control' group [2, 19, 25, 26]. It may therefore be suggested that identifying the appropriate calorie balance (i.e. calorie intake that matches calorie expenditure) in order to reach and maintain an ideal BCS throughout the lifespan of Labrador retrievers and adhering to this feeding level may be essential in achieving a long, healthy life.

There was a slower loss of total and significantly slower loss of percentage lean body mass in the Exceptional group versus the Expected group together with a slower increase in total body fat and a significantly slower increase in percentage body fat and a significantly lower change in fat to lean ratio. This is similar to the findings of another study in which body composition was measured from 6 years of age where the mean total lean mass was significantly greater in the 'Control' group compared to the 'Restricted' group; additionally, there was a progressive decline in total lean mass after 9 years of age in the 'Control' group but not in the 'Restricted' group until after 11 years of age [2, 19]. Furthermore, although mean percentage lean mass decreased significantly in both groups from 6 to 12 years of age it was always significantly higher among the 'Restricted' dogs than the 'Control' dogs [19]. Mean total and percentage body fat mass increased significantly in both groups from 6 to 12 years of age and was always significantly higher in the 'Control' group. There was no correlation between total lean and fat mass in the 'Restricted' group and this may suggest underlying processes that drive the beneficial longevity response in these dogs may be multiple and driven independently [2]. Somewhat paradoxically, the dogs in the Long lifespan group of the current study lost weight between the ages of 9 and 13 years whilst the Exceptional lifespan dogs maintained or slightly gained weight during this time period. Body mass and body composition are related to an individual dog's size and they may also independently influence the rate of ageing and longevity. The risks of an increase in the incidence and severity of chronic disease associated with high body fat has been reported in other studies [27–29]. In adult nonhuman primates, lower morbidity rates also have been reported in studies comparing calorie-restriction versus ad lib

Table 5 Cause of death for 34 dogs by gender and lifespan category as of 31 July 2014

Cancer	Expected: ≥9 to ≤12.9 years		Long: ≥13 to ≤15.5 years		Exceptional: ≥15.6 years		Total
Female	3 =	Haemangiosarcoma unspecified type/location Haemangiosarcoma splenic with metastasis Lymphosarcoma	3 =	Plasma cell tumour Haemangiosarcoma Osteosarcoma	2 =	Haemangiosarcoma splenic Adenocarcinoma pulmonary	8
Male	4 =	Haemangiosarcoma prostate/bladder Prostatic cancer Mast cell tumour metastasis Urinary tract cancer—TCC	1 =	Urinary tract cancer bladder	0		5
Sub-total	7 (54 %)		4 (27 %)		2 (33 %)		13 (38 %)
Other							
Female	4 =	Intervertebral disc disease Mega-oesophagus causing chronic vomiting Seizures—unresponsive to medication Osteoarthritis (CHD)	7 =	Gastric dilatation volvulus Chronic kidney disease (asymptomatic)[a] Progressive seizures Septicaemia Osteoarthritis (2) Quality of life	4 =	Osteoarthritis (2) Quality of life (2)	15
Male	2 =	Osteoarthritis	4 =	Found deceased in kennel (enteritis, colitis and PLE)[b] Gastro-intestinal inflammation[c] Chronic kidney disease (end stage) Myocardial fibrosis	0		6
Sub-total	6 (46 %)		11 (73 %)		4 (67 %)		21 (62 %)
Total	13 (100 %)		15 (100 %)		6 (100 %)		34 (100 %)

33 dogs underwent euthanasia due to deteriorating quality of life and one dog found dead in the morning[b]

[a] Histopathology revealed inflammatory process in kidney indicating chronic infection (asymptomatic)

[b] Post-mortem examination revealed enteritis and colitis with evidence of protein-losing enteropathy and mild multifocal glomerulosclerosis

[c] Histopathology revealed inflammatory changes in gastro-intestinal tract

Table 6 Body weight change (slope) for three age categories of Labrador retrievers up to death/censor date 31 July 2014

Longevity category	Up to 9 years			9–13 years			After 13 years		
	N	Mean (in kg/dog/year)	SEM	N	Mean (in kg/dog/year)	SEM	N	Mean (in kg/dog/year)	SEM
Expected (≥9 to ≤12.9 years)	13	0.59	0.3	13	−0.15	0.31		N/A	
Long (≥13 to ≤15.5 years)	15	0.52	0.28	15	−0.91*	0.28	15	−1.41	0.68
Exceptional (>15.6 years)	11	0.4	0.36	11	0.53*	0.32	11	−1.31	0.74

Means within the 9–13 years column which share an asterisk (*) are significantly different ($P = 0.007$); none of the means within the other two columns (up to 9 years, after 13 years) show any significant differences among them ($P > 0.05$)

N number of dogs, *SEM* standard error of the mean

feeding. In the calorie-restriction primates (fed 30–40 % less calories than their ad lib pair mate) the body fat content was within the normal range of 10–22 % [30]. Typically, the body fat in ad lib fed primates can range from 17–44 % [31]. This calorie-restriction induced prevention of morbidity does not therefore require excessive leanness.

A comparison between the dogs in the current study and those from the calorie restricted study [2, 19, 25] shows that energy intake per unit of body weight kcal/kg/day for the 'Restricted' group (≈46.5) was very close to the 46.2–48 kcal/kg/day of dogs in the current study (Table 8). Therefore, on an energy intake basis, we can consider these groups of dogs to be similar. This is reflected by the 'Restricted' group having a BCS in the ideal range of 4–6 on a 9-point scale from 6 to 12 years of age. However, the oldest dog in the 'Restricted' group died at 14.5 years of age whilst a female in the current study was still alive on July 31, 2014 at 17.5 years of age. We can only speculate why we had dogs showing much

Table 7 Results of linear mixed regression for average changes in body composition determined by DEXA scans performed annually up to 13 years of age

DEXA variable	Longevity category								
	Expected (≥9 to ≤12.9 years)			Long (≥13 to ≤15.5 years)			Exceptional (≥15.6 years)		
	N	Mean[a]	SEM[b]	N	Mean[a]	SEM[b]	N	Mean[a]	SEM[b]
Total fat mass (g)	13	1000*	165	15	320*	152	11	625	170
Total lean mass (g)	13	−593	127	15	−461	80	11	−269	165
Body fat (%)	13	2.69*#	0.35	15	1.25*	0.31	11	1.55#	0.36
Body lean (%)	13	−2.69*#	0.33	15	−1.31*	0.29	11	−1.58#	0.34
Fat:Lean[b]	13	0.06*#	0.01	15	0.03*	0.01	11	0.04#	0.01
Total BMC (g)	13	10	3.2	15	18	3.1	11	16.6	3.2
Total BMD (g)	13	0.0061*#	0.0022	15	0.0123*	0.0019	11	0.0131#	0.0024

Means within a row that share an asterisk (*) or a hash (#) are significantly different ($P < 0.05$); means within a row with no asterisk or hash are not significantly different ($P > 0.05$)

DEXA Dual-energy x-ray absorptiometer scans obtained using DXA Model Delphi-A, Serial No. 70852; Bedford, MA, USA

N number

[a] Means and standard errors of the mean (SEM) for changes in body composition (slope) as g/dog/year or %/dog/year up to 13 years

[b] The fat to lean ratio was determined as total fat mass (g)/total lean mass (g)

Table 8 Energy intake of Labrador retrievers in the current study and a previous calorie restricted study

Average daily intake of energy[b]	Current study			Calorie 'restricted' group[a]
	Expected	Long	Exceptional	
MJ/day	5.88	5.84	5.56	5.15
kcal/day	1405	1397	1329	1230
Energy intake kcal/kg/day	46.2	46.2	48	≈46.5

[a] Group of Labrador retrievers fed 25 % less than their 'Control' fed pair; Kealy et al. [19, 25] and Lawler et al. [2]

[b] Metabolic energy of the test diet fed was 3669 kcal/kg based on a Modified Atwater calculation

longer lifespan than the dogs in the other study despite being on the same calorie intake and BCS level. The detailed data on body composition is providing a potential in investigating reasons related to increased healthspan beyond the BCS and calorie intake. As well, the overall median lifespan was 13.0 years for the 48 dogs in the calorie restricted study whilst the median age (at death and for those still alive) was 14.01 years for the 39 dogs reported here. One important difference between the Labradors reported in this study and those in the calorie restricted study is that all the dogs in the present study were kept at a BCS between two and four throughout the study. The classic calorie restriction model used to examine the effects of feeding on the ageing process is often described as one of undernutrition without malnutrition. This usually involves control animals that are fed ad libitum (free choice with no or little restriction) as in the studies by Kealy, Lawler et al. [2, 19, 25, 26] and comparing these to animals fed a set restricted number of calories (i.e. not free choice). However, the energy intake of such 'control fed' animals often significantly exceeds the amount expended, resulting in a substantial gain in body weight, or positive energy balance, which is often associated with the early onset of disease [19, 32–34]. As the majority of dogs were recruited from the same breeder, the variation in environmental exposures among these dogs is reduced even if those dogs did not share the exact same habitat (for example due to temporal differences among litters). With regards to the genetic background, the dogs in this study were not as closely related as the dogs in the restricted feeding study. We recognise that the longevity effect seen in this study could be partly or wholly explained by the relatedness/line breeding of the dogs. However, dogs from the one breeder were found in all three longevity categories so although there might be a genetic predisposition for longevity, not all dogs expressed this characteristic.

As the mean body weights for the three longevity groups at the start of the study were not significantly different, we suggest that body weight alone, and particularly during middle age (5–8 years) is not predictive of longevity. The association over time between changes in different body mass components and health may provide key insights into future recommendations on how to manage our ageing dogs more successfully to achieve an improved healthspan. One key body mass component is skeletal muscle. A number of age-related changes may contribute to the gradual age-related loss of skeletal muscle which is reported in humans and dogs [35]. This loss of lean body mass in the absence of disease is termed 'sarcopenia' and it is important to differentiate this from 'cachexia' which is the loss of lean body mass with disease [36]. Sarcopenia is defined in humans as "a syndrome characterised by progressive and generalised loss of skeletal muscle mass and strength with a risk of adverse outcomes such as physical disability, poor quality of life and death" [37]. Sarcopenia in humans usually begins early in life and between the ages of 20 and 60 years there is on average a loss of 40 % of lean muscle mass [38]. In sarcopenia, the loss of lean body mass often is accompanied by an increase in fat mass so the total weight may not change (or may even increase), thus masking the sarcopenia [36]. Previous studies in dogs have shown that a high percentage of lean mass was associated with a protective effect from death whilst declining grams of lean body mass as well as a high percentage and absolute (grams) of fat mass predicted death [26]. The present study is the first published study to show an association between a slower rate of loss of lean body mass and exceptional longevity in dogs. The polynomial smooth plot (Fig. 2) revealed that the oldest dogs in the Exceptional group had an initial peak in body weight at 12 years of age and then re-gained weight after 16 years of age following a period of weight loss. This weight re-gain could represent a longevity advantage for these 'oldest of the old' dogs, however due to the small number of dogs included in this category, results need to be interpreted with caution. Further evaluation of what contributes to this late weight gain (e.g. slower loss of lean body mass combined with an increase in fat mass) could provide information on preferable body composition changes that would confer a longevity advantage to dogs.

Among human centenarians, women outlive men by four to one and, like women, female Rottweilers were more likely to achieve exceptional longevity (age at death $\geq$13 years) than males of this breed in a large retrospective study that examined the effect of ovary exposure up to 8 years of age [16]. However, this survival advantage was lost if the dogs underwent ovariectomy during the first 4 years of life. In females that retained their ovaries for more than 4 years, the likelihood of reaching exceptional longevity increased to more than three times that of males. Additional data from female Rottweiler dogs revealed that the number of years of ovary exposure was associated with exceptional longevity [39]. Females with the longest ovary exposure (6.1–8.0 years) were 3.2 times more likely to reach exceptional longevity than females spayed during the first 2 years of life ($P = 0.002$). Furthermore, there was no evidence of a female's physiological investment in offspring (number of litters, total number of pups, age at first reproduction, mean interbirth interval, age at last reproduction) being associated with a reduced longevity [18]. These findings suggest that the ovaries participate in functions beyond reproduction which may include a role in the orchestration of exceptional longevity. Contrastingly, there was no effect of gender or the age at neutering on the risk of death for the dogs in the present study. The discrepancies between the Rottweiler study and our study may be related to the small sample producing a low statistical power as supported by the finding that whilst female Labrador retrievers tended to live longer than males, there was no statistically significant effect of gender on risk of death and age at death.

Whilst these dogs were not housed in a natural pet environment (such as in a household with human 'companions'), they were housed in compatible social groups and also had regular daily interaction with people much as a household pet might. Although there may be large differences between the structured management of the study dogs and typical household/family dogs, the benefit of keeping the study dogs under very similar conditions throughout the study removes the effect of many potential confounding variables that could change over time in a household environment. A study of family-owned dogs would require a much larger sample size when investigating associations between risk factors and outcomes. Such a large sample would not only be very expensive but is likely to suffer from participants leaving the study due to the long time commitment. The decision not to treat any cancer diagnosis with chemotherapy or radiotherapy, and to manage the dog through palliative care with other medications, was due to an ethical position by the company as well as representing a choice that dog owners might make if their own pet was diagnosed with cancer, particularly at an older age. All dogs with cancer and other chronic medical conditions had quality of life assessments initiated at the time of diagnosis to ensure that their health and well-being was managed ethically and appropriately (see footnote 4). Other medical issues such as ear and skin conditions were managed by the healthcare staff under veterinary supervision. The radiation risk associated with the annual general anaesthetic for the DEXA scans was assumed to be negligible based on published information about DEXA scans in people [40].

Conducting breed-specific longevity studies is both a strength and a limitation; initially, it may seem to potentially limit the understanding of healthy ageing. For instance, it has been shown that the median lifespan of crossbreds is greater than purebred dogs [12, 41] and that even within a set weight range of breeds there can be differences in the median age of death [8, 12]. However, by evaluating a single breed, rather than multiple breeds, then the influence on longevity by factors such as obesity and ovary exposure, as well as the age at onset of specific age-related disease might become clearer [42] as variation on other factors is reduced. When multiple breeds are evaluated together, such associations may be disguised or distorted. A limitation of this study is the absence of a control group fed a different diet as a result of a business decision in 2008 to discontinue the third study group. However, the strength of the cohort approach taken in this longitudinal study is that it allows further work using survival analysis to examine the effects of the time-varying measurements on longevity and development of disease. Whilst this was not a birth cohort and the results may be confounded by early life experiences, previous work has shown that deaths in Labrador retrievers less than 6 years of age were mostly due to trauma [43] and in the aforementioned calorie restriction study only two dogs from the original 48 died before 6 years of age [26]. There are many factors that may have contributed to the ability of these dogs to exceed a typical lifespan and reach exceptional longevity. These include genetics, husbandry, preventative healthcare, socialisation, housing and environmental enrichment. Longevity is generally accepted as having a heritability of approximately 25–30 %, with the effect of the environment having a much larger influence [44]. Nutrition is part of this environmental influence and therefore has a potentially significant role to play in longevity. Many of the probable environmental influences that could impact successful ageing and longevity were maintained as constant as possible for all the dogs in the current study. The nutritional matrix fed to all dogs incorporated key nutritional components that have been shown to benefit canine health and well-being based on results of short-term research studies. This longitudinal study is the first to incorporate all of these nutritional components into the same dietary matrix consistently fed over an extended period of time. As dogs pass through the ageing process their nutritional requirements change reflecting a normal response to age-related metabolic and physiologic responses. The dietary matrix fed was designed to address recognised changes that take place as dogs pass from adulthood into their senior years. The test diet (Table 2) was a matrix based on animal protein ingredients, balanced omega-6/3 fatty acids with a blend of low glycaemic index carbohydrates alongside L-carnitine. Antioxidants vitamin E and beta-carotene, the moderately fermentable beet pulp and the prebiotic fructooligosaccharide were also incorporated. Finally, the outside of the dry food was coated with sodium hexametaphosphate to help with reduction of tartar build-up. It is likely that there are many dietary factors including total energy intake relative to energy needs, specific nutrients and other non-nutrient bioactive substances that, individually or collectively, influence the ageing process.

Highly successful ageing can be considered as being robust in an age-specific way and which translates into being resilient to disease, including cancer. For humans it has been hypothesised that centenarians either markedly delay or escape age-associated morbidity such as heart disease, stroke, diabetes, cancer, and Alzheimer's disease [45]. Consistent with this idea is the proposition from James Fries, known as the compression of morbidity hypothesis which states that individuals who reach the limits of human lifespan compress the onset and duration of illnesses toward the end of life [46, 47]. This hypothesis predicts that, in order to achieve their extreme old age, centenarians markedly delay or even escape diseases that would otherwise be lethal at younger ages. A retrospective cohort study of 424 human centenarians examining the ages of onset for 10 age-associated diseases and excluding cognitive impairment, found that the centenarians fitted into three morbidity profiles; Survivors, Delayers, and Escapers [48]. Survivors (38 % of study population) had a diagnosis of an age-associated illness prior to the age of 80, Delayers (43 %) were individuals who delayed the onset of age-associated illness until at least the age of 80 and Escapers (19 %) were individuals who attained their 100th year of life without the diagnosis of common age-associated illnesses. Centenarians have, therefore, shown successful ageing and have in some way developed an age-related robustness and resilience to disease. This resilience includes cancer, where proportional mortality rates increase with age during most of adulthood but decline in advanced age from nearly 40 % of all deaths between the ages of 50 and 69 to only 4 % of all deaths in patients older than age 100 years [49]. These data suggest that the oldest-old humans have a cancer-resistant phenotype compared to the general population. In the current study, cancer was the cause of euthanasia in 54 % of the dogs that lived to an Expected age, 27 % in the Long group and 33 % in the Exceptional group, suggesting that the longer-living dogs may have been less likely to experience cancer although this was not statistically significant. We were not able to show any association of cause of death with lifespan group or gender although this is likely due to the small numbers of dogs in each group.

Conclusions

The findings of this study indicate that the life-long maintenance of lean body mass and an attenuated accumulation of body fat are key factors influencing successful ageing as reflected by longer healthspan. In the current study, the combination of a high quality plane of nutrition with appropriate husbandry and veterinary care resulted in 28 % of the dogs reaching an Exceptional lifespan of ≥15.6 years and almost 90 % of the dogs exceeded the typical lifespan of 12 years. Future work includes further analysis of the data from this 10+ year study using survival analysis and other techniques to look at how variables change over time. The long-term objective is to provide clear and practical recommendations for both dog owners and veterinarians so that all dogs can live to their full genetic potential.

Abbreviations

BCS: body condition score; BW: body weight; C: celsius; Cox: cox proportional hazards regression; DEXA: dual-energy x-ray absorptiometer; IACUC: Institutional Animal Care and Use Committee; KM: Kaplan–Meier survival analysis; MH: mannoheptulose; MST: median survival time; P&G: Procter & Gamble Pet Care.

Authors' contributions

DMM was involved in data acquisition. VJA, SG and JP were responsible for data analysis and interpretation. DMM, PW and SC contributed to interpretation of data. All authors contributed to and approved of the writing of the final manuscript. The authors also wish to make a statement that this analysis was carried out in good faith that the data used were accurate to the best of their knowledge. All authors read and approved the final manuscript.

Author details

[1] Vet Epi, White Cottage, Dickleburgh, Norfolk IP21 4NT, UK. [2] Department of Veterinary Medicine, University of Cambridge, Madingley Road, Cambridge CB3 OES, UK. [3] University of Surrey, Vet School Main Building, Daphne Jackson Road, Guildford GU2 7AL, UK. [4] Nuffield Department of Orthopaedics, Centre for Statistics in Medicine, Rheumatology and Musculoskeletal Sciences, University of Oxford, Oxford OX3 7LD, UK. [5] School of Veterinary Medicine, Faculty of Health and Medical Sciences, University of Surrey, Vet School Main Building, Daphne Jackson Road, Guildford GU2 7AL, UK. [6] Spectrum Brands Schweiz GmbH, Stationsstrasse 3, Brüttisellen, 8306 Zurich, Switzerland.

Acknowledgements

The authors wish to thank all the former P&G Research & Development team involved for their assistance in this study since its inception over 10 years ago. The authors also wish to acknowledge the role of P&G for their financial support of this study and Spectrum Brands for supporting the analysis and preparation of this manuscript.

Competing interests

VJA, SG and JP received payment from Spectrum Brands (and formerly of P&G) for provision of analytical services and interpretation of data. DMM is an employee of Spectrum Brands (and formerly of P&G). The remaining authors declare that they did not receive payment for any services pertaining to the conduct of this study, interpretation of data or writing of this manuscript. The study was initially conceived and carried out by the Research & Development division of P&G, Cincinnati, Ohio, USA. This organization had no role in the data analysis, decision to publish or preparation of the manuscript. None of the authors of this article has a personal relationship with other people or organisations that could inappropriately influence or bias the content of the paper.

References

1. Sunvold GD, Bouchard GF. The glycemic response to dietary starch. In: Reinhart GA, Carey DP, editors. 1998 Iams nutrition symposium proceedings. Recent advances in canine and feline nutrition. Wilmington: Orange Frazer Press; 1998. p. 123–32.
2. Lawler DF, Larson BT, Ballam JM, Smith GK, Biery DN, Evans RH, et al. Diet restriction and ageing in the dog: major observations over two decades. Brit J Nutr. 2008;99:793–805.
3. Bellows J, Colitz CMH, Daristotle L, Ingram DK, Lepine A, Marks SL, et al. Common physical and functional changes associated with aging in dogs. J Am Vet Med Assoc. 2015;246:67–75.
4. Bellows J, Colitz CMH, Daristotle L, Ingram DK, Lepine A, Marks SL, et al. Defining healthy aging in older dogs and differentiating healthy aging from disease. J Am Vet Med Assoc. 2015;246:77–89.
5. Waters DJ. Aging research: exploring the pet dog paradigm. ILAR J. 2011;52(1):97–105.
6. Michell AR. Longevity of British breeds of dog and its relationships with sex, size, cardiovascular variables and disease. Vet Rec. 1999;145:625–9.
7. Proschowsky HF, Rugbjerg H, ErsbØll AK. Mortality of purebred and mixed-breed dogs in Denmark. Prev Vet Med. 2003;58:63–74.
8. Adams VJ, Evans KM, Sampson J, Wood JLN. Methods and mortality results of a health survey of purebred dogs in the UK. J Sm An Pract. 2010;51:512–24.
9. Kraus C, Pavard S, Promislow DEL. The size-lifespan trade off decomposed: why large dogs die young. Am Nat. 2013;181(4):492–505.
10. Galis F, Van Der Sluijs I, Van Dooren TJM, Metz JAJ, Nussbaumer M. Do large dogs die young? J Exp Zool B Mol Dev Evol. 2007;308B:119–26.
11. Greer KA, Canterberry SC, Murphy KE. Statistical analysis regarding the effects of height and weight on lifespan of the domestic dog. Res Vet Sci. 2007;82:208–14.
12. O'Neill DG, Church DB, McGreevy PD, Thomson PC, Brodbelt DC. Longevity and mortality of owned dogs in England. Vet J. 2013;198:638–43.
13. Moore GE, Burkman KD, Carter MN, Peterson MR. Causes of death or reasons for euthanasia in military working dogs: 927 cases (1993–1996). J Am Vet Med Assoc. 2001;219:209–14.
14. Hoffman J Creevy, Promislow DEL KE. Reproductive Capability is associated with lifespan and cause of death in companion dogs. PLoS One. 2013;8(4):e61082. doi:10.1371/journal.pone.006108.
15. Selman C, Nussey DH, Monaghan P. Ageing: it's a dog's life. Curr Biol. 2013;23:R451–3.
16. Waters DJ, Kengeri SS, Clever B, Booth JA, Maras AH, Schlittler DL, et al. Exploring mechanisms of sex differences in longevity: lifetime ovary exposure and exceptional longevity in dogs. Aging Cell. 2009;8:752–5.
17. Cooley DM, Schlittler DL, Glickman LT, Hayek MG, Waters DJ. Exceptional longevity in pet dogs is accompanied by cancer resistance and delayed onset of major disease. J Geron. 2003;58A(12):1078–84.
18. Kengeri SS, Maras AH, Suckow CL, Chiang EC, Waters DJ. Exceptional longevity in female Rottweiler dogs is not encumbered by investment in reproduction. Age (Dordr). 2013;35:2503–13.
19. Kealy RD, Lawler DF, Ballam JM, Mantz SL, Biery DN, Greeley EH, et al. Effects of diet restriction on lifespan and age-related changes in dogs. J Am Vet Med Assoc. 2002;220:1315–20.
20. Davenport G, Massimino S, Hayek M, Burr J, Ceddia M, Yeh CH, et al. Biological activity of avocado-derived mannoheptulose in dogs. FASEB J. 2010;24(Meeting abstract suppl):725.4.
21. McKnight LL, Flickinger EA, France J, Davenport GM, Shoveller AK. Mannoheptulose has differential effects on fasting and postprandial energy expenditure and respiratory quotient in adult Beagle dogs fed diets of different macronutrient contents. J Nutr Sci. 2014;3:e17.
22. Davenport G, Massimino S, Hayek M, Ceddia M, Burr J, Yeh CH, et al. Bioavailability of avocado-derived mannoheptulose in dogs. FASEB J. 2010;24(Meeting abstract suppl):725.3.
23. Boss N, Holmstrom S, Vogt AH, Jonas L, Krauter E, Moyer M, et al. Development of new canine and feline preventive healthcare guidelines designed to improve pet health (AVMA). J Am Vet Med Assoc. 2011;239:625–9.
24. Case LP, Daristotle L, Hayek MG, Raasch MF. Canine and Feline nutrition: a resource for companion animal professionals. Maryland Heights: Mosby Elsevier; 2011.

25. Kealy RD, Lawler DF, Ballam JM, Lust G, Biery DN, Smith GK, et al. Evaluation of the effect of limited food consumption on radiographic evidence of osteoarthritis in dogs. J Am Vet Med Assoc. 2000;217:1678–80.
26. Lawler DF, Evans RH, Larson BT, Spitznagel EL, Ellersieck MR, Kealy RD. Influence of lifetime food restriction on causes, time, and predictors of death in dogs. J Am Vet Med Assoc. 2005;226:225–31.
27. Schwartz MW, Brunzell JD. Regulation of body adiposity and the problem of obesity. Arterioscler Thromb Vasc Biol. 1997;17:233–8.
28. Barzilai N, Gupta G. Revisiting the role of fat mass in the life extension induced by caloric restriction. J Gerontol A Biol Sci Med Sci. 1999;54:B89–96.
29. Fisler JS. Cardiac effects of starvation and semi starvation diets: safety and mechanisms of action. Am J Clin Nutr. 1992;56:230s–4s.
30. Hansen BC, Bodkin NL, Ortmeyer HK. Calorie restriction in nonhuman primates: mechanism of reduced morbidity and mortality. Toxicol Sci. 1999;52(suppl):56–60.
31. Gresl TA, Colman RJ, Havighurst TC, Byerley LO, Allison DB, Schoeller DA, et al. Insulin sensitivity and glucose effectiveness from three minimal models: effects of energy restriction and body fat in adult male rhesus monkeys. Am J Physiol Regul Integr Comp Physiol. 2003;285:R1340–54.
32. Sohal RS, Forster MJ. Caloric restriction and the aging process: a critique. Free Radic Biol Med. 2014;73:366–82.
33. Weindruch R, Walford RL. The retardation of aging and disease by dietary restriction. Springfield: Thomas; 1988.
34. Warner HR, Fernandes G, Wang E. A unifying hypothesis to explain the retardation of aging and tumorigenesis by caloric restriction. J Gerontol A Biol Sci Med Sci. 1995;50:B107–9.
35. Zoran DL. Obesity in dogs and cats: a metabolic and endocrine disorder. Vet Clin N Am Small Anim Pract. 2010;40:221–39.
36. Freeman LM. Cachexia and sarcopenia: emerging syndromes of importance in dogs and cats. J Vet Intern Med. 2012;26:3–17.
37. Cruz-Jentoft AJ, Baeyens JP, Bauer JM, Boirie Y, Cederholm T, Land F, et al. Sarcopenia: European consensus on definition and diagnosis: report of the European Working Group on sarcopenia in older people. Age Ageing. 2010;39:412–23.
38. Lang T, Streeper T, Cawthon P, Baldwin K, Taffe DR, Harris TB. Sarcopenia: etiology, clinical consequences, intervention, and assessment. Osteoporos Int. 2009;21:543–59.
39. Waters DJ, Kengeri SS, Maras AH, Chiang EC. Probing the perils of dichotomous binning: how categorizing female dogs as spayed or intact can misinform our assumptions about the lifelong health consequences of ovariohysterectomy. Theriogenology. 2011;76:1496–500.
40. Njeh CF, Samat SB, Nightingale A, McNeil EA, Boivin CM. Radiation dose and in vitro precision in paediatric bone mineral density measurement using dual X-ray absorptiometry. Br J Radiol. 1997;70:719–27.
41. Patronek GJ, Waters DJ, Glickman LT. Comparative longevity of pet dogs and humans: implications for gerontology research. J Gerontol A Biol Sci Med Sci. 1997;52:B171–8.
42. Waters DJ. Longevity in pets; understanding what's missing. Vet J. 2014;200:3–5.
43. Anonymous. Summary results of the Purebred Dog Health Survey for Labrador Retrievers. In: report from the Kennel Club/British Small Animal Veterinary Association Scientific Committee. The Kennel Club. 2006. http://www.thekennelclub.org.uk/media/16574/labradorretriever.pdf. Accessed 13 Oct 2015.
44. Herskind AM, McGue M, Holm NV, SØrensen TIA, Harvald B, Vaupel JW. The heritability of human longevity: a population-based study of 2872 Danish twin pairs born 1870–1900. Hum Genet. 1996;97:319–23.
45. Perls TT, Kunkel L, Puca AA. The genetics of exceptional human longevity. J Am Geriatr Soc. 2002;50:359–68.
46. Perls TT. The oldest old. Sci Am. 1995;272:70–5.
47. Vita AJ, Terry RB, Hubert HB, Fries JF. Aging, health risks, and cumulative disability. N Engl J Med. 1998;338:1035–41.
48. Evert J, Lawler E, Bogan H, Perls T. Morbidity profiles of centenarians: survivors, delayers, and escapers. J Geront. 2003;58A(3):232–7.
49. Smith DWE. Cancer mortality at very old age. Cancer. 1996;77:1367–72.

17

Excretory/secretory products of anisakid nematodes: biological and pathological roles

Foojan Mehrdana[*] and Kurt Buchmann

Abstract

Parasites from the family Anisakidae are widely distributed in marine fish populations worldwide and mainly nematodes of the three genera *Anisakis, Pseudoterranova* and *Contracaecum* have attracted attention due to their pathogenicity in humans. Their life cycles include invertebrates and fish as intermediate or transport hosts and mammals or birds as final hosts. Human consumption of raw or underprocessed seafood containing third stage larvae of anisakid parasites may elicit a gastrointestinal disease (anisakidosis) and allergic responses. Excretory and secretory (ES) compounds produced by the parasites are assumed to be key players in clinical manifestation of the disease in humans, but the molecules are likely to play a general biological role in invertebrates and lower vertebrates as well. ES products have several functions during infection, e.g. penetration of host tissues and evasion of host immune responses, but are at the same time known to elicit immune responses (including antibody production) both in fish and mammals. ES proteins from anisakid nematodes, in particular *Anisakis simplex*, are currently applied for diagnostic purposes but recent evidence suggests that they also may have a therapeutic potential in immune-related diseases.

Keywords: Allergy, Anisakidosis, Anisakids, Excretory/secretory products

Background

Anisakid nematode larvae of the genera *Anisakis, Pseudoterranova,* and *Contracaecum* (family: Anisakidae; superfamily: Ascaridoidea; order: Ascaridida) are common parasites in a variety of marine fish species worldwide (Table 1). Different species of these parasites have been recognized, while some of them include sibling species within a particular morphospecies, e.g. *Contracaecum osculatum* complex [A, B, C, D, and E] [1], *Anisakis simplex* s.l. [*A. simplex* sensu stricto (s.s.), *A. berlandi* (formerly termed *A. simplex* sp. C) and *A. pegreffii*] [2, 3], and *Pseudoterranova decipiens* complex [*P. decipiens* (sensu stricto), *P. krabbei*, *P. bulbosa* (previously termed *P. decipiens* C) and *P. azarasi* (formerly termed *P. decipiens* D)] [4, 5]. Infection with these parasites is considered a threat to public health due to their zoonotic potential, and the presence of larvae in fish products reduces their commercial value. Free or encapsulated larvae are present within the body cavity, in the visceral organs or in the musculature of the fish host [6] whereby larvae may accidentally be ingested by consumers. The term anisakidosis refers to the disease in humans caused by any member of the family Anisakidae, whereas anisakiasis (or anisakiosis) is specifically caused by members of the genus *Anisakis*, pseudoterranoviasis (or pseudoterranovosis) by the genus *Pseudoterranova* [7, 8] and contracaeciasis (or contracaecosis) is caused by members of the genus *Contracaecum* [9]. Recent studies have revealed that a series of allergens in *Anisakis* play a major role in the progression and clinical picture of the disease. These allergens are a part of a rich series of excretory and secretory (ES) worm products, which may play profound biological roles in the life cycle of these helminths. Research on anisakid ES products has so far mainly focused on *Anisakis* spp., in particular *A. simplex*, owing to its frequent occurrence and cause of anisakiasis. In the present work, we review the biological and pathological role of anisakid ES products with a main focus on the compounds released from the genus *Anisakis*.

Search strategy

A literature search was conducted in PubMed (http://www.ncbi.nlm.nih.gov/pubmed) and ScienceDirect (http://www.sciencedirect.com) using the terms "excretory and

*Correspondence: foojan@sund.ku.dk
Laboratory of Aquatic Pathobiology, Department of Veterinary and Animal Sciences, Faculty of Health and Medical Sciences, University of Copenhagen, 1870 Frederiksberg C, Denmark

Table 1 Occurrence of anisakids in fish and humans worldwide

Location	Recorded parasites			Disease form	Ab(s)	Allergen(s) detected	References
	Anisakis simplex s.l.	*Pseudoterranova decipiens*	*Contracaecum* sp.				
Spain	+/++	++	+	GA, IA, GAL, AL	mAb UA3 mAb mouse anti-human IgE Rabbit anti-human IgE Goat anti-human IgE	Ani s 1, Ani s 3, Ani s 4, Ani s 5, Ani s 7, Ani s 8, Ani s 9, Ani s 10, Ani s troponin	[54, 62, 64, 65, 68, 69, 75, 76, 77, 85, 86, 94, 115, 120, 121, 148, 149*, 150, 151, 152*, 153*, 154]
Italy	++	++	–	GA, IA, GAL, AL	Goat anti-human IgE mAb mouse anti-human IgE	Ani s 1, Ani s 4, Ani s 5, Ani s 9, Ani s 10	[23, 24, 105, 116, 155, 156]
Norway	+/++	+	+	AL	mAb mouse anti-human IgE	Ani s 1, Ani s 7	[122, 157*, 158*, 159*]
Denmark	+/++	+	+	IA	–	–	[146*, 160, 161*, 162*]
Sweden	–	+	–		–	–	[163*]
Iceland	–	++	–	GA	–	–	[31]
Germany	++	–	++	GA, GIA	–	–	[27, 164]
Netherlands	++	–	–	GA	–	–	[165]
Poland	+	+	+		–	–	[147*]
Croatia	++	–	–	AL	NA	Ani s 1, Ani s 7	[166]
Portugal	+	–	–		–	–	[167*]
France	++	–	–	GIA	–	–	[168]
Japan	+/++	++	+/++	GA, AL	Goat anti-human IgE	Ani s 8, Ani s 9, Ani s 11, Ani s 12	[29, 57, 66, 83, 169, 170*, 171*]
Korea	++	++	–	GA, GIA, AL, GAL	NA	NA	[21, 25, 89, 172, 173]
Taiwan	++	–	–	GA	–	–	[129]
Canada	++	+	–	IA	–	–	[174*, 175]
USA	++	++	+	GA, IA	–	–	[176, 177, 178*]
Brazil	+	+	+		HRP-mouse anti-human IgE	NA	[179, 180*, 181*]
Chile	+	+/++	–	GA	–	–	[26, 182*, 183]
Argentina	–	–	+		–	–	[184*]
Australia	+	–	+/++	GIA	–	–	[28, 185*]
Egypt	+	+	+		–	–	[6*]
South Africa	++	–	–	AL	NA	NA	[52]

+ infection recorded in fish, ++ infection recorded in humans, *Asterisk sign* (*) studies reporting on occurrence of the parasites in fish populations, *GA* gastric anisakidosis, *IA* intestinal anisakidosis, *GIA* gastrointestinal anisakidosis, *AL* allergy, *GAL* gastro-allergic anisakiasis, *NA* not available, *Ab(s)* antibodies used for *Anisakis*-specific IgE detection in patients sera secretory products" AND "allergy" OR "anisakidosis" combined with anisakid parasites names *"Anisakis"* OR *"Pseudoterranova"* OR *"Contracaecum"*. The title and abstract of resulted hits were evaluated and the most relevant articles were assessed in detail. Our own archives were also used as an additional source of information. The papers included in this systematic review have been published between 1960 and 2016.

General biology of anisakids

The life cycles of anisakid nematodes comprise adult worms in marine mammals, e.g. seals, sea lions, dolphins, whales [7, 10, 11] and/or piscivorous birds [12–14] and hatched larvae which are free-living until they are ingested by an invertebrate host (e.g. a crustacean) whereafter they are transferred to a teleost transport host by predation. Humans act only as accidental hosts for anisakids. They obtain infection through consumption of raw or underprocessed seafood, but the nematodes do not reach the adult stage in humans whereby human hosts cannot transmit the infection further by releasing parasite eggs with feces. In contrast, marine mammalian hosts (pinnipeds and cetaceans) allow maturation of the anisakid worms in their gastrointestinal tract. Following copulation between adult male and female worms, parasite eggs are released by the adult female worm and leave the host with faeces to the marine environment where they develop and subsequently hatch [15]. The released free third stage larvae (L3) become ingested by the first invertebrate hosts (including crustaceans, cephalopods and polychaetes) in which they reach extra-intestinal sites such as the hemocoel, a process which must involve enzymatic activity. Following ingestion by the fish, the worm larvae penetrate the fish gut and reach internal organs such as body cavity, viscera or musculature. The fish host range depends to some extent on the anisakid species [2, 13, 16] but their geographical distribution is also limited by the availability of the intermediate and final hosts [17]. Therefore, the presence of the parasite in a host implies the co-presence of all the required host species for completing the parasitic life cycle at the same time in the same area and indicates that ES genes encoding products needed for all steps in the life cycle are present in that particular strain of the parasite [18].

Human infections

Humans are accidental hosts of anisakid parasites, and acquire L3 through consumption of raw or inadequately processed seafood. Ingestion may cause anisakidosis, which is manifested by distinct gastrointestinal symptoms, e.g. vomiting, diarrhoea, and epigastric pain [19, 20]. *Anisakis simplex* s.s. (Rudolphi, 1809) is the most frequently reported causative agent for anisakiasis [8] but recently *Anisakis pegreffii* was reported to cause anisakiasis in the Republic of Korea [21], Croatia [22], and Italy [23, 24]. Infections caused by *P. decipiens* (Krabbe, 1878) [25, 26] and *C. osculatum* (Rudolphi, 1802) [27–29] have been reported at a lower frequency (Table 1). Infections with *Pseudoterranova* may in certain cases cause asymptomatic infections and come to medical attention only when worms are recovered following vomiting, coughing or defecating [30, 31]. The few cases of contracaeciasis reported severe abdominal pain associated with the infection [27, 28].

Production of ES compounds

During all stages of the life cycle, nematodes produce and release a series of excretory and secretory molecules (ES compounds) which may be key players in parasite-host interactions including host-specificity. However, this does not necessarily mean that the composition of compounds or the individual molecules are identical at all stages [32]. It may be suggested that production of ES compounds in the third stage larvae varies (quantitatively and qualitatively) depending on the type of host (crustaceans, fish and mammals) due to the different structural and physiological conditions in these host groups. The habitat of poikilothermic organisms, such as crustaceans and fish, may reach near zero degree in certain marine areas whereas marine mammals are homoiothermic animals with body temperatures near 40 °C, which challenges the temperature optima of enzymatic systems differently. Thus, the temperature-dependent production of ES compounds in *Anisakis* was shown by Bahlool et al. [33]. In addition, the chemical interactions (such as receptor-ligand binding) between host and parasite must differ due to conformational changes of proteins at different temperatures. A number of genes encoding central immune factors have been partly conserved throughout evolution from invertebrates via fish to mammals, but the variation is high [34, 35] and thereby it should be expected that host evasion mechanisms in different animal groups differ. It has also been suggested that differences among life cycles of different parasite species and even sibling species [11, 36] may be attributed to the relative abundance and function of these bioactive molecules influencing host specificity [37].

Biochemical composition of ES products

The ES molecules can be released from parasite organs including glands, oesophagus, ventricle, intestine and outer surfaces. In the final host, adult male and female worms mate and it is believed that during this phase chemical communication occurs between sexes which may add sex pheromones to the list of possible ES products. At all stages various enzyme activities have been associated with the released materials. Enzymes serving a basic metabolic role in the parasite, acid and alkaline phosphatases are found [33] and together with enzymes connected to infectivity, immune evasion and pathogenicity (proteases, nucleotidases, esterases, glycases, dismutases) they may serve roles at all life cycle stages. However, no studies have as yet been presented showing the action of ES products in invertebrate hosts and it cannot be excluded that different isotypes are expressed to different degrees in intermediate and final hosts. It is known that hydrolytic enzymes enable the worm to penetrate and migrate in fish tissues [33] and several other functions have also been suggested for secreted proteins from nematodes. For example, some anticoagulant activities are recorded from larval *A. simplex* ES products causing prolongation of partial thromboplastin time (PTT) which may have a key role in human anisakiasis regarding larval penetration into the gastrointestinal mucosa [38]. Moreover, a number of ES compounds from *A. simplex* larvae ranging from 66 to 95 kDa may have a cytostatic inhibitory effect on lymphocyte blastogenesis [39]. Acetylcholinesterase (AChE) released by some gastrointestinal nematodes may play an important role in altering permeability of host intestinal cells to secure parasite feeding and therefore survival. This enzyme may also adversely affect coagulation and glycogenesis in the host [40]. Podolska and Nadolna [41] speculated that increased secretion of AChE from *A. simplex* larvae in herring should be considered an adaptive response to neurotoxic compounds released by the host. In general, nematode secretions have immunomodulatory effects interfering with host immune responses. AChE, glutathione-*S*-transferase (GST), and superoxide dismutase (SOD) secreted by the hookworm *Necator americanus* are known to suppress host inflammatory responses [42]. This is in line with secreted AChE from the filarial nematode *Wuchereria bancrofti* where the suppressive effect is due to degradation of acetylcholine, a neurotransmitter, which is responsible for releasing lysosomal enzymes and phagocytosis in the host [43]. AChE produced by the ruminant nematodes *Ostertagia* and *Haemonchus* has been assumed to affect host responses by controlling gastric acid secretion [40]. GST has been identified in secretions from the swimbladder nematode *Anguillicoloides crassus* in European eels and its function was suggested to quench reactive oxygen radicals released as part of the host innate responses toward the infection [44]. Proteolytic enzymes produced by *A. simplex* larvae are likely to target central proteins in the teleost immune system, e.g. antibodies and complement factors, and thereby enhance the parasite survival in the fish [33].

Future proteomic studies are likely to extend the list of annotated molecules in the ES molecule mixture of anisakids but it may be worthwhile to search molecules already described from a range of parasites (see the review [37]). Thus, apart from a range of enzymes and antioxidants, functional effector molecules including protease inhibitors, lectins, heat shock proteins, mucins and cytokine regulators may be detected.

Immunogenicity of ES products

Many of the *A. simplex* ES molecules are highly immunogenic and can provoke antibody production both in fish and mammals. Serum obtained from infected saithe (*Pollachius virens*) were found to react with larval *A. simplex* molecules in an enzyme linked immunosorbent assay (ELISA) [45], and specific antibodies from European eel (*Anguilla anguilla*) reacting against GST in ES isolated from *A. crassus* were detected by western blotting [44]. ES molecules in other anisakid larvae have not been studied to the same extent, but several proteins from *Contracaecum* species have been isolated and shown to elicit a humoral response in Antarctic teleosts [46]. Seals also produce antibodies with affinity to anisakid antigens. In a study focusing on seal serum antibody reactivity against the adult lungworm *Otostrongylus circumlitus*, it was found that the sera also reacted with whole body extract of other nematodes including *Pseudoterranova* sp. and *Anisakis* sp. [47]. This corresponds to the well-studied antibody production in mammals against nematode antigens, which even has been found associated with protective immunity [48, 49]. The humoral immune reactions against ES products from *A. simplex* in accidentally infected humans have been intensely investigated. Several immunoglobulin classes may be involved, but worm specific IgE has attracted considerable interest because it is associated with disease progression and allergic responses to the parasite.

Allergenicity of ES products

Symptoms associated with anisakid nematode larvae present in human tissues may—at least in some cases—be due to allergic responses. Allergens in *A. simplex* comprise both somatic antigens (SA) and ES molecules and several have been shown to be resistant to various freeze-, heat- and digestive processes. It is believed, based on empirical data, that allergy towards *A. simplex* must be induced by an active infection by a live worm but then subsequent exposure to allergens including ES products is sufficient to elicit an allergic response [50]. However, ingestion of larvae is not the only possibility to acquire anisakid-related disease. Occupational exposure to the parasitized fish containing anisakid allergens can elicit allergic reactions, e.g. bronchial hyperreactivity and dermatitis [51–53].

Anisakis allergens

Anisakis simplex has so far been described as the only anisakid parasite responsible for allergic reactions in humans. Different groups of allergenic molecules have been isolated from L3 larvae; (1) ES proteins secreted by the parasite, (2) SA of the larval organs, and (3) cuticular proteins [8]. Allergenic proteins (Ani s1 to Ani s12, Ani s 13, Ani s 14, Ani s 24 kDa, Ani s CCOS3, Ani s cytochrome B, Ani s FBPP, Ani s NADHDS4L, Ani s NARaS, Ani s PEPB, and Ani s troponin) have been described in *A. simplex*, of which Ani s 1, Ani s 2, Ani s 7, Ani s 12, Ani s 13, Ani s 14, and an Ani S 11-like protein (Ani s 11.0201) are identified as major allergens [54–60]. Allergens Ani s 7 and Ani s 10–12 are still uncharacterized with unknown functions [54]. A number of putative novel allergens (cyclophilin and two proteins with unknown function) have recently been characterized for the first time from *A. simplex* transcriptomes by comparing predicted amino acid sequences with homologous known allergenic proteins [61]. In general, *A. simplex* ES allergens are known to be more potent which could be a result of their higher affinity to specific IgE compared to the somatic antigens [62].

Allergen persistence

Despite the fact that anisakid larvae lose their infectivity by adequate food preparation, it should be noted that parasite allergens (SA or ES products) may be resistant to heat, freezing, and pepsin (Ani s 1, Ani s 4, Ani s 5, Ani s 8, Ani s 9, Ani s 10, Ani s 11.0201) as they preserve the antigenicity and may trigger allergic responses in sensitized persons following consumption of well-cooked or canned fish [60, 63–70].

Allergen cross-reactivity

IgE raised in patients against SA and ES antigens of *A. simplex* may cross-react with homologous antigens of other ascarid nematodes (e.g. *Ascaris suum, Ascaris lumbricoides, Toxocara canis, Hysterothylacium aduncum*), or arthropods (German cockroach, chironomids) [71–73]. However, somatic proteins are more likely to cross-react, while ES antigens are more specific. For example, Ani s 2 (paramyosin, a somatic antigen) has been shown to have high similarity and, therefore, high degree of cross-reactivity with some dust mites, e.g. *Acarus siro* and *Tyrophagus putrescentiae.* Ani s 3 (tropomyosin), another somatic allergen, is also suggested to have the potential to cross-react with molecules from crustaceans, e.g. *Homarus americanus* (American lobster), and *Metapenaeus ensis* (greasyback shrimp), molluscs, e.g. *Perna viridis* (green mussel), and *Crassostrea gigas* (giant Pacific oyster), and also with the insect American cockroach (*Periplaneta americana*) [74]. The allergen Ani s 1, an ES protein, is generally considered to have no cross-reaction with other allergens, which make it a suitable candidate for diagnosis of hypersensitivity and intestinal anisakiasis [75, 76]. Using this allergen along with Ani s 4 has been shown to achieve a diagnostic sensitivity of 95% by IgE immunoblotting [77]. Further precision of diagnosis may be achieved if combined with detection of Ani s 5, another ES antigen, which also has demonstrated its utility for serodiagnosis of the *Anisakis* larvae sensitization [68].

Allergens in other anisakids

The allergenic potential of other anisakids, e.g. *P. decipiens,* molecules has not been studied to the same extent as *A. simplex.* A number of somatic antigens in *C. osculatum* larvae have been isolated with the molecular weight of 47, 63, and mainly 91 kDa [46], but a recent study using experimental infection of mice with live *Contracaecum* sp. larvae did not show IgG or IgE antibody responses specific to SA or ES antigens [78]. However, the *Contracaecum* body structure and migratory strategy in the fish host are partly similar to those of *Anisakis* larvae [79] suggesting that further genomic and proteomic analysis of SA and ES molecules of *Contracaecum* L3 should be conducted.

Pathology and ES products

Pathological changes associated with anisakidosis may result from the direct tissue invasion by the larva into the gastric or intestinal mucosa, but immunological reactions (cellular and humoral) towards worm constituents are likely to play a major role. It has been suggested that the parasite pathogenicity may vary among closely related species and geographic strains [80–82] which may at least partly explain differential occurrence of disease. In addition, the infection dosage may be expected to influence the host reaction. In many cases of anisakidosis a single larva is responsible for infection. However, a total of 56 *A. simplex* larvae were recovered in a patient in Japan [83], and another human case in Spain was diagnosed infected with more than 200 *A. simplex* larvae accumulated in the gastric mucosa [84].

Clinical symptoms are partly connected to allergic reactions involving IgE-mediated hypersensitivity with resulting acute urticaria, angioedema, and anaphylaxis occasionally accompanied by gastroallergic anisakidosis [8, 85–89]. However, specific anti-*Anisakis* IgE is still detectable in patients over the years after the allergic episodes with a declining trend [90].

Cellular reactions with partial remodeling of tissues involving infiltration with macrophages, eosinophils, mast cells, neutrophils and lymphocytes at the penetration site are known to occur both in fish and pigs [33, 91]. Furthermore, in a recent in vitro study exposure of human fibroblast cell line HS-68 to *A. pegreffii* ES compounds led to elevation in reactive oxygen species (ROS) levels causing oxidative stress and also activation of kinases and subsequent inflammation, cell proliferation, inhibition of apoptosis and DNA damage [92].

In the case of invasive anisakidosis, ulcerations and hemorrhages are found in the intestinal or stomach wall. Even if worm larvae die in the human host, it should be noted that antigens released from the remains of the worm may induce inflammatory responses eliciting symptoms which cannot be differentiated from other disorders, e.g. cholecystitis, neoplasia, gastritis, peritonitis [93], appendicitis [94], eosinophilic gastroenteritis, and Crohn's disease [95].

Diagnosis and ES products

Diagnosis of anisakidosis initially relies on a detailed history of recent seafood consumption and may be confirmed by direct visualization and examination of the larvae. Removal of the worm by endoscopy/colonoscopy [96] or surgery [97] allows concurrent diagnosis and treatment of gastric/intestinal form of the disease, but non-invasive methods such as sonography and X-ray have also been proven as valuable diagnostic tools [98–100]. Haematological evaluations may show leukocytosis, e.g. mild to moderate eosinophilia, and mast-cell degranulation [93, 101, 102]. Diagnosis of anisakiasis can be conducted with serologic tests which are partly based on reactions towards ES products of the worm. ELISA, IgE immunoblotting and ImmunoCAP can detect *Anisakis*-specific IgE reactivity to a complete extract of *Anisakis* L3 larvae which supports diagnosis of intestinal and allergic diseases [75, 103–105]. However, interpretation of results may not be clear-cut due to cross-reactivity of the *A. simplex* antigens with other antigens such as products from *Ascaris* spp., *T. canis*, insects (cockroaches) or crustaceans (shrimps) and care should be taken to omit false-positive serology results [106–108]. Since it has been shown that detection of specific IgG4 raised in the infected human host against *A. simplex* is likely to be more specific than specific IgE in diagnosis of gastro-allergic anisakiasis [88, 109], detection of this Ig subclass is relevant to include in serological tests. Flow cytometry has also been applied as a tool for diagnosing allergy to *Anisakis* products activating basophils [110]. Skin prick tests (SPTs), inserting *Anisakis* products into the skin of the patient, may assist diagnosis of the allergic form of the disease mediated by cellular immune responses, but the test has a low specificity and high rate of false positives due to cross reactivity with other allergens from seafood and mites [111], and from *A. lumbricoides* [112, 113]. This frames the necessity of improving diagnostic kits based on specific *Anisakis* antigens, e.g. purified natural or recombinant allergens [114–116] and has accelerated immunoscreening of protein-expressing cDNA libraries [117], phage display system [118], and mass spectrometry-based proteomics [54] to identify novel allergen candidates.

It has been shown that the application of recombinant allergens of *A. simplex*, expressed in *Escherichia coli* or *Pichia pastoris*, can improve diagnostic assays by increasing specificity and avoid misdiagnosis caused by cross-reactions [115]. Measuring IgE reactivity to recombinant Ani s 1 (rAni s 1) and Ani s 7 (rAni s 7) allergens has been suggested as the most efficient serodiagnostic means for anisakiasis, when combining sensitivity and specificity. However, Ani s 1 is considered the major allergen in gastro-allergic anisakiasis, while Ani s 7 can be recognized independently of the amount of specific IgE production, i.e. in the case of chronic urticaria with lower serum specific IgE values [119, 120]. Furthermore, an internal fragment of the rAni s 7 (435Met-713Arg), known as t-Ani s 7, is shown to have the potential to improve serodiagnostic specificity [121]. In a recent survey of two groups of subjects in Norway, including recruited blood donors (BDO) and patients with total IgE levels $\geq$1000 kU/l (IGE+), the prevalence of anti-*Anisakis* IgE antibodies was 0.4 and 16.2% in the BDO and IGE+ groups, respectively. However, further analyses of *Anisakis* positive sera by ELISA against recombinant allergens rAni s 1 and rAni s 7 showed a seroprevalence of 0.0 and 0.2%, respectively, and it cannot be excluded that false-positivity occurs due to cross-reactivity to other allergens such as shrimp and house dust mite [122]. Gamboa et al. [123] also emphasized the value of rAni s 1 for diagnosing allergy to *Anisakis* both in vivo (SPT) and in vitro [specific IgE and basophil activation test (BAT)]. Both natural and recombinant Ani s 10 have also shown positive reactivity with 39% of *Anisakis*-allergic patients' sera [69]. Besides high specificity, there are other advantages using recombinant allergens. For example, the yield of purified recombinant *Anisakis* proteins from bacterial cultures is higher compared to the yield of the natural protein from *Anisakis* larvae, while they show equivalent immunochemical properties [124, 125]. Asturias et al. [126] reported a high yield of 6.6 mg/L culture of a purified recombinant tropomyosin from *A. simplex* (*As*-TPM), whereas the final yield of the purified natural *As*-TPM was only 0.36 mg/g of *Anisakis* larvae, which advocates for inclusion of recombinant allergens in allergy diagnostic tests.

Treatment and ES products

There is no standard medication available to treat anisakiasis. However, benzimidazoles such as the anthelmintic albendazole (400–800 mg daily for 6–21 days) have been suggested as a possible therapy [127–129]. It has also been shown that administration of corticosteroids like 6-methylprednisolone (1 mg/kg/24 h for 5 days) may be a useful option to treat the acute intestinal anisakiasis as an alternative to surgical resection [130]. Moreover, prednisolone (5 mg/day for 10 days) and olopatadine hydrochloride (10 mg/day for 6 weeks) have demonstrated promising results to resolve intestinal anisakiasis symptoms [100].

In addition, novel treatment options are likely to follow. Thus, in vitro studies on larvicidal activities of natural terpenes, e.g. geraniol, citronella essential oil, and tea tree essential oil [131, 132], *Matricaria chamomilla* essential oil (including α-bisabolol) and in vivo work on administration of the aldehydic monoterpene citral and the alcoholic citronellol suggested that these compounds may be effective against infections caused by *A. simplex* and/or *Contracaecum* sp. [133–136]. Medical treatment leading to killing worm larvae in tissues may result in significant release of worm antigens (SA and/or ES products) which could exacerbate disease symptoms and it may be necessary to combine treatment with immune-moderating drugs such as corticosteroids.

Therapeutic potential of anisakid molecules

Ascarid nematode larvae carry genes encoding various immunoregulatory products which ensure the survival of the parasite in the host immune environment [137, 138] and ES products of anisakids are expected to have similar properties. In a mouse experimental model of asthma, induced by an *A. suum* allergen (APAS-3), it was shown that an ES protein, PAS-1, could reduce Th2 responses, inhibit cellular migration, suppress cytokine expression (IL-4, IL-5), and reduce chemokine production in bronchoalveolar lavage (BAL) fluid [139]. Similarly, PAS-1 has in a mouse model been shown to have an inhibitory effect (probably mediated by IL-10 and TGF-β secretion) on *E. coli* LPS (lipopolysaccharide)-induced inflammation via suppression of TNF-α, IL-1β and IL-6 [140, 141]. Lung allergic inflammation in mice induced by ovalbumin (OVA) was inhibited by PAS-1 immunization mediated by stimulation of IL-10 and IFN-γ production and subsequent suppression of cytokine and antibody reactions [142, 143]. An anaphylactic immune response to peanut in a mouse model has also been inhibited partially by *A. simplex* or *A. lumbricoides* somatic extracts through reduction of specific IgG1 and subsequently inhibition of anaphylactic symptoms score [144]. It was also shown by Bahlool et al. [33] that *Anisakis* ES compounds decreased expression of genes encoding inflammatory cytokines. In addition, a recent study has demonstrated immunoregulatory effects of *A. simplex* ES antigens in a colitis zebrafish model [145]. These findings suggest that by appropriate biochemical techniques the immunoregulatory potential of anisakid ES molecules may be further characterized and exploited for prevention and/or treatment of inflammatory diseases.

Conclusion and perspectives

Increasing population of anisakid final hosts (marine mammals) and thereby their endoparasitic anisakid nematodes may lead to elevated infection levels in fish [146, 147]. This may together with the increasing trend of raw or undercooked seafood consumption explain increasing occurrence of anisakidosis and infection-induced allergies. ES products released by the anisakid nematodes have been shown to play a central role not only in the general biology of the parasite but also in human disease. Some ES products elicit allergic responses in humans but as in other helminths, other ES products may modify host immunity and suppress immune responses which open alternative usage of anisakid parasite products as therapeutics. In this review, we have focused on *A. simplex* allergens and the associated allergy, since our current knowledge is mainly limited to this species. The immunomodulatory activities of other relevant anisakids, particularly *P. decipiens* and *C. osculatum*, are still inadequately described and further investigations using in vitro and in vivo techniques are necessary to identify the allergenic or immunosuppressive properties of anisakid-originated components and elucidate the mechanisms involved in immunoregulations.

Abbreviations

AChE: acetylcholinesterase; As-TPM: *Anisakis simplex* tropomyosin; BAL: bronchoalveolar lavage; BAT: basophil activation test; BDO: blood donors; ELISA: enzyme linked immunosorbent assay; ES: excretory and secretory; GST: glutathione-S-transferase; L3: third stage larvae; LPS: lipopolysaccharide; OVA: ovalbumin; PTT: partial thromboplastin time; rAni s 1: recombinant Ani s 1; ROS: reactive oxygen species; SA: somatic antigens; SOD: superoxide dismutase; SPT: skin prick test.

Authors' contributions

FM drafted the manuscript. KB shared his valuable comments and finalized the manuscript structure and contents. Both authors read and approved the final manuscript.

Authors' information

KB is a professor in fish pathobiology investigating infectious diseases in fish with a particular focus on parasitic infections and fish–parasite interactions. FM is a Ph.D. candidate investigating zoonotic parasites in fish for the last 6 years and is the author of six original publications and a review in this field together with KB.

Acknowledgements

This study was supported by the European Union's Horizon 2020 research and innovation programme through the Grant Agreement No. 634429 (ParaFishControl).

Competing interests

Both authors declare that they have no competing interests.

Funding

This study has received funding from the European Union's Horizon 2020 research and innovation programme under Grant Agreement No. 634429 (ParaFishControl). This output reflects only the authors' view and the European Union cannot be held responsible for any use that may be made of the information contained herein.

References

1. Orecchia P, Mattiucci S, D'Amelio S, Paggi L, Plötz J, Cianchi R, Nascetti G, Arduino P, Bullini L. Two new members in the *Contracaecum osculatum* complex (Nematoda, Ascaridoidea) from the Antarctic. Int J Parasitol. 1994;24:367–77.
2. Mattiucci S, Nascetti G, Clanchi R, Paggi L, Arduino P, Margolis L, Brattey J, Webb S, D'Amelio S, Orecchia P, Bullini L. Genetic and ecological data on the *Anisakis simplex* complex, with evidence for a new species (Nematoda, Ascaridoidea, Anisakidae). J Parasitol. 1997;83:401–16.
3. Mattiucci S, Cipriani P, Webb SC, Paoletti M, Marcer F, Bellisario B, Gibson DI, Nascetti G. Genetic and morphological approaches distinguish the three sibling species of the *Anisakis simplex* species complex, with a species designation as *Anisakis berlandi* n. sp. for *A. simplex* sp. C (Nematoda: Anisakidae). J Parasitol. 2014;100:199–214.
4. Mattiucci S, Paggi L, Nascetti G, Ishikura H, Kikuchi K, Sato N, Cianchi R, Bullini L. Allozyme and morphological identification of *Anisakis*, *Contracaecum* and *Pseudoterranova* from Japanese waters (Nematoda, Ascaridoidea). Syst Parasitol. 1998;40:81–92.
5. Paggi L, Mattiucci S, Gibson DI, Berland B, Nascetti G, Cianchi R, Bullini L. *Pseudoterranova decipiens* species A and B (Nematoda, Ascaridoidea): nomenclatural designation, morphological diagnostic characters and genetic markers. Syst Parasitol. 2000;45:185–97.
6. El-Asely AM, El Madawy RS, El Tanany MA, Afify GS. Prevalence and molecular characterization of anisakidosis in both European (*Merluccius merluccius*) and lizard head (*Saurida undosquamis*) hakes. GSTF J Vet. 2015;1(2). doi:10.7603/s40871-014-0001-8.
7. Margolis L. Public health aspects of "codworm" infection: a review. J Fish Res Board Can. 1977;34:887–98.
8. Audicana MT, Kennedy MW. *Anisakis simplex*: from obscure infectious worm to inducer of immune hypersensitivity. Clin Microbiol Rev. 2008;21:360–79.
9. Buchmann K, Mehrdana F. Effects of anisakid nematodes *Anisakis simplex* (s.l.), *Pseudoterranova decipiens* (s.l.) and *Contracaecum osculatum* (s.l.) on fish and consumer health. FAWPAR. 2016;4:13–22.
10. Ishikura H, Kikuchi K, Nagasawa K, Ooiwa T, Takamiya H, Sato N, Sugane K. Anisakidae and anisakidosis. In: Sun T, editor. Progress in clinical parasitology, vol. 3. New york: Springer; 1993. p. 43–102.
11. Skrzypczak M, Rokicki J, Pawliczka I, Najda K, Dzido J. Anisakids of seals found on the Southern coast of Baltic Sea. Acta Parasitol. 2014;59:165–72.
12. Barus V, Sergeeva TP, Sonin MD, Ryzhikov KM. Nematoda. In: Rysavy B, Ryzhikov KM, editors. Helminths of fish-eating birds of the palearctic region. Moscow: USSR Academy of Sciences; 1978.
13. Anderson RC. Nematode parasites of vertebrates: their development and transmission, Chapter 5: order Ascaridida. Wallingford, Oxfordshire, England: CABI; 2000. p. 270-88.
14. Sanmartín ML, Cordeiro JA, Alvarez MF, Leiro J. Helminth fauna of the yellow-legged gull *Larus cachinnans* in Galicia, Northwest Spain. J Helminthol. 2005;79:361–71.
15. Køie M, Fagerholm HP. The life cycle of *Contracaecum osculatum* (Rudolphi, 1802) sensu stricto (Nematoda, Ascaridoidea, Anisakidae) in view of experimental infections. Parasitol Res. 1995;81:481–9.
16. Paggi L, Nascetti G, Cianchi R, Orecchia P, Mattiucci M, D'Amelio S, Berland B, Brattey J, Smith JW, Bullini L. Genetic evidence for three species within *Pseudoterranova decipiens* (Nematoda, Ascaridida, Ascaridoidea) in the North Atlantic and Norwegian and Barents Seas. Int J Parasitol. 1991;21:195–212.
17. Mattiucci S, Nascetti G. Advances and trends in the molecular systematics of anisakid nematodes, with implications for their evolutionary ecology and host-parasite co-evolutionary process. Adv Parasitol. 2008;66:47–148.
18. Culurgioni J, Figus V, Cabiddu S, De Murtas R, Cau A, Sabatini A. Larval helminth parasites of fishes and shellfishes from Santa Gilla lagoon (Sardinia, Western Mediterranean), and their use as bioecological indicators. Estuaries Coasts. 2015;38:1505–19.
19. Chai YL, Murrel KD, Lymbery AJ. Fish-born parasitic zoonoses: status and issues. Int J Parasitol. 2005;35:1233–54.
20. Dorny P, Praet N, Deckers N, Gabriel S. Emerging food-borne parasites. Vet Parasitol. 2009;163:196–206.
21. Lim H, Jung BK, Cho J, Yooyen T, Shin EH, Chai JY. Molecular diagnosis of cause of anisakiasis in humans, South Korea. Emerg Infect Dis. 2015;21:342–4.
22. Mladineo I, Popović M, Drmić-Hofman I, Poljak V. A case report of *Anisakis pegreffii* (Nematoda, Anisakidae) identified from archival paraffin sections of a Croatian patient. BMC Infect Dis. 2016;16:42.
23. Fumarola L, Monno R, Ierardi E, Rizzo G, Giannelli G, Lalle M, Pozio E. *Anisakis pegreffi* etiological agent of gastric infections in two Italian women. Foodborne Pathog Dis. 2009;6:1157–9.
24. Mattiucci S, Paoletti M, Borrini F, Palumbo M, Palmieri RM, Gomes V, Casati A, Nascetti G. First molecular identification of the zoonotic parasite *Anisakis pegreffii* (Nematoda: Anisakidae) in a paraffin-embedded granuloma taken from a case of human intestinal anisakiasis in Italy. BMC Infect Dis. 2011;11:82.
25. Yu JR, Seo M, Kim YW, Oh MH, Sohn WM. A human case of gastric infection by *Pseudoterranova decipiens* larva. Korean J Parasitol. 2001;39:193–6.
26. Torres P, Jercic MI, Weitz JC, Dobrew EK, Mercado RA. Human pseudoterranovosis, an emerging infection in Chile. J Parasitol. 2007;93:440–3.
27. Schaum E, Müller W. Heterocheilidiasis (case report). DMW. 1967;92:2230–3.
28. Shamsi S, Butcher AR. First report of human anisakidosis in Australia. MJA. 2011;194:199–200.
29. Nagasawa K. The biology of *Contracaecum osculatum* sensu lato and *C. osculatum* A (Nematoda: Anisakidae) in Japanese waters: a review. Biosph Sci. 2012;51:61–9.
30. McCarthy J, Moore TA. Emerging helminth zoonoses. Int J Parasitol. 2000;30:1351–60.
31. Skirnisson K. *Pseudoterranova decipiens* (Nematoda, Anisakidae) larvae reported from humans in Iceland after consumption of insufficiently cooked fish. Laeknabladid. 2006;92:21–5 **(in Icelandic)**.
32. Kim JS, Kim KH, Cho S, Park HY, Cho SW, Kim YT, Joo KH, Lee JS. Immunochemical and biological analysis of allergenicity with excretory-secretory products of *Anisakis simplex* third stage larva. Int Arch Allergy Immunol. 2005;136:320–8.
33. Bahlool QZM, Skovgaard A, Kania PW, Buchmann K. Effects of excretory/secretory proteins from *Anisakis simplex* (Nematoda) on immune gene expression in rainbow trout (*Oncorhynchus mykiss*). Fish Shellfish Immunol. 2013;35:734–9.
34. Buchmann K. Fish immune responses against endoparasitic nematodes—experimental models. J Fish Dis. 2012;35:623–35.
35. Buchmann K. Evolution of innate immunity: clues from invertebrates via fish to mammals. Front Immunol. 2014;5:459.
36. Kuhn T, Hailer F, Palm HW, Klimpel S. Global assessment of molecularly identified *Anisakis* Dujardin, 1845 (Nematoda: Anisakidae) in their teleost intermediate hosts. Folia Parasitol. 2013;60:123–34.
37. Hewitson JP, Grainger JR, Maizels RM. Helminth immunoregulation: the role of parasite secreted proteins in modulating host immunity. Mol Biochem Parasitol. 2009;167:1–11.
38. Perteguer MJ, Raposo R, Cuellar C. In vitro study on the effect of larval excretory/secretory products and crude extracts from *Anisakis simplex* on blood coagulation. Int J Parasitol. 1996;26:105–8.

39. Raybourne R, Deardorff TL, Bier JW. *Anisakis simplex*: larval excretory secretory protein production and cytostatic action in mammalian cell cultures. Exp Parasitol. 1986;62:92–7.
40. Lee DL. Why do some nematode parasites of the alimentary tract secrete acetylcholinesterase? Int J Parasitol. 1996;26:499–508.
41. Podolska M, Nadolna K. Acetylcholinesterase secreted by *Anisakis simplex* larvae (Nematoda: Anisakidae) parasitizing herring, *Clupea harengus*: an inverse relationship of enzyme activity in the host–parasite system. Parasitol Res. 2014;113:2231–8.
42. Pritchard DI. The survival strategies of hookworms. Parasitol Today. 1995;11:255–9.
43. Bhattacharya C, Singh RN, Misra S, Rathaur S. Diethylcarbamazine: effect on lysosomal enzymes and acetylcholine in *Wuchereria bancrofti* infection. Trop Med Int Health. 1997;2:686–90.
44. Nielsen ME, Buchmann K. Glutathione-s-transferase is an important antigen in the eel nematode *Anguillicola crassus*. J Helminthol. 1997;71:319–24.
45. Priebe K, Huber C, Märtlbauer E, Terplan G. Detection of antibodies against the larva of *Anisakis simplex* in the pollock *Pollachius virens* using ELISA. Zentralbl Veterinarmed B. 1991;38:209–14.
46. Coscia MR, Oreste U. Presence of antibodies specific for proteins of *Contracaecum osculatum* (Rudolphi, 1908) in plasma of several Antarctic teleosts. Fish Shellfish Immunol. 1998;8:295–302.
47. Elson-Riggins JG, Riggins SA, Gulland FM, Platzer EG. Immunoglobulin responses of northern elephant and Pacific harbor seals naturally infected with *Otostrongylus circumlitus*. J Wildl Dis. 2004;40:466–75.
48. Dopheide TA, Tachedjian M, Phillips C, Frenkel MJ, Wagland BM, Ward CW. Molecular characterisation of a protective, 11-kDa excretory-secretory protein from the parasitic stages of *Trichostrongylus colubriformis*. Mol Biochem Parasitol. 1991;45:101–7.
49. McKeand JB, Knox DP, Duncan JL, Kennedy MW. Protective immunisation of guinea pigs against *Dictyocaulus viviparus* using excretory/secretory products of adult parasites. Int J Parasitol. 1995;25:95–104.
50. Alonso-Gómez A, Moreno-Ancillo A, López-Serrano MC, Suarez-de-Parga JM, Daschner A, Caballero MT, Barranco P, Cabañas R. *Anisakis simplex* only provokes allergic symptoms when the worm parasitises the gastrointestinal tract. Parasitol Res. 2004;93:378–84.
51. Purello-D'Ambrosio F, Pastorello E, Gangemi S, Lombardo G, Ricciardi L, Fogliani O, Merendino RA. Incidence of sensitivity to *Anisakis simplex* in a risk population of fisherman/fishmongers. Ann Allergy Asthma Immunol. 2000;84:439–44.
52. Nieuwenhuizen N, Lopata AL, Jeebhay MF, Herbert DR, Robins TG, Brombacher F. Exposure to the fish parasite *Anisakis* causes allergic airway hyperreactivity and dermatitis. J Allergy Clin Immunol. 2006;117:1098–105.
53. Ventura MT, Tummolo RA, Di Leo E, D'Ersasmo M, Arsieni A. Immediate and cell-mediated reactions in parasitic infections by *Anisakis simplex*. J Investig Allergol Clin Immunol. 2008;18:253–9.
54. Fæste CK, Jonscher KR, Dooper MMWB, Egge-Jacobsen W, Moen A, Daschner A, Egaas E, Christians U. Characterisation of potential novel allergens in the fish parasite *Anisakis simplex*. EuPA Open Proteom. 2014;4:140–55.
55. Pérez-Pérez J, Fernandez-Caldas E, Marañón F, Sastre J, Bernal ML, Rodríguez J, Bedate CA. Molecular cloning of paramyosin, a new allergen of *Anisakis simplex*. Int Arch Allergy Immunol. 2000;123:120–9.
56. Anadón AM, Romarís F, Escalante M, Rodríguez E, Gárate T, Cuéllar C, Ubeira FM. The *Anisakis simplex* Ani s 7 major allergen as an indicator of true *Anisakis* infections. Clin Exp Immunol. 2009;156:471–8.
57. Kobayashi Y, Ohsaki K, Ikeda K, Kakemoto S, Ishizaki S, Shimakura K, Nagashima Y, Shiomi K. Identification of novel three allergens from *Anisakis simplex* by chemiluminescent immunoscreening of an expression cDNA library. Parasitol Int. 2011;60:144–50.
58. González-Fernández J, Daschner A, Nieuwenhuizen NE, Lopata AL, Frutos CD, Valls A, Cuéllar C. Haemoglobin, a new major allergen of *Anisakis simplex*. Int J Parasitol. 2015;45:399–407.
59. Kobayashi Y, Kakemoto S, Shimakura K, Shiomi K. Molecular cloning and expression of a new major allergen, Ani s 14, from *Anisakis simplex*. Shokuhin Eiseigaku Zasshi. 2015;56:194–9.
60. Carballeda-Sangiao N, Rodríguez-Mahillo AI, Careche M, Navas A, Caballero T, Dominguez-Ortega J, Jurado-Palomo J, González-Muñoz M. Ani s 11-like protein is a pepsin- and heat-resistant major allergen of *Anisakis* spp. and a valuable tool for *Anisakis* allergy component-resolved diagnosis. Int Arch Allergy Immunol. 2016;169:108–12.
61. Baird FJ, Su X, Aibinu I, Nolan MJ, Sugiyama H, Otranto D, Lopata AL, Cantacessi C. The *Anisakis* transcriptome provides a resource for fundamental and applied studies on allergy-causing parasites. PLoS Negl Trop Dis. 2016;10:e0004845.
62. Baeza ML, Rodríguez A, Matheu V, Rubio M, Tornero P, de Barrio M, Herrero T, Santaolalla M, Zubeldia JM. Characterization of allergens secreted by *Anisakis simplex* parasite: clinical relevance in comparison with somatic allergens. Clin Exp Allergy. 2004;34:296–302.
63. Audicana L, Audicana MT, de Corres LF, Kennedy MW. Cooking and freezing may not protect against allergic reactions to ingested *Anisakis simplex* antigens in humans. Vet Rec. 1997;140:235.
64. Caballero ML, Moneo I. Several allergens from *Anisakis simplex* are highly resistant to heat and pepsin treatments. Parasitol Res. 2004;93:248–51.
65. Moneo I, Caballero ML, Gónzalez-Muñoz M, Rodriguez-Mahillo AI, Rodriguez-Perez R, Silva A. Isolation of a heat-resistant allergen from the fish parasite *Anisakis simplex*. Parasitol Res. 2005;96:285–9.
66. Kobayashi Y, Shimakura K, Ishizaki S, Nagashima Y, Shiomi K. Purification and cDNA cloning of a new heat stable allergen from *Anisakis simplex*. Mol Biochem Parasitol. 2007;155:138–45.
67. Rodriguez-Perez R, Moneo I, Rodriguez-Mahillo A, Caballero ML. Cloning and expression of Ani s 9, a new *Anisakis simplex* allergen. Mol Biochem Parasitol. 2008;159:92–7.
68. Caballero ML, Moneo I, Gómez-Aguado F, Corcuera MT, Casado I, Rodríguez-Pérez R. Isolation of Ani s 5, an excretory–secretory and highly heat-resistant allergen useful for the diagnosis of *Anisakis* larvae sensitization. Parasitol Res. 2008;103:1231–3.
69. Caballero ML, Umpierrez A, Moneo I, Rodriguez-Perez R. Ani s 10, a new *Anisakis simplex* allergen: cloning and heterologous expression. Parasitol Int. 2011;60:209–12.
70. Carballeda-Sangiao N, Olivares F, Rodriguez-Mahillo AI, Careche M, Tejada M, Moneo I, González-Muñoz M. Identification of autoclave-resistant *Anisakis simplex* allergens. J Food Prot. 2014;77:605–9.
71. Pascual CY, Crespo JF, San Martin S, Ornia N, Ortega N, Caballero T, Muñoz-Pereira M, Martin-Esteban M. Cross-reactivity between IgE-binding proteins from *Anisakis*, German cockroach, and chironomids. Allergy. 1997;52:514–20.
72. Fernández-Caldas E, Quirce S, Marañón F, Diez Gómez ML, Gijón Botella H, López Román R. Allergenic cross-reactivity between third stage larvae of *Hysterothylacium aduncum* and *Anisakis simplex*. J Allergy Clin Immunol. 1998;101:554–5.
73. Lozano MJ, Martín HL, Díaz SV, Mañas AI, Valero LA, Campos BM. Cross-reactivity between antigens of *Anisakis simplex* s.l. and other ascarid nematodes. Parasite. 2004;11:219–23.
74. Guarneri F, Guarneri C, Benvenga S. Cross-reactivity of *Anisakis simplex*: possible role of Ani s 2 and Ani s 3. Int J Dermatol. 2007;46:146–50.
75. Caballero ML, Moneo I. Specific IgE determination to Ani s 1, a major allergen from *Anisakis simplex*, is a useful tool for diagnosis. Ann Allergy Asthma Immunol. 2002;89:74–7.
76. Moneo I, Caballero ML, Gómez F, Ortega E, Alonso MJ. Isolation and characterization of a major allergen from the fish parasite *Anisakis simplex*. J Allergy Clin Immunol. 2000;106:177–81.
77. Moneo I, Caballero ML, Rodriguez-Perez R, Rodriguez-Mahillo AI, Gonzalez-Muñoz M. Sensitization to the fish parasite *Anisakis simplex*: clinical and laboratory aspects. Parasitol Res. 2007;101:1051–5.
78. Vericimo MA, Figueiredo I Jr, Teixeira GAPB, São Clemente SC. Experimental anisakid infections in mice. J Helminthol. 2015;89:620–4.
79. Laffon-Leal SM, Vidal-Martínez VM, Arjona-Torres G. 'Cebiche'—a potential source of human anisakiasis in Mexico? J Helminthol. 2000;74:151–4.
80. Desowitz RS. Human and experimental anisakiasis in the United States. Hokkaido Igaku Zasshi. 1986;61:358–71.
81. Suzuki J, Murata R, Hosaka M, Araki J. Risk factors for human *Anisakis* infection and association between the geographic origins of *Scomber japonicus* and anisakid nematodes. Int J Food Microbiol. 2010;137:88–93.
82. Klimpel S, Palm HW. Anisakid nematode (Ascaridoidea) life cycles and distribution: Increasing zoonotic potential in the time of climate change? In: Mehlhorn H, editor. Progress in parasitology, parasitology

research monographs 2, Chapter 11. 2011. p. 201–22.

83. Kagei N, Isogaki H. A case of abdominal syndrome caused by the presence of a large number of *Anisakis* larvae. Int J Parasitol. 1992;22:251–3.
84. Jurado-Palomo J, López-Serrano MC, Moneo I. Multiple acute parasitization by *Anisakis simplex*. J Investig Allergol Clin Immunol. 2010;20:437–41.
85. Moreno-Ancillo A, Caballero MT, Cabañas R, Contreras J, Martin-Barroso JA, Barranco P, López-Serrano MC. Allergic reactions to *Anisakis simplex* parasitizing seafood. Ann Allergy Asthma Immunol. 1997;79:246–50.
86. López-Serrano MC, Gomez AA, Daschner A, Moreno-Ancillo A, de Parga JM, Caballero MT, Barranco P, Cabañas R. Gastroallergic anisakiasis: findings in 22 patients. J Gastroenterol Hepatol. 2000;15:503–6.
87. Audicana MT, Ansotegui IJ, de Corres LF, Kennedy MW. *Anisakis simplex*: dangerous—dead and alive? Trends Parasitol. 2002;18:20–4.
88. Daschner A, Pascual CY. *Anisakis simplex*: sensitization and clinical allergy. Curr Opin Allergy Clin Immunol. 2005;5:281–5.
89. Choi SJ, Lee JC, Kim MJ, Hur GY, Shin SY, Park HS. The clinical characteristics of *Anisakis* allergy in Korea. Korean J Intern Med. 2009;24:160–3.
90. Carballeda-Sangiao N, Rodríguez-Mahillo AI, Careche M, Navas A, Moneo I, González-Muñoz M. Changes over time in IgE sensitization to allergens of the fish parasite *Anisakis* spp. PLoS Negl Trop Dis. 2016;10:e0004864.
91. Strøm SB, Haarder S, Korbut R, Mejer H, Thamsborg SM, Kania PW, Buchmann K. Third stage nematode larvae of *Contracaecum osculatum* from Baltic cod (*Gadus morhua*) elicit eosinophilic granulomatous reactions when penetrating the stomach mucosa of pigs. Parasitol Res. 2015;114:1217–20.
92. Messina CM, Pizzo F, Santulli A, Bušelić I, Boban M, Orhanović S, Mladineo I. *Anisakis pegreffii* (Nematoda: Anisakidae) products modulate oxidative stress and apoptosis-related biomarkers in human cell lines. Parasites Vectors. 2016;9:607.
93. Acha P, Szyfres B. Zoonoses and communicable diseases common to man and animals. Vol. 3: Parasitoses. 3rd ed. Washington, DC: Pan American Health Organisation; 2003. p. 231–6.
94. Repiso OA, Alcántara TM, González FC, Artaza VT, Rodríguez MR, Valle MJ, Martínez PJL. Gastrointestinal anisakiasis. Study of a series of 25 patients. Gastroenterol Hepatol. 2003;26:341–6 **(in spanish)**.
95. Montalto M, Miele L, Marcheggiano A, Santoro L, Curigliano V, Vastola M, Gasbarrini G. *Anisakis* infestation: a case of acute abdomen mimicking Crohn's disease and eosinophilic gastroenteritis. Dig Liver Dis. 2005;37:62–4.
96. Tsukui M, Morimoto N, Kurata H, Sunada F. Asymptomatic anisakiasis of the colon incidentally diagnosed and treated during colonoscopy by retroflexion in the ascending colon. J Rural Med. 2016;11:73–5.
97. Caramello P, Vitali A, Canta F, Caldana A, Santi F, Caputo A, Lipani F, Balbiano R. Intestinal localization of anisakiasis manifested as acute abdomen. Clin Microbiol Infect. 2003;9:734–7.
98. Matsumoto T, Iida M, Kimura Y, Tanaka K, Kitada T, Fujishima M. Anisakiasis of the colon: radiologic and endoscopic features in six patients. Radiology. 1992;183:97–9.
99. Ido K, Yuasa H, Ide M, Kimura K, Toshimitsu K, Suzuki T. Sonographic diagnosis of small intestinal anisakiasis. J Clin Ultrasound. 1998;26:125–30.
100. Toyoda H, Tanaka K. Intestinal anisakiasis treated successfully with prednisolone and olopatadine hydrochloride. Case Rep Gastroenterol. 2016;10:30–5.
101. Balows A, Hausler WJ Jr, Ohashi M, Turano A. Laboratory diagnosis of infectious diseases: principles and practice. Vol. 1. Bacterial, mycotic, and parasitic diseases. Berlin: Springer; 1988.
102. Ko RC. Fish-borne parasitic zoonoses. In: Woo PTK, editor. Fish diseases and disorders. Vol. 1: Protozoan and metazoan infections. Chapt. 16. Wallingford, Oxfordshire, England: CABI; 2006. p. 611–615.
103. García M, Moneo I, Audicana MT, del Pozo MD, Muñoz D, Fernández E, Díez J, Etxenagusia MA, Ansotegui IJ, de Corres LF. The use of IgE immunoblotting as a diagnostic tool in *Anisakis simplex* allergy. J Allergy Clin Immunol. 1997;99:497–501.
104. Rodero M, Cuellar C, Chivato T, Mateos JM, Laguna R. Western blot antibody determination in sera from patients diagnosed with *Anisakis* sensitization with different antigenic fractions of *Anisakis simplex* purified by affinity chromatography. J Helminthol. 2007;81:307–10.
105. Mattiucci S, Fazii P, De Rosa A, Paoletti M, Megna AS, Glielmo A, De Angelis M, Costa A, Meucci C, Calvaruso V, Sorrentini I, Palma G, Bruschi F, Nascetti G. Anisakiasis and gastroallergic reactions associated with *Anisakis pegreffii* infection, Italy. Emerg Infect Dis. 2013;19:496–9.
106. Iglesias R, Leiro J, Ubeiro FM, Santamarina MT, Navarrete I, Sanmartin ML. Antigenic cross-reactivity in mice between third-stage larvae of *Anisakis simplex* and other nematodes. Parasitol Res. 1996;82:378–81.
107. Perteguer MJ, Chivato T, Montoro A, Cuellar C, Mateos JM, Laguna R. Specific and total IgE in patients with recurrent, acute urticarial caused by *Anisakis simplex*. Ann Trop Med Parasitol. 2000;94:259–68.
108. Hochberg NS, Hamer DH. Anisakidosis: perils of the deep. Clin Infect Dis. 2010;51:806–12.
109. Daschner A, Vega de La Osada F, González Leza B. Specific IgG and IgG4 in patients with IgE-antibodies against *Anisakis simplex*: acute urticaria in gastro-allergic anisakiasis versus chronic urticarial. J Allegy Clin Immunol. 2002;109:126.
110. Gónzalez-Muñoz M, Luque R, Nauwelaers F, Moneo I. Detection of *Anisakis simplex*-induced basophil activation by flow cytometry. Cytom B Clin Cytom. 2005;68:31–6.
111. Bernardini R, Lombardi E, Novembre E, Ingargiola A, Pucci N, Favilli T, Vierucci A. Predictors of *Anisakis simplex* symptoms. Allergy. 2000;55:979–80.
112. García Ara MC, Alonso Gómez A, Martín Muñoz MF, Díaz Pena JM, Daschner A, Ojeda JA. *Anisakis simplex* (AS) sensitization in children: frequency study. Allergy. 1997;2:67.
113. Weiler CR. *Anisakis simplex* and cross-reacting antigens. Int J Dermatol. 2007;46:224–5.
114. Valls A, Pascual CY, Martín Esteban M. Anisakis allergy: an update. Rev Fr Allergol. 2005;45:108–13.
115. Caballero ML, Umpierrez A, Perez-Piñar T, Moneo I, de Burgos C, Asturias JA, Rodríguez-Pérez R. *Anisakis simplex* recombinant allergens increase diagnosis specificity preserving high sensitivity. Int Arch Allergy Immunol. 2012;158:232–40.
116. Caballero ML, Asero R, Antonicelli L, Kamberi E, Colangelo C, Fazii P, de Burgos C, Rodriguez-Perez R. *Anisakis* allergy component-resolved diagnosis: clinical and immunologic differences between patients from Italy and Spain. Int Arch Allergy Immunol. 2013;162:39–44.
117. Kobayashi Y, Ishizaki S, Shimakura K, Nagashima Y, Shiomi K. Molecular cloning and expression of two new allergens from *Anisakis simplex*. Parasitol Res. 2007;100:1233–41.
118. López I, Pardo MA. A phage display system for the identification of novel *Anisakis simplex* antigens. J Immunol Methods. 2011;373:247–51.
119. Anadón AM, Rodríguez E, Gárate MT, Cuéllar C, Romarís F, Chivato T, Rodero M, González-Díaz H, Ubeira FM. Diagnosing human anisakiasis: recombinant Ani s 1 and Ani s 7 allergens versus the UniCAP 100 fluorescence enzyme immunoassay. Clin Vaccine Immunol. 2010;17:496–502.
120. Cuéllar C, Daschner A, Valls A, De Frutos C, Fernández-Fígares V, Anadón AM, Rodríguez E, Gárate T, Rodero M, Ubeira FM. Ani s 1 and Ani s 7 recombinant allergens are able to differentiate distinct *Anisakis simplex*-associated allergic clinical disorders. Arch Dermatol Res. 2012;304:283–8.
121. Rodríguez E, Anadón AM, García-Bodas E, Romarís F, Iglesias R, Gárate T, Ubeira FM. Novel sequences and epitopes of diagnostic value derived from the *Anisakis simplex* Ani s 7 major allergen. Allergy. 2008;63:219–25.
122. Lin AH, Nepstad I, Florvaag E, Egaas E, Van Do T. An extended study of seroprevalence of anti-*Anisakis simplex* IgE antibodies in Norwegian blood donors. Scand J Immunol. 2014;79:61–7.
123. Gamboa PM, Asturias J, Martínez R, Antépara I, Jáuregui I, Urrutia I, Fernández J, Sanz ML. Diagnostic utility of components in allergy to *Anisakis simplex*. J Investig Allergol Clin Immunol. 2012;22:13–9.
124. Rodriguez-Mahillo AI, Gonzalez-Muñoz M, Gomez-Aguado F, Rodriguez-Perez R, Corcuera MT, Caballero ML, Moneo I. Cloning and characterisation of the *Anisakis simplex* allergen Ani s 4 as a cysteine-protease inhibitor. Int J Parasitol. 2007;37:907–17.
125. Ibarrola I, Arilla MC, Herrero MD, Esteban MI, Martínez A, Asturias JA. Expression of a recombinant protein immunochemically equivalent to the major *Anisakis simplex* allergen Ani s 1. J Investig Allergol Clin Immunol. 2008;18:78–83.
126. Asturias JA, Eraso E, Martínez A. Cloning and high level expression in *Escherichia coli* of an *Anisakis simplex* tropomyosin isoform. Mol Biochem Parasitol. 2000;108:263–7.
127. Moore DAJ, Girdwood RWA, Chiodini PL. Treatment of anisakiasis with albendazole. Lancet. 2002;360:54.

128. Pacios E, Arias-Diaz J, Zuloaga J, Gonzalez-Armengol J, Villarroel P, Balibrea JL. Albendazole for the treatment of anisakiasis ileus. Clin Infect Dis. 2005;41:1825–6.
129. Li SW, Shiao SH, Weng SC, Liu TH, Su KE, Chen CC. A case of human infection with *Anisakis simplex* in Taiwan. Gastrointest Endosc. 2015;82:757–8.
130. Ramos L, Alonso C, Guilarte M, Vilaseca J, Santos J, Malagelada JR. *Anisakis simplex*-induced small bowel obstruction after fish ingestion: preliminary evidence for response to parenteral corticosteroids. Clin Gastroenterol Hepatol. 2005;3:667–71.
131. Hierro I, Valero A, Pérez P, González P, Cabo MM, Montilla MP, Navarro MC. Action of different monoterpenic compounds against *Anisakis simplex* s.l. L3 larvae. Phytomedicine. 2004;11:77–82.
132. Gómez-Rincón C, Langa E, Murillo P, Valero MS, Berzosa C, López V. Activity of tea tree (*Melaleuca alternifolia*) essential oil against L3 larvae of *Anisakis simplex*. Biomed Res Int. 2014;2014:549510.
133. da Silva Justino CH, Barros LA. In vitro evaluation of the resistence of the *Contracaecum* sp. larvae (Railliet & Henry, 1912) (Nematoda: Anisakidae), to the essential oil of citronella (Cymbopogon sp.) (Poaceae). R bras Ci Vet. 2008;15:122–5.
134. Barros LA, Yamanaka AR, Silva LE, Vanzeler MLA, Braum DT, Bonaldo J. In vitro larvicidal activity of geraniol and citronellal against *Contracaecum* sp. (Nematoda: Anisakidae). Braz J Med Biol Res. 2009;42:918–20.
135. Hierro I, Valero A, Navarro MC. In vivo larvicidal activity of monoterpenic derivatives from aromatic plants against L3 larvae of *Anisakis simplex* s. l. Phytomedicine. 2006;13:527–31.
136. Romero Mdel C, Valero A, Martín-Sánchez J, Navarro-Moll MC. Activity of *Matricaria chamomilla* essential oil against anisakiasis. Phytomedicine. 2012;19:520–3.
137. Maizels RM, Tetteh KK, Loukas A. *Toxocara canis*: genes expressed by the arrested infective larval stage of a parasitic nematode. Int J Parasitol. 2000;30:495–508.
138. Jex AR, Liu S, Li B, Young ND, Hall RS, Li Y, et al. *Ascaris suum* draft genome. Nature. 2011;479:529–33.
139. Itami DM, Oshiro TM, Araujo CA, Periniz A, Martinsz MA, Macedow MS, Macedo-Soares MF. Modulation of murine experimental asthma by *Ascaris suum* components. Clin Exp Allergy. 2005;35:873–9.
140. Oshiro TM, Macedo MS, Macedo-Soares MF. Anti-inflammatory activity of PAS-1, a protein component of *Ascaris suum*. Inflamm Res. 2005;54:17–21.
141. Antunes MF, Titz TO, Batista IF, Marques-Porto R, Oliveira CF, Alves de Araujo CA, Macedo-Soares MF. Immunosuppressive PAS-1 is an excretory/secretory protein released by larval and adult worms of the ascarid nematode *Ascaris suum*. J Helminthol. 2015;89:367–74.
142. Araújo CA, Perini A, Martins MA, Macedo MS, Macedo-Soares MF. PAS-1, a protein from *Ascaris suum*, modulates allergic inflammation via IL-10 and IFN-γ, but not IL-12. Cytokine. 2008;44:335–41.
143. Araújo CAA, Perini A, Martins MA, Macedo MS, Macedo-Soares MF. PAS-1, an *Ascaris suum* protein, modulates allergic airway inflammation via $CD8^+$ $\gamma\delta TCR^+$ and $CD4^+$ $CD25^+$ $FoxP3^+$ T cells. Scand J Immunol. 2010;72:491–503.
144. La Rotta A, Higaki Y, Marcos G, Kilimajer J, Zubeldia JM, Baeza ML. *Anisakis simplex* and *Ascaris lumbricoides* inhibit the allergic response to peanut in a murine model of anaphylaxis. J Allergy Clin Immunol. 2010;125:AB28.
145. Haarder S, Kania PW, Holm TL, Jørgensen LvG, Buchmann K. Effect of ES-products from *Anisakis* (Nematoda: Anisakidae) on experimentally induced colitis in adult zebrafish. Parasite Immunol. 2016 (**unpublished data**).
146. Buchmann K, Kania P. Emerging *Pseudoterranova decipiens* (Krabbe, 1878) problems in Baltic cod, *Gadus morhua* L., associated with grey seal colonization of spawning grounds. J Fish Dis. 2012;35:861–6.
147. Nadolna K, Podolska M. Anisakid larvae in the liver of cod (*Gadus morhua*) L. from the Southern Baltic Sea. J Helminthol. 2014;88:237–46.
148. Valiñas B, Lorenzo S, Eiras A, Figueiras A, Sanmartín ML, Ubeira FM. Prevalence of and risk factors for IgE sensitization to *Anisakis simplex* in a Spanish population. Allergy. 2001;56:667–71.
149. Adroher FJ, Valero A, Ruiz-Valero J, Iglesias L. Larval anisakids (Nematoda: Ascaridoidea) in horse mackerel (*Trachurus trachurus*) from the fish market in Granada, Spain. Parasitol Res. 1996;82:319–22.
150. Del Rey Moreno A, Valero A, Mayorga C, Gómez B, Torres MJ, Hernández J, Ortiz M, Lozano Maldonado J. Sensitization to *Anisakis simplex* s.l. in a healthy population. Acta Trop. 2006;97:265–9.
151. Puente P, Anadón A, Rodero M, Romarís F, Ubeira F, Cuéllar C. *Anisakis simplex*: the high prevalence in Madrid (Spain) and its relation with fish consumption. Exp Parasitol. 2008;118:271–4.
152. Rello FJ, Valero A, Adroher FJ. Anisakid parasites of the pouting (*Trisopterus luscus*) from the Cantabrian Sea coast, Bay of Biscay, Spain. J Helminthol. 2008;82:287–91.
153. Pulleiro-Potel L, Barcala E, Mayo-Hernández E, Muñoz P. Survey of anisakids in commercial teleosts from the western Mediterranean Sea: infection rates and possible effects of environmental and ecological factors. Food Control. 2015;55:12–7.
154. López-Vélez R, García A, Barros C, Manzarbeitia F, Oñate JM. Anisakiasis in Spain. Report of 3 cases. Enferm Infecc Microbiol Clin. 1992;10:158–61.
155. Pampiglione S, Rivasi F, Criscuolo M, De Benedittis A, Gentile A, Russo S, Testini M, Villan M. Human anisakiasis in Italy: a report of eleven new cases. Pathol Res Pract. 2002;198:429–34.
156. Cavallero S, Scribano D, D'Amelio S. First case report of invasive pseudoterranoviasis in Italy. Parasitol Int. 2016;65:488–90.
157. Levsen A, Lunestad BT. *Anisakis simplex* third stage larvae in Norwegian spring spawning herring (*Clupea harengus* L.), with emphasis on larval distribution in the flesh. Vet Parasitol. 2010;171:247–53.
158. Karpiej K, Dzido J, Rokicki J, Kijewska A. Anisakid nematodes of Greenland halibut *Reinhardtius hippoglossoides* from the Barents Sea. J Parasitol. 2013;99:650–4.
159. Levsen A, Karl H. *Anisakis simplex* (s.l.) in Grey gurnard (*Eutrigla gurnardus*) from the North Sea: food safety considerations in relation to fishing ground and distribution in the flesh. Food Control. 2014;36:15–9.
160. Andreassen J, Jörring K. Anisakiasis in Denmark. Infection with nematode larvae from marine fish. Nord Med. 1970;84:1492–5 **(in Danish)**.
161. Mehrdana F, Bahlool QZ, Skov J, Marana MH, Sindberg D, Mundeling M, Overgaard BC, Korbut R, Strøm SB, Kania PW, Buchmann K. Occurrence of zoonotic nematodes *Pseudoterranova decipiens*, *Contracaecum osculatum* and *Anisakis simplex* in cod (*Gadus morhua*) from the Baltic Sea. Vet Parasitol. 2014;205:581–7.
162. Haarder S, Kania PW, Galatius A, Buchmann K. Increased *Contracaecum osculatum* infection in Baltic cod (*Gadus morhua*) livers (1982–2012) associated with increasing grey seal (*Halichoerus gryphus*) populations. J Wildl Dis. 2014;50:537–43.
163. Lunneryd SG, Boström MK, Aspholm PE. Sealworm (*Pseudoterranova decipiens*) infection in grey seals (*Halichoerus grypus*), cod (*Gadus morhua*) and shorthorn sculpin (*Myoxocephalus scorpius*) in the Baltic Sea. Parasitol Res. 2015;114:257–64.
164. Möller H, Schröder S. Neue aspekte der anisakiasis in Deutschland (New aspects of anisakidosis in Germany). Arch Lebensmittelhyg. 1987;38:123–8 **(in German)**.
165. van Thiel P, Kuipers FC, Roskam RT. A nematode parasitic to herring, causing acute abdominal syndromes in man. Trop Geogr Med. 1960;12:97–113.
166. Mladineo I, Poljak V, Martínez-Sernández V, Ubeira FM. Anti-*Anisakis* IgE seroprevalence in the healthy Croatian coastal population and associated risk factors. PLoS Negl Trop Dis. 2014;8:e2673.
167. Marques JF, Cabral HN, Busi M, D'Amelio S. Molecular identification of *Anisakis* species from Pleuronectiformes off the Portuguese coast. J Helminthol. 2006;80:47–51.
168. Bourree P, Paugam A, Petithory JC. Anisakidosis: report of 25 cases and review of the literature. Comp Immunol Microbiol Infect Dis. 1995;18:75–84.
169. Umehara A, Kawakami Y, Araki J, Uchida A. Molecular identification of the etiological agent of the human anisakiasis in Japan. Parasitol Int. 2007;56:211–5.
170. Umehara A, Kawakami Y, Ooi HK, Uchida A, Ohmae H, Sugiyama H. Molecular identification of *Anisakis* type I larvae isolated from hairtail fish off the coasts of Taiwan and Japan. Int J Food Microbiol. 2010;143:161–5.
171. Quiazon KM, Yoshinaga T, Ogawa K. Distribution of *Anisakis* species larvae from fishes of the Japanese waters. Parasitol Int. 2011;60:223–6.
172. Im KI, Shin H, Kim B, Moon S. Gastric anisakiasis in Cheju-do, Korea. Korean J Parasitol. 1995;33:179–86.

173. Na HK, Seo M, Chai JY, Lee EK, Jeon SM. A Case of anisakidosis caused by *Pseudoterranova decipiens* larva. Korean J Parasitol. 2013;51:115–7.
174. McClelland G, Martell DJ. Surveys of larval sealworm (*Pseudoterranova decipiens*) infection in various fish species sampled from Nova Scotian waters between 1988 and 1996, with an assessment of examination procedures. NAMMCO Sci Publ. 2001;3:57–76.
175. Couture C, Measures L, Gagnon J, Desbiens C. Human intestinal anisakiosis due to consumption of raw salmon. Am J Surg Pathol. 2003;27:1167–72.
176. Pinkus GS, Coolidge C, Little MD. Intestinal anisakiasis. First case report from North America. Am J Med. 1975;59:114–20.
177. Amin OM, Eidelman WS, Domke W, Bailey J, Pfeifer G. An unusual case of anisakiasis in California, USA. Comp Parasitol. 2000;67:71–5.
178. Bergmann GT, Motta PJ. Infection by anisakid nematodes *Contracaecum* spp. in the Mayan cichlid fish *Cichlasoma* (*Nandopsis*) *urophthalmus* (Günther 1832). J Parasitol. 2004;90:405–7.
179. Figueiredo Junior I, Vericimo MA, Cardoso LR, São Clemente SC, do Nascimento ER, Teixeira GA. Cross-sectional study of serum reactivity to *Anisakis simplex* in healthy adults in Niterói, Brazil. Acta Parasitol.
180. Luque JL, Poulin R. Use of fish as intermediate hosts by helminth parasites: a comparative analysis. Acta Parasitol. 2004;49:353–61.
181. Eiras JC, Pavanelli GC, Takemoto RM, Yamaguchi MU, Karkling LC, Nawa Y. Potential risk of fish-borne nematode infections in humans in Brazil—current status based on a literature review. FAWPAR. 2016;5:1–6.
182. Torres P, Moya R, Lamilla J. Nematodos anisákidos de interés en salud pública en peces comercializados en Valdivia, Chile. Arch Med Vet. 2000;32:107–13.
183. Mercado R, Torres P, Munoz V, Apt W. Human infection by *Pseudoterranova decipiens* in Chile: report of seven cases. Mem Inst Oswald Cruz. 2001;96:653–5.
184. Garbin LE, Mattiucci S, Paoletti M, Diaz JI, Nascetti G, Navone GT. Molecular identification and larval morphological description of *Contracaecum pelagicum* (Nematoda: Anisakidae) from the anchovy *Engraulis anchoita* (Engraulidae) and fish-eating birds from the Argentine North Patagonian Sea. Parasitol Int. 2013;62:309–19.
185. Jabbar A, Fong RW, Kok KX, Lopata AL, Gasser RB, Beveridge I. Molecular characterization of anisakid nematode larvae from 13 species of fish from Western Australia. Int J Food Microbiol. 2013;161:247–53.

18

Seroprevalence of 12 serovars of pathogenic *Leptospira* in red foxes (*Vulpes vulpes*) in Poland

Jacek Żmudzki[1*], Zbigniew Arent[2], Artur Jabłoński[1], Agnieszka Nowak[1], Sylwia Zębek[1], Agnieszka Stolarek[3], Łukasz Bocian[3], Adam Brzana[4] and Zygmunt Pejsak[1]

Abstract

Background: *Leptospira* spp. infect humans and a wide range of domestic and wild animals, but certain species such as small rodents and red foxes (*Vulpes vulpes*) play a particular role as reservoirs and transmission of leptospirosis as they easily adapt to many habitats including human environments. To investigate the significance of red foxes in the epidemiology of leptospirosis in Poland, a seroprevalence survey was conducted. During the 2014–2015 hunting season, blood samples of 2134 red foxes originating from the central-eastern part of Poland were collected. Serum samples were tested by a microscopic agglutination test for the presence of specific antibodies to *Leptospira* serovars Icterohaemorrhagiae, Grippotyphosa, Sejroe, Tarassovi, Pomona, Canicola, Hardjo, Ballum, Australis, Bataviae, Saxkoebing and Poi.

Results: Antibodies to at least one serovar were detected in 561 sera (26.3%). The highest seroprevalence was found in the Subcarpathia (41.6%) and Warmia-Masuria (40.3%) provinces. Antibodies were mainly directed against serovars Poi (12.4%), Saxkoebing (11.3%), and Sejroe (6.0%).

Conclusions: Exposure of red foxes to certain *Leptospira* serovars seems to be common in central and eastern Poland. In addition, the high prevalence of antibodies against *Leptospira* spp. in foxes may indicate a potential risk of infection for humans and other species coming into contact with these animals.

Keywords: Leptospirosis, Prevalence, Red fox, Serology, *Vulpes vulpes*, Zoonosis

Background

Leptospirosis caused by pathogenic spirochetes of the genus *Leptospira* is an important but sometimes neglected infection that affects people and animals worldwide. Leptospirosis is a re-emerging major public health problem in many countries and is one of the most widespread zoonoses. It is an excellent example validating the "One Health" approach, where the relationship between humans, animals and ecosystems needs to be considered in order to better understand and manage a disease [1]. Some serovars of *Leptospira* can chronically infect domestic and wild animals and in particular small rodents. In addition to rodents, other wild animal species such as the red fox (*Vulpes vulpes*) may act as a reservoir [2]. The bacteria are occasionally transmitted through direct contact with mammal hosts, but the majority are usually transmitted via contact with contaminated soil and water [3], where leptospires' survival outside the host is favoured by warm moist conditions [4]. The red fox lives throughout Europe, mainly inhabiting forests, meadows, coastal dunes and urbanized areas [5]. The Polish hunting statistics for 2015 indicate that the population of red foxes in Poland is 190,000–200,000 individuals, with a tendency to remain stable [6]. Red foxes prey upon small rodents, among other animals and the red fox may transmit leptospirosis to humans. A recent study indicate that small mammals might be an important source of human leptospirosis as both rodents and

*Correspondence: jaca@piwet.pulawy.pl
[1] Swine Diseases Department, National Veterinary Research Institute, Partyzantow 57, 24-100 Pulawy, Poland

humans share infections caused by *Leptospira* spp. from the same serogroups [7]. The aim of the present study was to determine the seroprevalence for *Leptospira* spp. in red foxes from central and eastern Poland.

Methods

Sample collection and study area

Blood samples from red foxes (n = 2134) were collected during the 2014–2015 hunting seasons in Poland. Blood was taken from the thoracic cavity or heart of animals culled primarily through the rabies monitoring program. Sex and geographic location were recorded and age was determined by the degree of dentine surface wear and tooth eruption (juveniles: < 1 year; mature > 1 year) (Table 1). The samples originated from 134 counties of nine provinces of Poland and were mainly collected from the central and eastern (49–55°N, 17–23°E) parts of the country (Fig. 1). Blood samples were centrifuged at 4500 *g* for 30 min and serum stored at − 20 °C until analysis.

Microscopic agglutination test

Serum samples were tested by a microscopic agglutination test (MAT) using a range of 12 *Leptospira* serovars representative of 10 serogroups found in Europe: Icterohaemorrhagiae (RGA strain, representing the Icterohaemorrhagiae serogroup), Grippotyphosa (Moskva V strain, Grippotyphosa serogroup), Sejroe (M84 strain, Sejroe serogroup), Tarassovi (Perepelicyn strain, Tarassovi serogroup), Pomona (Pomona strain, Pomona serogroup), Canicola (Hond Utrecht IV strain, Canicola serogroup), Hardjo (Hardjoprajitno strain, Sejroe serogroup), Ballum (MUS127 strain, Ballum serogroup), Australis (Ballico strain, Australis serogroup), Bataviae (Swart strain, Bataviae serogroup), Saxkoebing (MUS 24 strain, Sejroe serogroup) and Poi (Poi strain, Javanica serogroup) [8, 9]. The selection of the serovars used was based on their common identification in previous European studies [10–13] reporting *Leptospira* spp. in wild carnivores.

Each serovar was grown in 10 mL of Ellinghausen–McCullough–Johnson–Harris (EMJH) medium, at 30 ± 1 °C for at least 4 but no more than 8 days depending on the serovar. The concentration of bacteria was adjusted to $1–2 \times 10^8$ cells/mL using a Helber counting chamber. The sera were initially diluted 1:50 and screened for antibodies to the 12 serovars. A volume of each antigen equal to the diluted serum volume was added to each well with a final serum dilution of 1:100 in the screening test. The final concentration of antigen after mixing with the diluted serum was $1–2 \times 10^4$ cells/mL. The plates were incubated at 30 ± 1 °C for 2–4 h and subsequently examined by dark-field microscopy. The titre was defined as the highest dilution where ≥ 50% of the antigen suspension added to the tested serum was agglutinated. When agglutination was observed, the relevant sera were end-point tested using twofold dilutions ranging from 1:100 to 1:25,600.

The quality control of the MAT was performed by using certified reference *Leptospira* strains and anti-*Leptospira* rabbit antisera (Veterinary Sciences Division, AFBI, OIE Leptospira Reference Laboratories, Belfast, and the WHO/FAO and National Collaborating Centre for Reference and Research on Leptospirosis, Royal Tropical Institute (KIT), Amsterdam, the Netherlands). Testing of the samples was conducted at the National Reference Laboratory of Leptospirosis, National Veterinary Research Institute in Pulawy, Poland using an accredited method according to PN/EN ISO/IEC 17025-2005.

Statistical analysis

Statistical analysis was used to study the impact of the season, sex, age, region and population density of foxes on *Leptospira* seroprevalence. It was based on logistic regression models to describe the influence of several variables $X_1, X_2, \ldots, X_n$ on the dichotomous variable Y:

$$P(Y = 1|x_1, x_2, \ldots, x_n) = \frac{e^{(\beta_0 + \sum_{i=1}^{n} \beta_i x_i)}}{1 + e^{(\beta_0 + \sum_{i=1}^{n} \beta_i x_i)}}$$

where β_i is the regression coefficient for $i = 0, \ldots, n$, χ_i are independent variables (measurable or qualitative) for $i = 1, 2, \ldots, n$.

The maximum likelihood method was used to estimate the model's coefficients. The Wald test was used to evaluate the significance of individual variables. Evaluation of model fit to data was performed using the likelihood ratio (LR) test.

Five predictors (4 qualitative and 1 quantitative) were included in the modelling:

- *sampling season* (spring: March–May, summer: June–August, autumn: September–November, or winter: December–Feburary);
- *sex* (male, female);
- *age* (young, adult);
- *province* (LD: Łódzkie; MP: Lesser Poland; MA: Masovia; OP: Opolskie; PK: Subcarpathia; PM: Pomerania; SL: Silesia; SW: Świętokrzyskie; WM: Warmia-Masuria); (Fig. 1) and
- *fox density in counties in 2015* (No/km^2).

The dependent variable was the qualitative result of the study. Analysis was performed for results without distinguishing between serovars (*Leptospira* spp.: positive/

Table 1 Total number of red foxes from Poland hunted in 9 Polish provinces between 2014 and 2015

Sex	Females						Males						Unknown	Total	No of seropositive	% of anti-*Leptospira* sp. antibodies positive (95% CI)
Age	Adult		Young		Unknown		Adult		Young		Unknown		Unknown			
Result (*Leptospira* sp.)	−	+	−	+	−	+	−	+	−	+	−	+	−			
Province/season																
LD	45	14	35	14			81	27	26	12				254	67	26.4 (21.1–32.3)
Spring	12	4	3				11	4	4	1				39	9	
Autumn	12	2	9	1			15	3	7					49	6	
Winter	21	8	23	13			55	20	15	11				166	52	
MP	56	18	60	8			92	23	51	12				320	61	19.1 (14.9–23.8)
Unknown	36	10	37	3			75	13	28	5				207	31	
Spring	17	6	5	2			12	6	7	2				57	16	
Autumn	3	2	18	3			5	4	16	5				56	14	
MA					47	30					80	42		199	72	36.2 (29.5–43.3)
Unknown					47	30					80	42		199	72	
OP	25	13	29	6			42	24	25	9				173	52	30.1 (23.3–37.5)
Summer	4	1	11	3			7	5	11	3				45	12	
Autumn	21	12	18	3			35	19	14	6				128	40	
PK			19	17		1			38	24	2			101	42	41.6 (31.9–51.8)
Unknown			19	17		1			38	24	2			101	42	
PM	43	17	7	4			36	16	3	5				131	42	32.1 (24.2–40.8)
Winter	43	17	7	4			36	16	3	5				131	42	
SL	61	11	62	8			106	8	55	9			1	321	36	11.2 (8.0–15.2)
Spring	7	2	3				9	2	5	1			1	30	5	
Summer	13	2	22	4			18	3	17	5				84	14	
Autumn	23	5	28	1			48	2	22	2				131	10	
Winter	18	2	9	3			31	1	11	1				76	7	
SW	40	8	73	11			73	14	36	5				260	38	14.6 (10.6–19.5)
Spring	8	1	5				5	2						21	3	
Summer	5	2	13				10	3	9					42	5	
Autumn	3	1	27	7			15	3	10	3				69	14	
Winter	24	4	28	4			43	6	17	2				128	16	
WM	73	36	30	26			87	70	34	19				375	151	40.3 (35.3–45.4)
Winter	73	36	30	26			87	70	34	19				375	151	
Total	343	117	315	94	47	31	517	182	268	95	82	42	1	2134	561	26.3 (24.4–28.2)

LD Łódzkie, *MP* Leser Poland, *MA* Masovia, *OP* Opolskie, *PK* Subcarpathia, *PM* Pomerania, *SL* Silesia, *SW* Świętokrzyskie, *WM* Warmia-Masuria

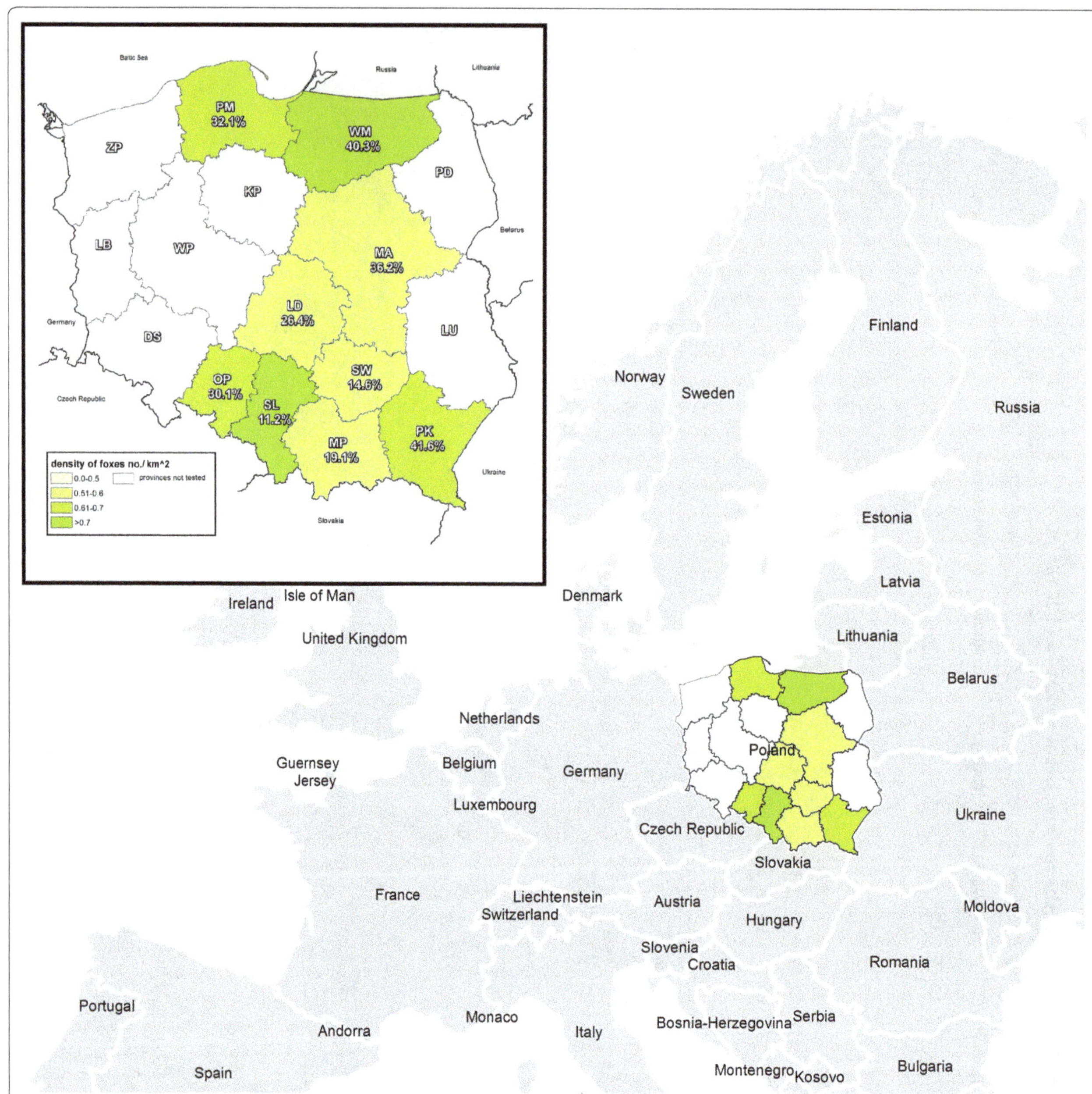

Fig. 1 Geographic distribution of red foxes seropositive for pathogenic *Leptospira* in Poland. *LD* Łódzkie, *MP* Lesser Poland, *MA* Masovia, *OP* Opolskie, *PK* Subcarpathia, *PM* Pomerania, *SL* Silesia, *SW* Świętokrzyskie, *WM* Warmia-Masuria, *DS* Lower Silesia, *KP* Kuyavian-Pomerania, *LB* Lubuskie, *LU* Lubelskie, *PD* Podlaskie, *WP* Greater Poland, *ZP* West Pomerania

negative) and for each serovar separately. The selection of variables for modelling was based on analytical stepping methods (step-wise). For qualitative variables, 0–1 coding for k − 1 variables was used (Table 2).

The following classes of variables were reference classes in models: 'summer' for *sampling season*, 'female' for *sex*, 'young' for *age* and 'SL' for province. Parameters of significant and best fit logistic regression models obtained for each analysis are shown in Table 3. The accepted

Table 2 Dichotomous coding for qualitative variables with an example of sampling season

Sampling season	Spring	Autumn	Winter
Spring	1	0	0
Summer	0	0	0
Autumn	0	1	0
Winter	0	0	1

Table 3 Results of the best fit logistic regression models obtained for each analysis

Significance assessment of model (*P* value of LR test)	Independent variable	Coefficient (β_i)	Std. error	P value (Wald)	Odds ratio	Confidence OR − 95%	Confidence OR + 95%
Models for infection of *Leptospira* sp. (without distinction of serovars)							
< 0.001	Absolute term (β_0)	− 2.92912	0.296482	< 0.001	0.05	0.03	0.10
	LD	1.216036	0.233494	< 0.001	3.37	2.13	5.33
	MP	0.671037	0.228562	0.003	1.96	1.25	3.06
	MA	1.68051	0.237135	< 0.001	5.37	3.37	8.55
	OP	1.388372	0.247953	< 0.001	4.01	2.46	6.52
	PK	1.769046	0.269941	< 0.001	5.87	3.45	9.96
	PM	1.534127	0.265823	< 0.001	4.64	2.75	7.81
	SW	0.555254	0.259964	0.03	1.74	1.05	2.90
	WM	1.630786	0.20659	< 0.001	5.11	3.41	7.66
	Fox density (No/km^2)	1.142803	0.307487	< 0.001	3.14	1.72	5.73
< 0.001	Absolute term (β_0)	− 1.50766	0.198255	< 0.001	0.22	0.15	0.33
	Spring	0.267965	0.280004	0.34	1.31	0.75	2.26
	Autumn	0.0834	0.232275	0.72	1.09	0.69	1.71
	Winter	0.688467	0.211402	0.001	1.99	1.31	3.01
Model for Icterohaemorrhagiae							
0.003	Absolute term (β_0)	− 6.41457	0.839692	< 0.001	0.002	0.0003	0.008
	Fox density (No/km^2)	2.913659	0.989553	0.003	18.42	2.65	128.30
	Adult	− 1.18961	0.553268	0.03	0.30	0.10	0.90
Model for Grippotyphosa							
0.001	Absolute term (β_0)	− 5.71115	0.543301	< 0.001	0.003	0.001	0.01
	Fox density (No/km^2)	2.364823	0.677533	< 0.001	10.64	2.82	40.19
Model for Sejroe							
0.015	Absolute term (β_0)	− 3.43721	0.318798	< 0.001	0.03	0.02	0.06
	LD	1.130284	0.386552	0.003	3.10	1.45	6.61
	MP	0.35268	0.419714	0.40	1.42	0.62	3.24
	MA	0.85591	0.422493	0.04	2.35	1.03	5.39
	OP	0.110974	0.514159	0.83	1.12	0.41	3.06
	PK	1.228934	0.461089	0.008	3.42	1.38	8.44
	PM	1.047612	0.44818	0.02	2.85	1.18	6.87
	SW	0.408686	0.434724	0.35	1.50	0.64	3.53
	WM	0.880843	0.376223	0.02	2.41	1.15	5.05
Model for Australis							
< 0.001	Absolute term (β_0)	− 6.36907	0.610643	< 0.001	0.002	0.0005	0.01
	Fox density (No/km^2)	2.843724	0.730836	< 0.001	17.18	4.10	72.02
Models for Saxkoebing							
0.024	Absolute term (β_0)	− 2.77882	0.325736	< 0.001	0.06	0.03	0.12
	Spring	0.445929	0.436438	0.31	1.56	0.66	3.68
	Autumn	0.408323	0.368228	0.27	1.50	0.73	3.10
	Winter	0.806557	0.34165	0.02	2.24	1.15	4.38

Table 3 (continued)

Significance assessment of model (*P* value of LR test)	Independent variable	Coefficient (β_i)	Std. error	P value (Wald)	Odds ratio	Confidence OR −95%	Confidence OR +95%
< 0.001	Absolute term (β_0)	−2.94772	0.25661	< 0.001	0.05	0.03	0.09
	LD	1.010782	0.318737	0.002	2.75	1.47	5.13
	MP	0.715284	0.318663	0.03	2.04	1.09	3.81
	MA	1.257746	0.322546	< 0.001	3.52	1.87	6.62
	OP	1.021486	0.343397	0.003	2.78	1.42	5.45
	PK	1.939495	0.341159	< 0.001	6.96	3.56	13.58
	PM	1.452948	0.341859	< 0.001	4.28	2.19	8.36
	SW	−0.63976	0.461137	0.17	0.53	0.21	1.30
	WM	1.121314	0.296979	< 0.001	3.07	1.71	5.49
Models for Poi							
< 0.001	Absolute term (β_0)	−5.45234	0.689411	< 0.001	0.004	0.001	0.02
	LD	2.814176	0.617742	< 0.001	16.68	4.97	56.01
	MP	1.032509	0.682165	0.13	2.81	0.74	10.70
	MA	3.445862	0.612244	< 0.001	31.37	9.44	104.22
	OP	3.293047	0.618209	< 0.001	26.92	8.01	90.51
	PK	2.239957	0.687842	0.001	9.39	2.44	36.19
	PM	2.960175	0.643965	< 0.001	19.30	5.46	68.24
	SW	2.610502	0.629299	< 0.001	13.61	3.96	46.74
	WM	3.666819	0.591781	< 0.001	39.13	12.26	124.88
	Fox density (No/km^2)	1.043369	0.476866	0.03	2.84	1.11	7.23
< 0.001	Absolute term (β_0)	−2.89037	0.342638	< 0.001	0.06	0.03	0.11
	Spring	0.375612	0.464447	0.42	1.46	0.59	3.62
	Autumn	0.519876	0.383324	0.18	1.68	0.79	3.57
	Winter	1.368756	0.353764	< 0.001	3.93	1.96	7.87
0.003	Absolute term (β_0)	−2.30544	0.125369	0	0.10	0.08	0.13
	Adult	0.437116	0.152208	0.004	1.55	1.15	2.09

LD Łódzkie, *MP* Leser Poland, *MA* Masovia, *OP* Opolskie, *PK* Subcarpathia, *PM* Pomerania, *SW* Świętokrzyskie, *WM* Warmia-Masuria

significance level was alpha = 0.05. STATISTICA data analysis software in version 10 (StatSoft, Inc.) and ArcGIS 10.4.1 for Desktop Standard (ESRI, Inc.) were used for statistical and spatial data analysis. Red fox demographics were derived from the Polish Hunting Association-PZL [6].

Results

Antibodies against a *Leptospira* serovar was found in 561 serum samples (26.3%). The highest seroprevalence was observed in foxes hunted in the Subcarpathia (41.6%) and Warmia-Masuria provinces (40.3%) (Table 1, Fig. 1). Specific antibodies were mainly directed against Poi (12.4%), Saxkoebing (11.3%), and Sejroe (6.0%) serovars with serum antibody titres up to 1:25,600 in individual animals (Table 4). When analysing the logistic regression model of positive and negative serostatus (excluding data related to individual *Leptospira* serovars), a significant influence of the area (province) and associated density of foxes on the serostatus was found. The model showed that all provinces had significantly greater odds for having seropositive foxes than the reference SL province, in which the lowest percentage of seropositive foxes was observed. The highest odds ratio (OR = 5.87) with the highest seroprevalence was shown for the PK province. In addition, with an increase of fox density by one animal per km^2, the probability of detecting seropositive animals increased more than threefold and it almost doubled in winter when compared to summer. However due to data deficiencies e.g. sampling date, seasonal influence on the obtained serological results was analysed using a separate logistic regression model.

Based on analyses for individual serovars, an increase of fox density by one animal per km^2 increased the risk of being seropositive by 2.8, 10.6, 17.2 and 18.4 times for the serovars Poi, Grippotyphosa, Australis and Icterohaemorrhagiae, respectively. The models also show a significant influence of the province on the proportion of seropositive samples. A significantly higher risk of being seropositive to Sejroe serovar was observed in the LD

Table 4 Distribution of pathogenic *Leptospira* antibody titers for 561 positive red foxes hunted during season 2014–2015 in Poland

Serovar	No of antibody-positive samples (%)										Prevalence of serovar (95% CI) (%)
	1:100	1:200	1:400	1:800	1:1600	1:3200	1:6400	1:12800	1:25600	Total	
Icterohaemorrhagiae	8 (0.4)	3 (0.1)	3 (0.1)	1 (0.05)	2 (0.1)	1 (0.05)	0	0	0	18	0.8 (0.5–1.3)
Grippotyphosa	6 (0.3)	16 (0.75)	8 (0.4)	4 (0.2)	1 (0.05)	2 (0.1)	0	0	0	37	1.7 (1.2–2.4)
Sejroe	39 (1.8)	37 (1.7)	30 (1.4)	16 (0.75)	2 (0.1)	2 (0.1)	0	0	1 (0.05)	127	6.0 (5.0–7.0)
Tarassovi	0	1 (0.05)	0	0	0	0	0	0	0	1	0.1 (0.0–0.3)
Pomona	7 (1.5)	7 (1.5)	8 (0.4)	8 (0.4)	2 (0.1)	2 (0.1)	0	0	0	34	1.6 (1.1–2.2)
Canicola	0	2 (0.1)	1 (0.05)	0	0	0	0	0	0	3	0.1 (0.0–0.4)
Australis	7 (1.5)	11 (0.5)	1 (0.05)	7 (1.5)	2 (0.1)	0	0	0	0	28	1.3 (0.9–1.9)
Saxkoebing	63 (3.0)	55 (2.6)	66 (3.1)	44 (2.1)	8 (0.4)	3 (0.1)	2 (0.1)	0	1 (0.05)	242	11.3 (10.0–12.8)
Ballum	0	1 (0.05)	1 (0.05)	1 (0.05)	0	0	0	0	0	3	0.1 (0.0–0.4)
Poi	64 (3.0)	68 (3.2)	63 (3.0)	34 (1.6)	11 (0.5)	19 (0.9)	4 (0.2)	1 (0.05)	1 (0.05)	265	12.4 (11.1–13.9)
Bataviae	1 (0.05)	1 (0.05)	3 (0.1)	3 (0.1)	0	1 (0.05)	0	0	0	9	0.4 (0.2–0.8)
Hardjo	0	2 (0.1)	0	1 (0.05)	0	0	1 (0.05)	0	0	4	0.2 (0.1–0.5)

(OR = 3.1), MA (OR = 2.4), PK (OR = 3.4), PM (OR = 2.9) and WM (OR = 2.4) provinces compared to the SL province.

When compared to the reference SL province, antibodies to the Saxkoebing and Poi serovars were more prevalent in foxes from all provinces except SW (OR from 2.0 to 7.0), and MP province (OR from 9.4 to 39.1) respectively. An impact of the season on the seroprevalence to particular serovars was observed. Antibodies against serovars Saxkoebing and Poi were ~2 and 4 times more frequent, respectively, during the winter period than during summer. The age of the foxes influenced the serostatus for some serovars such as Icterohaemorrhagiae that was detected more frequently in young foxes (OR = 3.3) and Poi found more often in adults (OR = 1.5) (Table 3). Using a one-factor model the association between influence of sex on serostatus was not significant (LR-test P = 0.0525, OR = 1.44, 95% CI 0.99–2.09).

Discussion

Other serological surveys have shown that red foxes are frequently exposed to *Leptospira* spp. of different serovars [10, 11, 13]. However this is the first prevalence study on the occurrence of antibodies to a broad range of *Leptospira* serovars in a red fox population in eastern Europe. The high seroprevalence (26.3%) in red foxes in Poland is comparable to that found in Spain (47.1%) [10] and Croatia (31.3%) [13] but higher than in other European countries such as Germany (1.9%) [14] and Norway (9.9%) [11]. Hypothetically any pathogenic *Leptospira* may infect domestic and wild animals, but in practice only a small number of serovars are endemic in any particular region.

Antibodies against serovar Poi were the most commonly detected. Exposure of foxes to this serovar is not surprising given the results of previous Polish studies where serogroup Javanica (to which serovar Poi belongs) was also reported in horses, goats, and sheep [15–17]. Besides serovar Poi, antibodies against serovar Sejroe were also prevalent in foxes. This is consistent with other studies as serovars Hardjo, Sejroe and Saxkoebing (all belonging to the Sejroe serogroup) are widely prevalent in animals in Europe [18–21]. MAT reactions to serovar Hardjo commonly detected in sheep and cattle [18–20, 22, 23] were not common in foxes. The presence of seropositive animals to this serogroup could be mainly attributed to Sejroe or Saxkoebing serovars (Table 4). It may be associated with fox diet as the main source of food for red foxes are wild small mammals, which are known reservoirs of Saxkoebing and Sejroe serovars [24]. Antibodies to Sejroe serogroup were previously detected in pigs, dogs, horses and cattle in Poland confirming a widespread exposure of different animal species to leptospires from this serogroup [15, 25–28]. In addition, this indicates an endemic occurrence of this serovar and a possible role of the environment in pathogen transmission. The observed regional differences in exposure to different *Leptospira* serovars may be related to active circulation of *Leptospira* spp. in the environment [12].

Studies conducted in other European countries provide scientific evidences that the most common serovar among red foxes is serovar Icterohaemorrhagiae [10, 11, 13], which however seems to be rare in the Polish red fox population (Table 4). As leptospires are sensitive to desiccation, the regional differences in climate conditions may have a significant influence on seroprevalence in general or for some serovars in particular. In that aspect, Poland differs from other countries such as Spain and Croatia where the seroprevalence of *Leptospira* spp. in foxes has been investigated [10, 13].

Although the studies were conducted on a reasonable number of hunted animals originating from different locations across the country, the number of tested serum samples of red foxes did not fully reflect the size of the animal population present in the studied provinces. It could be taken as a major limitation to interpretation of the occurrence and prevalence of tested *Leptospira* serovars in the Polish population of red foxes. Nevertheless, the findings still provide useful data on the seroepidemiology of red foxes exposed to different *Leptospira* serovars in this part of Europe and their role as an important source of zoonotic *Leptospira* spp. for humans.

Conclusions

Red foxes of central and eastern Poland, particularly in the Subcarpathia and Warmia-Masuria regions, are highly exposed to *Leptospira* spp. Due to the high prevalence of foxes, their predatory behaviour and their varied diet mainly composed of small mammals, they could be considered as sentinel animals of environmental contamination with leptospires. Interactions between animals require further epidemiological investigations to elucidate the role of wild carnivores as a reservoir of rarely occurring *Leptospira* serovars pathogenic for other animals and humans.

Abbreviations

DS: Lower Silesia; EMJH: Ellinghausen–McCullough–Johnson–Harris medium; KP: Kuyavian-Pomerania; LB: Lubuskie; LD: Łódzkie; LR: likelihood ratio; LU: Lubelskie; MA: Masovia; MAT: microscopic agglutination test; MP: Lesser Poland; OP: Opolskie; OR: odds ratio; PD: Podlaskie; PK: Subcarpathia; PM: Pomerania; SL: Silesia; SW: Świętokrzyskie; WM: Warmia-Masuria; WP: Greater Poland; ZP: West Pomerania.

Authors' contributions

JZ designed and coordinated the study. SZ and AN were responsible for the laboratory work and preliminary data analysis under the supervision of JZ, AJ and ZP. AS was involved in the analyses of epidemiological data. LB performed the statistical analyses. ZA, AJ and AB had the main responsibility of checking and authoring the manuscript. All authors read and approved the final manuscript.

Author details

[1] Swine Diseases Department, National Veterinary Research Institute, Partyzantow 57, 24-100 Pulawy, Poland. [2] University Centre of Veterinary Medicine UJ-UR, University of Agriculture in Krakow, Mickiewicza 24/28, 30-059 Krakow, Poland. [3] Epidemiology and Risk Assessment Department, National Veterinary Research Institute, Partyzantow 57, 24-100 Pulawy, Poland. [4] Veterinary Hygiene Research Station, Wroclawska 170, 45-836 Opole, Poland.

Acknowledgements

We are grateful to the hunters of all nine provinces. Many thanks to Jolanta Sajna from the Warsaw Veterinary Hygiene Research Station (Ostrołęka field division) and to Zofia Klimczak from the Bydgoszcz Veterinary Hygiene Research Station for data and serum samples from foxes; without their help this investigation would not have been possible. The authors would like to warmly thank Artur Rzeżutka for useful comments and editing of the manuscript.

Competing interests

The authors declare that they have no competing interests.

Funding

This study was supported by the Polish National Science Centre (Grant No. 2013/09/B/NZ7/02563). The open access publication fee was funded by the KNOW (Leading National Research Centre) Scientific Consortium "Healthy Animal—Safe Food", Ministry of Science and Higher Education resolution no. 05-1/KNOW2/2015".

References

1. Jancloes M, Bertherat E, Scheider C, Belmain S, Munoz-Zanzi C, Hartskeerl R, et al. Towards a "one health" strategy against leptospirosis. Planet@Risk. 2014;2:204–6 **(Special Issue on One Health (Part I/II): GRF Davos)**.
2. Levett PN. Leptospirosis. Clin Microbiol Rev. 2001;14:296–326.
3. Bharti AR, Nally JE, Ricaldi JN, Matthias MA, Diaz MM, Lovett MA, et al. Leptospirosis: a zoonotic disease of global importance. Lancet Infect Dis. 2003;3:757–71.
4. Ellis WA. Leptospirosis: Leptospira spp. serovars Pomona, Kennewicki, Bratislava, Muenchen, Tarassovi, Canicola, Grippotyphosa, Hardjo, others—abortion and stillbirths. In: Zimmerman JJ, Karriker LA, Ramirez A, Schwartz KJ, Stevenson GW, editors. Diseases of swine. 10th ed. New York: Wiley; 2012. p. 770–8.
5. National Geographic. Animals. Washington, D.C. 2017. https://www.nationalgeographic.com/animals/mammals/r/red-fox/. Accessed 04 Mar 2018.
6. Polish Hunting Association-PZL. Warsaw. 2015. http://www.czempin.pzlow.pl/palio/html.run?_Instance=pzl_www&_PageID=21&_CAT=CZEMPIN.MATERIALY. Accessed 04 Mar 2018.
7. Stritof Majetic Z, Galloway R, Ruzic Sabljic E, Milas Z, Mojcec Perko V, Habus J, et al. Epizootiological survey of small mammals as *Leptospira* spp. reservoirs in Eastern Croatia. Acta Trop. 2014;131:111–6.
8. OIE Terrestrial Manual 2014. Chapter 2.1.12. Leptospirosis. http://www.oie.int/fileadmin/Home/eng/Health_standards/tahm/2.01.12_LEPTO.pdf. Accessed 04 Mar 2018.
9. Wolff JW. The laboratory diagnosis of leptospirosis. Illinois: Charles C. Thomas Publishers; 1954. p. 31–51.
10. Millán J, Candela MG, López-Bao JV, Pereira M, Jiménez MA, León-Vizcaíno L. Leptospirosis in wild and domestic carnivores in natural areas in Andalusia, Spain. Vector Borne Zoonotic Dis. 2009;9:549–54.
11. Akerstedt J, Lillehaug A, Larsen IL, Eide NE, Arnemo JM, Handeland K. Serosurvey for canine distemper virus, canine adenovirus, *Leptospira interrogans*, and *Toxoplasma gondii* in free-ranging canids in Scandinavia and Svalbard. J Wildl Dis. 2010;46:474–80.
12. Moinet M, Fournier-Chambrillon C, André-Fontaine G, Aulagnier S, Mesplède A, Blanchard B. Leptospirosis in free-ranging endangered European mink (*Mustela lutreola*) and other small carnivores (*Mustelidae, Viverridae*) from southwestern France. J Wildl Dis. 2010;46:1141–51.
13. Slavica Ž, Cvetnić Z, Milas Z, Janicki Z, Turk N, Konjević D, et al. Incidence of leptospiral antibodies in different game species over a 10-year period (1996–2005) in Croatia. Eur J Wildl Res. 2008;54:305–11.
14. Müller H, Winkler P. Results of serological studies of *Leptospira* antibodies in foxes. Berl Munch Tierarztl Wochenschr. 1994;107:90–3.
15. Arent ZJ, Kedzierska-Mieszkowska S. Seroprevalence study of leptospirosis in horses in northern Poland. Vet Rec. 2013;172:269.
16. Czopowicz M, Kaba J, Smith L, Szalus-Jordanow O, Nowicki M, Witkowski L. Leptospiral antibodies in the breeding goat population of Poland. Vet Rec. 2011;169:230–4.
17. Krawczyk M. Serological studies on leptospirosis in sheep. Med Weter. 1999;55:397–9.
18. Little TW, Stevens AE, Hathaway SC. Serological studies on British isolates of the Sejroe serogroup I. The identification of British isolates of the Sejroe serogroup by the cross agglutinin absorption test. J Hyg (Lond). 1986;97:123–31.
19. Little TW, Stevens AE, Hathaway SC. Serological studies on British isolates of the Sejroe serogroup of leptospira II. An evaluation of the factor analysis method of identifying leptospires using strains belonging to the Sejroe serogroup. Epidemiol Infect. 1987;99:107–15.

20. Slavica A, Dezdek D, Konjevic D, Cvetnic Z, Sindicic M, Stanin D. Prevalence of leptospiral antibodies in the red fox (*Vulpes vulpes*) population of Croatia. Vet Med (Praha). 2011;56:209–13.
21. Lange S. Seroepidemiological studies of the detection of leptospires of the Sejroe group in cattle in middle Thuringia. Berl Munch Tierarztl Wochenschr. 1992;105:374–7.
22. Arent Z, Frizzell C, Gilmore C, Mackie D, Ellis WA. Isolation of leptospires from genital tract of sheep. Vet Rec. 2013;173:582.
23. Ellis WA. Animal leptospirosis. In: Adler B, editor. Leptospira and leptospirosis, vol. 387., Current topics in microbiology and immunologyBerlin: Springer; 2015. p. 99–137. https://doi.org/10.1007/978-3-662-45059-8_1.
24. Sebek Z, Sixl W, Sixl-Voigt B, Köck M, Stünzner D, Valova M. First evidence of the leptospirosis natural foci of the serotype Saxkoebing in Austria. Geogr Med Suppl. 1989;2:17–22.
25. Krawczyk M. Serological evidence of leptospirosis in animals in northern Poland. Vet Rec. 2005;156:88–9.
26. Wasiński B. Occurrence of Leptospira sp. antibodies in swine in Poland. Bull Vet Inst Pulawy. 2007;51:225–8.
27. Wasiński B, Pejsak Z. Occurrence of leptospiral infections in swine population in Poland evaluated by ELISA and microscopic agglutination test. Pol J Vet Sci. 2010;13:695–9.
28. Wasiński B. Infections of swine caused by Leptospira serovars of serogroup Sejroe—possibilities of recognition with the use of PCR. Bull Vet Inst Pulawy. 2014;58:521–6.

19

Environmental resistance development to influenza antivirals: a case exemplifying the need for a multidisciplinary One Health approach including physicians

Josef D. Järhult*

Abstract

A multidisciplinary approach is a prerequisite for One Health. Physicians are important players in the One Health team, yet they are often hard to convince of the benefits of the One Health approach. Here, the case for multidisciplinarity including physicians is made using the example of environmental resistance development to influenza antivirals. Neuraminidase inhibitors are the major class of anti-influenza pharmaceuticals, and extensively stockpiled globally as a cornerstone of pandemic preparedness, especially important in the first phase before vaccines can be mass-produced. The active metabolite of oseltamivir that is excreted from treated patients degrades poorly in conventional sewage treatment processes and has been found in river waters. Dabbling ducks constitute the natural influenza A virus reservoir and often reside near sewage treatment plant outlets, where they may be exposed to neuraminidase inhibitor residues. In vivo experiments using influenza-infected Mallards exposed to neuraminidase inhibitors present in their water have shown resistance development and persistence, demonstrating that resistance may be induced and become established in the influenza strains circulating in natural hosts. Neuraminidase inhibitor resistance genes may become part of a human-adapted influenza virus with pandemic potential through reassortment or direct transmission. A pandemic caused by a neuraminidase inhibitor-resistant influenza virus is a serious threat as the first line defense in pandemic preparedness would be disarmed. To assess the risk for environmental influenza resistance development, a broad multidisciplinary team containing chemists, social scientists, veterinarians, biologists, ecologists, virologists, epidemiologists, and physicians is needed. Information about One Health early in high school and undergraduate training, an active participation of One Health-engaged physicians in the debate, and more One Health-adapted funding and publication possibilities are suggested to increase the possibility to engage physicians.

Keywords: Avian influenza, Drug residue, Influenza A virus, Lanamivir, Mallard, Neuraminidase inhibitor, Oseltamivir, Pandemic preparedness, Peramivir, Zanamivir

Introduction

Although the One Health approach has recently gained increasing traction, engaging physicians remains a challenge. Whereas veterinarians generally have a thorough understanding of the association of animal and human health—introduced already at an early stage of their training—physicians tend to struggle appreciating humans as yet another animal species and tend to have an overly anthropocentric view. A multitude of professionals need to work together in One Health and are equally important; the multidisciplinarity per se is an important feature of the One Health concept. Yet, engaging specifically physicians in One Health issues is important for several reasons such as: (1) their expertise is needed to plan and evaluate projects from a human health perspective; (2) the engagement of physicians is needed to underscore and give credibility to the human health impact of the

*Correspondence: josef.jarhult@medsci.uu.se
Zoonosis Science Center, Department of Medical Sciences, Uppsala University, 75185 Uppsala, Sweden

issue in question; (3) engagement of physicians can help bring the issue in question to the attention of policy makers and the general public; and (4) engagement of physicians can help open doors to funding aimed primarily at human health. Likely, engaging physicians in One Health is a long, multi-step process that involves interventions at an early phase of their training as well as making already practicing physicians aware of the concept and its importance. In this literature review, environmental resistance development to influenza antivirals will be used as an example to illustrate the importance of multidisciplinarity and engagement of physicians.

Influenza in the avian-human interface

Influenza A virus (IAV) is a pathogen with major economic and health implications in both human and veterinary medicine. Stamping out interventions cost animal lives and cause huge economic losses to the poultry industry, and seasonal as well as pandemic outbreaks in humans strain health care budgets and organizations. Though important to human health, IAV is a zoonotic virus; dabbling ducks and other waterfowl constitute the natural reservoir [1, 2]. Occasional spill-over events occur to other species, humans included. Thus, genetic material from avian IAVs is the basis for human IAVs. The transfer of IAV genetic material from avian sources to humans can occur through two entirely different routes, *direct transmission* and *reassortment*. Direct transmission means that an avian IAV infects humans without previous adaptation in a non-avian host. This is exemplified by transmission of highly-pathogenic avian influenza viruses (HPAIVs) such as H5N1 from infected poultry to humans. Reassortment on the other hand occurs when two or more IAVs infect the same host cell simultaneously. There is no proofing mechanism to sort genetic segments from the respective parental IAV strain into coherent viral offspring, and thus reassortants containing all different variations of the gene segments from each parental strain will be formed. In the context of avian-to-human spread, reassortment is mostly a slow and stepwise process involving several reassortment events over time. As an example, the 2009 pandemic H1N1 IAV was formed from genetic segments from three different IAVs circulating in swine, initially originating from avian sources 1918–1998 and formed through multiple reassortment events [3].

The potential for environmental resistance development in the natural influenza host

Given the connection of IAVs in the avian reservoir and in humans, resistance development to antiviral drugs in naturally circulating avian IAVs is a potential concern also for human health. Pandemic preparedness plans rely heavily on antivirals in the first phase before vaccines can be mass-produced, and antivirals are stockpiled extensively [4]. Experiences from the 2009 IAV pandemic demonstrate that the timely global production and distribution of vaccines was even more difficult to achieve that previously estimated [5]. Thus, antiviral drugs play a crucial role in the beginning of a new IAV outbreak, regardless if the origin is reassortment (like the last four pandemics) or direct transmission (e.g. a human-adapted HPAIV). To date, neuraminidase inhibitors (NAIs) constitute the absolute majority of anti-influenza drugs used. The other, older class of anti-influenza antivirals on the market, adamantanes, are largely abandoned due to side effects and resistance development [6]. The most used NAI, oseltamivir (Tamiflu ©), is administered as a prodrug, oseltamivir phosphate, and rapidly converted in the human body to oseltamivir carboxylate (OC), the active metabolite. OC is excreted mainly via urine and remains stable in surface water and sewage treatment processes [7]. Thus, there is a risk that discharge of OC from sewage treatment plants (STPs) pollutes water bodies downstream of the STP outlets. Dabbling ducks such as the Mallard constitute the natural influenza reservoir, and often reside in waters downstream of STPs. Therefore, dabbling ducks may be exposed to OC in their water environment. IAV is a gastrointestinal infection in Mallards [8] and hence replicating IAV and low levels of OC could co-exist in the intestine of the Mallard, creating a risk for resistance development. If OC-resistant- or NAI-resistant-strains are established among IAVs circulating in the natural reservoir, resistance could be an inherent property of newly human-introduced IAVs, either through reassortment or direct transmission. This is a worrisome scenario given the crucial importance of NAIs in pandemic preparedness. The environmental resistance development hypothesis and its potential connection to humans is depicted in Fig. 1, and has also previously been reviewed [9, 10].

Occurrence of neuraminidase inhibitors in the environment

Ample evidence has accumulated to demonstrate the poor degradation of NAIs in STPs, and the occurrence of NAIs in the environment. OC has been demonstrated in effluent water from STPs [11], as have the newer NAIs zanamivir (Relenza©) [12], peramivir [13], and lanamivir [13]. All four NAIs have also been detected in river water; OC up to 865 ng/L [12, 14], zanamivir 59 ng/L [12, 15], peramivir 11 ng/L [13], and lanamivir 9 ng/L [13]. The highest NAI levels have been found in Japan, the top world-wide per-capita consumer, but OC has also been found in river waters in Europe, e.g. in the UK up to 193 ng/L [16]. One study has also highlighted discharge

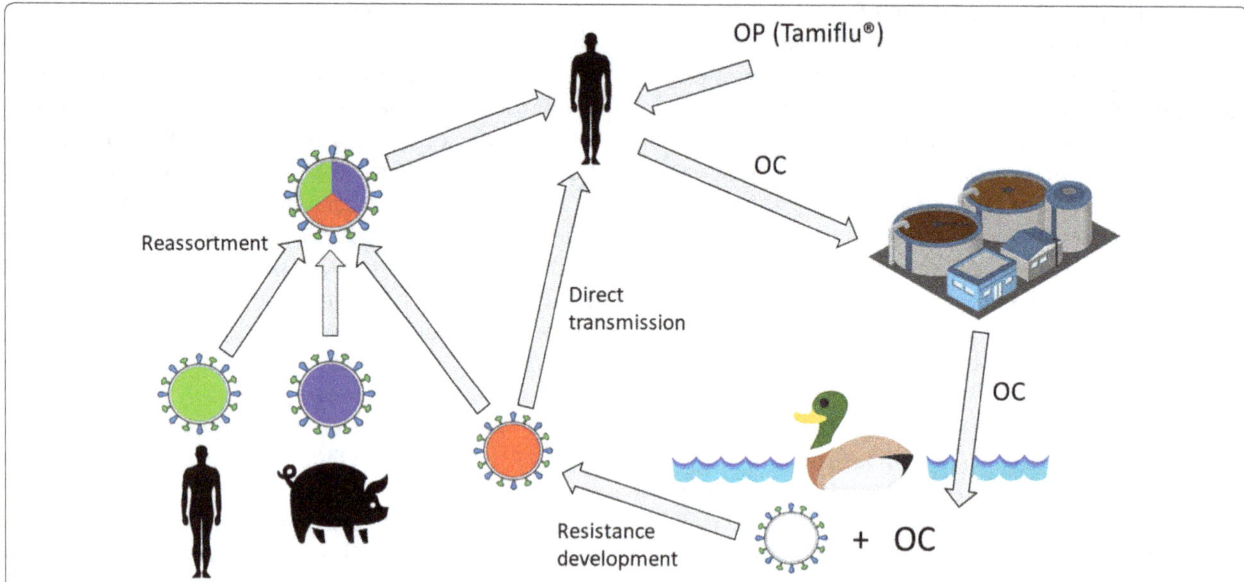

Fig. 1 As OC degrades poorly in STPs and surface waters, it can enter aquatic environments where dabbling ducks can be exposed to the substance. Dabbling ducks constitute the natural influenza reservoir and have a perpetual circulation of influenza A virus in their population. Thus, there is a risk of resistance development in the intestine of the ducks where replicating virus and OC co-exist. Through reassortment or direct transmission, an oseltamivir-resistant influenza virus could spread to humans. *OC* oseltamivir carboxylate, *OP* oseltamivir phosphate, *STP* sewage treatment plant

from drug production facilities as a potential contributing factor to environmental pollution of oseltamivir [17]. To analyze degradation and presence of antiviral drugs in the environment, as well as assessing the implications, environmental chemists are vital in understanding and combatting environmental IAV resistance.

A prerequisite for the occurrence of NAIs in the environment is that the drugs are being used. In most parts of the world, use is regulated through prescription by physicians. Thus, involvement of physicians in a One Health approach, enabling them to appreciate the risks with NAI prescription in a broader perspective, is important to obtain a prudent use of NAIs. Multiple studies, many of them drug company-sponsored, have failed to demonstrate effects of oseltamivir and zanamivir (the second most used NAI) on uncomplicated influenza in otherwise healthy patients than simply shortening of length of clinical disease (symptoms) by 1 day (e.g. [18]). Hence, liberal use of NAIs to for uncomplicated influenza can be questioned, and should definitely be avoided if symptoms have been present > 48 h before treatment, as the effect of NAIs is much dependent of early start of treatment. To implement these guidelines, participation of other health professionals such as nurses and medical practitioners is important. A special case is NAI use in parts of the world where antiviral drugs are sold over the counter (without prescription). Under these circumstances, self-medication with NAIs without previous medical consultation is likely a major driver for NAI pollution. Thus, educating the general public about One Health, as well as strengthening local health systems are important measures in this setting. Social science professionals, e.g. behavioral scientists, are especially important to help understand prescriptions/drug use in a cultural context.

Resistance development in LPAIVs infecting Mallards exposed to NAIs

As NAIs are present in river water, what is the risk of IAV resistance development in the natural reservoir? Mallards perpetuate low pathogenic IAVs (LPAIVs) with a pronounced spatial and temporal prevalence variation; in the Northern Hemisphere the prevalence is typically high (up to 60%) during fall migration and low (0.4–2%) at wintering grounds [19]. Several in vivo studies using LPAIV-infected Mallards subjected to low levels of OC in their water have demonstrated resistance development. Exposure of a H1N1 LPAIV to 0.95 μg/L of OC resulted in the well-known resistance mutation H275Y [20], H5N2 exposure to 1 μg/L in E199V [21], H6N2–12 μg/L in R292K [22], and H7N9–2.5 μg/L in I222T [23]. At least for the H1H1 and H5N2 IAVs, detected OC levels in river water are of the same magnitude as where resistance development occurred. Similar in vivo Mallard studies addressing the risk of resistance development to other NAIs are important, especially as these drugs may be more widely used in the future in case of oseltamivir resistance. To assess the risk for resistance development, several players in the One Health team are needed; bird ecologists to understand migration patterns and behavior of dabbling ducks, virologists to elucidate resistance development at a molecular and functional level, and veterinarians to investigate the aspect of influenza disease in birds.

Persistence of resistance without drug pressure

Once resistance is induced among LPAIVs circulating among wild birds, it is imperative to assess if the resistance can persist without drug pressure. Influenza outbreaks are sporadic, and thus NAIs are not constantly present in the environment. Further, the NAI resistance dogma has been that resistance can quite easily develop during treatment but that resistance development is of less concern, as mutants have decreased fitness—as noted in e.g. early in vitro oseltamivir studies [24]. However, a human seasonal H1N1 IAV strain resistant to oseltamivir through the H275Y mutation spread globally during the 2007–2009 influenza seasons, and the spread was not correlated to oseltamivir use [25]. This demonstrated that in certain genetic backgrounds, NAI resistance do not cause decreased IAV fitness. Several compensatory mutations likely contributed to the ability of the seasonal H1N1 IAV to harbor H275Y without fitness loss [26, 27]. Interestingly, Mallard in vivo experiments demonstrate that in a H1N1 LPAIV that acquired H275Y when infected Mallards were subjected to OC in their water [20], resistance persisted despite removal of OC from the water of the Mallards and subsequent IAV replication and transmission [28]. On the contrary, in a H6N2 virus harboring the R292K mutation from an in vivo experiment [22], resistance did not persist without drug pressure [29], illustrating the impact of different IAV genetic backgrounds. Thus, both from human epidemiological data and in vivo studies, there is evidence that in certain genetic backgrounds, IAV resistance mutations do not result in decreased viral fitness. Here, public health/epidemiology expertise is important to successfully assess spread of resistant strains in the human population and the relation to NAI use. Clinical pharmacists can contribute to NAI prescription analysis and physicians can provide expertise in human influenza disease and drug use from a prescriber's perspective.

Risk of resistance transmission to humans

Reassortment

If resistance to NAIs can develop in IAVs circulating in the natural host, and in certain genetic backgrounds persist without drug pressure, what is the risk that the resistant NA gene becomes part of a human IAV? All four pandemic IAVs seen during the last century were formed through reassortment and all of them were formed by genetic material of avian origin [30, 31]. Thus, it is possible that a NAI-resistant NA gene originating from the natural host can form part of a new pandemic IAV through reassortment. However several factors can influence the likelihood of this event: (1) How prevalent are NAI-resistance among IAVs circulating in the natural host? (2) Is there a loss of fitness when the NAI-resistant NA gene reassorts with other IAVs, i.e. is there a barrier for reassortment? (3) For how long is the NAI-resistant IAV circulating in other hosts (e.g. swine) before it spills over to humans, i.e. what delay is there from resistance development in the environment/natural host until human introduction? To start answering these questions several actions and professionals are needed – such as IAV surveillance in wild waterbirds by biologists and experimental studies regarding reassortment including a NAI-resistant NA gene by virologists. To keep the research questions linked to the human health perspective, involvement of physicians is important.

Direct transmission

There is a barrier for direct transmission of avian-adapted IAVs to humans. The virus must overcome several hurdles such as differences in host body temperature, receptor architecture, and immune response. To date, this has precluded efficient human-to-human transmission of directly transmitted IAVs. However, two research groups have found that small changes in a H5N1 HPAIV allowed for mammal-to-mammal transmission [32, 33]. In one of the studies five point mutations were sufficient to enable transmission, and a subsequent study demonstrated that some circulating H5N1 strains already carried two out of the five point mutations and has modelled factors that can increase the probability for acquisition of the last three [34]. Thus, the genetic barrier for direct transmission may not be as protective as previously thought, and given the high morbidity and mortality for H5N1 and H7N9 IAVs [35], sustained human-to-human transmission is a serious threat. NAI-resistance in such an IAV would make matters much worse; preparedness plans initially rely on stockpiles of NAIs and resistance could render them useless. To assess the risks for human health and to guide pandemic preparedness planning, physicians are crucial. Other important players include virologists to assess the genetic barrier for direct transmission in different IAV genetic backgrounds and environmental settings, immunologists to provide knowledge of human and avian immune defenses and their differences, and professionals with skills in logistics and societal structure to implement the findings into pandemic preparedness.

A summary of key players in a One Health team investigating environmental resistance development to influenza antivirals is depicted in Fig. 2.

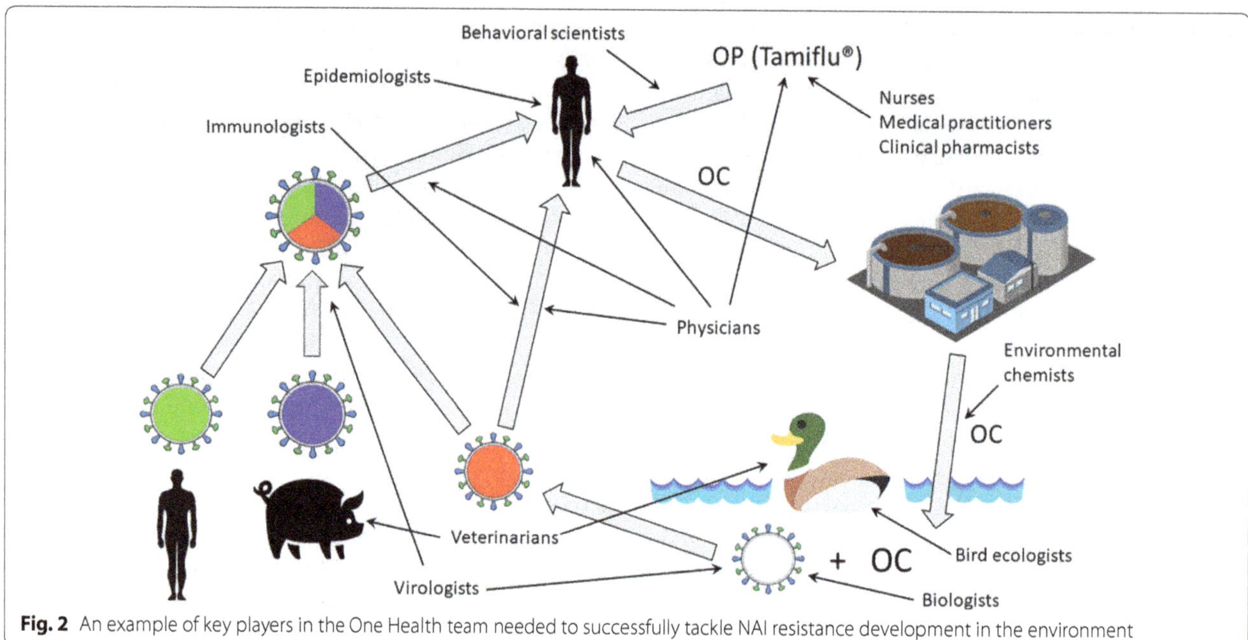

Fig. 2 An example of key players in the One Health team needed to successfully tackle NAI resistance development in the environment

Conclusions

Multidisciplinarity is a key element of the One Health approach, and it is imperative to engage physicians as one of several key players in One Health questions. The example of environmental resistance development in influenza demonstrates this, but it is true for most other One Health questions as well. Engaging physicians in One Health is a challenging task—it is the author's opinion that information and discussion activities early in high school and undergraduate training, a more active voice of One Health-engaged physicians, and funding and publication possibilities more suited to One Health research are important factors in the process.

Abbreviations

HPAIV: highly pathogenic avian influenza virus; IAV: influenza A virus; LPAIV: low-pathogenic avian influenza virus; NA: neuraminidase; NAI: neuraminidase inhibitor; OC: oseltamivir carboxylate; STP: sewage treatment plant.

Authors' information

JJ is an infectious disease physician and researcher in the field of antimicrobial resistance, with a focus on the animal/human/environment interface. He did his Ph.D. on resistance development to oseltamivir in the environment and has since mentored several Ph.D. students in further studies in the area of environmental resistance development to NAIs and the risk of transmission to humans. JJ works as a consultant in infectious diseases at Uppsala University Hospital, Sweden and an Associate Professor in infectious diseases at Uppsala University.

Acknowledgements

Not applicable.

Competing interests

The author declares that he has no competing interests.

Funding

Dr. Järhult's research is funded by the Swedish Research Council VR (Grant No. 2016-02606) and Swedish Research Council FORMAS (Grants Nos. 211-2013-1320 and 2016-00790).

References

1. Olsen B, Munster VJ, Wallensten A, Waldenstrom J, Osterhaus AD, Fouchier RA. Global patterns of influenza a virus in wild birds. Science. 2006;312:384–8.
2. Webster RG, Bean WJ, Gorman OT, Chambers TM, Kawaoka Y. Evolution and ecology of influenza A viruses. Microbiol Rev. 1992;56:152–79.
3. Garten RJ, Davis CT, Russell CA, Shu B, Lindstrom S, Balish A, et al. Antigenic and genetic characteristics of swine-origin 2009 A(H1N1) influenza viruses circulating in humans. Science. 2009;325:197–201.
4. Wan Po AL, Farndon P, Palmer N. Maximizing the value of drug stockpiles for pandemic influenza. Emerg Infect Dis. 2009;15:1686–7.
5. Partridge J, Kieny MP. Global production of seasonal and pandemic (H1N1) influenza vaccines in 2009–2010 and comparison with previous estimates and global action plan targets. Vaccine. 2010;28:4709–12.
6. Nelson MI, Simonsen L, Viboud C, Miller MA, Holmes EC. The origin and global emergence of adamantane resistant A/H3N2 influenza viruses. Virology. 2009;388:270–8.
7. Fick J, Lindberg RH, Tysklind M, Haemig PD, Waldenstrom J, Wallensten A, et al. Antiviral oseltamivir is not removed or degraded in normal sewage water treatment: implications for development of resistance by influenza A virus. PLoS ONE. 2007;2:e986.
8. Daoust PY, Kibenge FSB, Fouchier RAM, van de Bildt MWG, van Riel D, Kuiken T. Replication of low pathogenic avian influenza virus in naturally infected mallard ducks (Anas platyrhynchos) causes no morphologic lesions. J Wildl Dis. 2011;47:401–9.
9. Gillman A. Risk of resistant avian influenza A virus in wild waterfowl as a result of environmental release of oseltamivir. Infect Ecol Epidemiol. 2016;6:32870.
10. Järhult JD. Oseltamivir (Tamiflu(R)) in the environment, resistance development in influenza A viruses of dabbling ducks and the risk of transmission of an oseltamivir-resistant virus to humans—a review. Infect Ecol Epidemiol. 2012;2:18385.
11. Leknes H, Sturtzel IE, Dye C. Environmental release of oseltamivir from a Norwegian sewage treatment plant during the 2009 influenza A (H1N1) pandemic. Sci Total Environ. 2012;414:632–8.

12. Takanami R, Ozaki H, Giri RR, Taniguchi S, Hayashi S. antiviral drugs zanamivir and oseltamivir found in wastewater and surface water in Osaka, Japan. J Water Environ Technol. 2012;10:57–68.
13. Azuma T, Ishiuchi H, Inoyama T, Teranishi Y, Yamaoka M, Sato T, et al. Detection of peramivir and laninamivir, new anti-influenza drugs, in sewage effluent and river waters in Japan. PLoS ONE. 2015;10:e0131412.
14. Takanami R, Ozaki H, Giri RR, Taniguchi S, Hayashi S. Detection of antiviral drugs oseltamivir phosphate and oseltamivir carboxylate in Neya River, Osaka Japan. J Water Environ Technol. 2010;8:363–72.
15. Azuma T, Nakada N, Yamashita N, Tanaka H. Mass balance of anti-influenza drugs discharged into the Yodo River system, Japan, under an influenza outbreak. Chemosphere. 2013;93:1672–7.
16. Singer AC, Jarhult JD, Grabic R, Khan GA, Lindberg RH, Fedorova G, et al. Intra- and inter-pandemic variations of antiviral, antibiotics and decongestants in wastewater treatment plants and receiving rivers. PLoS ONE. 2014;9:e108621.
17. Prasse C, Schlusener MP, Schulz R, Ternes TA. Antiviral drugs in wastewater and surface waters: a new pharmaceutical class of environmental relevance? Environ Sci Technol. 2010;44:1728–35.
18. Jefferson T, Jones MA, Doshi P, Del Mar CB, Hama R, Thompson MJ, et al. Neuraminidase inhibitors for preventing and treating influenza in healthy adults and children. Cochrane Database Syst Rev. 2014:CD008965.
19. Latorre-Margalef N, Tolf C, Grosbois V, Avril A, Bengtsson D, Wille M, et al. Long-term variation in influenza A virus prevalence and subtype diversity in migratory mallards in northern Europe. Proc Biol Sci. 2014;281:20140098.
20. Järhult JD, Muradrasoli S, Wahlgren J, Söderström H, Orozovic G, Gunnarsson G, et al. Environmental levels of the antiviral oseltamivir induce development of resistance mutation H274Y in influenza A/H1N1 virus in mallards. PLoS ONE. 2011;6:e24742.
21. Achenbach JE, Bowen RA. Effect of oseltamivir carboxylate consumption on emergence of drug-resistant H5N2 avian influenza virus in Mallard ducks. Antimicrob Agents Chemother. 2013;57:2171–81.
22. Gillman A, Muradrasoli S, Soderstrom H, Nordh J, Brojer C, Lindberg RH, et al. Resistance mutation R292K is induced in influenza A(H6N2) virus by exposure of infected mallards to low levels of oseltamivir. PLoS ONE. 2013;8:e71230.
23. Gillman A, Nykvist M, Muradrasoli S, Soderstrom H, Wille M, Daggfeldt A, et al. Influenza A(H7N9) virus acquires resistance-related neuraminidase I222T substitution when infected mallards are exposed to low levels of oseltamivir in water. Antimicrob Agents Chemother. 2015;59:5196–202.
24. Xu KM, Li KS, Smith GJ, Li JW, Tai H, Zhang JX, et al. Evolution and molecular epidemiology of H9N2 influenza A viruses from quail in southern China, 2000 to 2005. J Virol. 2007;81:2635–45.
25. Moscona A. Global transmission of oseltamivir-resistant influenza. NEngl J Med. 2009;360:953–6.
26. Abed Y, Pizzorno A, Bouhy X, Boivin G. Role of permissive neuraminidase mutations in influenza A/Brisbane/59/2007-like (H1N1) viruses. PLoS Pathog. 2011;7:e1002431.
27. Bloom JD, Gong LI, Baltimore D. Permissive secondary mutations enable the evolution of influenza oseltamivir resistance. Science. 2010;328:1272–5.
28. Gillman A, Muradrasoli S, Soderstrom H, Holmberg F, Latorre-Margalef N, Tolf C, et al. Oseltamivir-resistant influenza A (H1N1) virus strain with an h274y mutation in neuraminidase persists without drug pressure in infected mallards. Appl Environ Microbiol. 2015;81:2378–83.
29. Gillman A, Muradrasoli S, Mardnas A, Soderstrom H, Fedorova G, Lowenthal M, et al. Oseltamivir resistance in influenza A(H6N2) Caused by an R292K substitution in neuraminidase is not maintained in mallards without drug pressure. PLoS ONE. 2015;10:e0139415.
30. Cox NJ, Subbarao K. Global epidemiology of influenza: past and present. Annu Rev Med. 2000;51:407–21.
31. Guan Y, Vijaykrishna D, Bahl J, Zhu H, Wang J, Smith GJ. The emergence of pandemic influenza viruses. Protein Cell. 2010;1:9–13.
32. Herfst S, Schrauwen EJ, Linster M, Chutinimitkul S, de Wit E, Munster VJ, et al. Airborne transmission of influenza A/H5N1 virus between ferrets. Science. 2012;336:1534–41.
33. Imai M, Watanabe T, Hatta M, Das SC, Ozawa M, Shinya K, et al. Experimental adaptation of an influenza H5 HA confers respiratory droplet transmission to a reassortant H5 HA/H1N1 virus in ferrets. Nature. 2012;486:420–8.
34. Russell CA, Fonville JM, Brown AE, Burke DF, Smith DL, James SL, et al. The potential for respiratory droplet-transmissible A/H5N1 influenza virus to evolve in a mammalian host. Science. 2012;336:1541–7.
35. WHO. Influenza at the human-animal interface. 2017. http://www.who.int/influenza/human_animal_interface/Influenza_Summary_IRA_HA_interface_09_27_2017.pdf?ua=1.

Monitoring variables affecting positron emission tomography measurements of cerebral blood flow in anaesthetized pigs

Aage Kristian Olsen Alstrup[1*], Nora Elisabeth Zois[2], Mette Simonsen[1] and Ole Lajord Munk[1]

Abstract

Background: Positron emission tomography (PET) imaging of anaesthetized pig brains is a useful tool in neuroscience. Stable cerebral blood flow (CBF) is essential for PET, since variations can affect the distribution of several radiotracers. However, the effect of physiological factors regulating CBF is unresolved and therefore knowledge of optimal anaesthesia and monitoring of pigs in PET studies is sparse. The aim of this study was therefore to determine if and how physiological variables and the duration of anaesthesia affected CBF as measured by PET using [^{15}O]-water in isoflurane–N_2O anaesthetized domestic female pigs. First, we examined how physiological monitoring parameters were associated with CBF, and which parameters should be monitored and if possible kept constant, during studies where a stable CBF is important. Secondly, we examined how the duration of anaesthesia affected CBF and the monitoring parameters.

Results: No significant statistical correlations were found between CBF and the nine monitoring variables. However, we found that arterial carbon dioxide tension ($PaCO_2$) and body temperature were important predictors of CBF that should be observed and kept constant. In addition, we found that long-duration anaesthesia was significantly correlated with high heart rate, low arterial oxygen tension, and high body temperature, but not with CBF.

Conclusions: The findings indicate that $PaCO_2$ and body temperature are crucial for maintaining stable levels of CBF and thus optimizing PET imaging of molecular mechanisms in the brain of anaesthetized pigs. Therefore, as a minimum these two variables should be monitored and kept constant. Furthermore, the duration of anaesthesia should be kept constant to avoid variations in monitoring variables.

Keywords: Animal, Brain research, CBF, [^{15}O]-water, Positron emission tomography, Swine

Background

Positron emission tomography (PET) scanning of the brain of pigs is a useful tool in neuroscience [1–5]. Often, cerebral blood flow (CBF) is measured by PET scans using [^{15}O]-water [5, 6]. CBF measurements are key parameters in pig studies of human conditions such as stroke [7], drug abuse [8] and brain stimulation [9]. In addition, [^{15}O]-water PET scans are performed in some animal studies to assess the degree in which anaesthesia-induced variations in CBF affect the kinetic parameters of PET tracers in the brain in vivo [10]. As an example, the pharmacokinetics of the dopamine D_1 tracer [11] C SCH23390 are affected depending on whether the pig is anaesthetized with isoflurane or propofol, which increase and decrease CBF, respectively [11]. Furthermore, CBF is tightly coupled to brain metabolism, and changes in CBF may therefore also affect results in studies of brain metabolism [12, 13]. Clearly, stable CBF is crucial in many PET studies of the brain, but little is currently known on how various physiological variables affect CBF in anaesthetized pigs.

Previously, we studied the effects of normocapnia *versus* hypercapnia on CBF in anaesthetized domestic pigs

*Correspondence: aagols@rm.dk
[1] Department of Nuclear Medicine and PET Centre, Faculty of Health, Aarhus University Hospital, Noerrebrogade 44, 10C, 8000 Aarhus C, Denmark

[6]. CBF increased markedly from a mean of 0.48 mL blood/min/mL brain tissue during normocapnia to 0.74 mL blood/min/mL brain tissue during hypercapnia. The result confirmed that arterial carbon dioxide tension ($PaCO_2$) plays a key role in regulating CBF in pigs, and indicates that control of $PaCO_2$ is a crucial factor for maintaining CBF within certain boundaries during PET studies of the brain. We needed to establish whether other physiological factors alter CBF in anaesthetized pigs in order to establish optimal experimental conditions for studying molecular mechanisms in the brain in vivo. Therefore, we carried out the present study to determine the role of arterial pH, $PaCO_2$, arterial oxygen tension (PaO_2), haematocrit (HCT), blood glucose (GLC), heart rate (HR), systolic blood pressure (SBP), diastolic blood pressure (DBP), body temperature (TEMP) and the duration of anaesthesia (TIME) on CBF in domestic pigs during isoflurane–N_2O anaesthesia.

Methods

Animals

All procedures involving animals were approved by the Danish Experimental Animal Inspectorate. The present study was based on data obtained from 37 female domestic pigs (Danish Landrace x Yorkshire) weighing 38.1 ± 2.2 kg (mean $\pm$ SD). The pigs were fed a restricted pellet diet (600 g per pig; DIA plus FI, DLG, Denmark) and iron-(II)-fumarate/iron-(III)-oxide (Grynt, DLG, Denmark), and they were group housed for at least 5 days in the animal facility prior to the study. They were fasted 16 h prior to the study, but had free access to tap water. The pigs were not subjected to any specific health-monitoring program, but had no clinical signs of disease. The environmental temperature in the animal facility was 20 °C, 51% relative humidity with no specific light cycles and with the air exchanged 8 times/h.

Anaesthesia and PET scanning

All pigs were pre-medicated with 50 mg (1.3 mg/kg) midazolam (Dormicum, Roche, Denmark) and 500 mg (13 mg/kg) ketamine (Ketalar, Pfizer, Denmark) intramuscularly. Anaesthesia was induced with 50 mg (1.3 mg/kg) midazolam and 250 mg (12.5 mg/kg) ketamine intravenously and was maintained with a vaporizer setting of 2.0% isoflurane in oxygen and N_2O (1:2). The pigs were mechanically ventilated with a tidal volume of approximately 8 mL/kg and a frequence of 15 times/min (minute volume: 4.5 L). Heart catheters (Johnson and Johnson, Miami, FL, USA) were surgically placed in a femoral artery and a femoral vein as described in [14]. Blood gases ($PaCO_2$ and PaO_2), pH, HCT, and GLC were monitored prior to the initial [^{15}O]-water PET scan, while HR, SBP, DBP, and rectal TEMP were continuously monitored using a six-channel device (Kivex, Bethesda, MD). The monitor was read immediately before the scan. Duration of anaesthesia was calculated as the time from the switching on of isoflurane and until the tracer was injected. Arterial blood samples were handled according to [15] and were analysed using an ABL 550 (Radiometer, Denmark). Isotonic saline was infused intravenously at a rate of 100–200 mL/h to prevent dehydration. After performing the baseline [^{15}O]-water PET scan, the pigs were scanned with other tracers not reported here. At the end of the study, the pigs were killed with an overdose of 100 mg/kg of pentobarbitone (Veterinærapoteket, Frederiksberg, Denmark) intravenously. Necropsy of thorax (e.g. bronchopneumonia) and abdomen (e.g. peritonitis) was performed in all pigs.

PET scan examination

The CBF was evaluated by using the radioactive PET tracer [^{15}O]-water and measurements of the radioactivity as a function of time both in brain and in the bloodstream [16]. PET imaging was performed using a Siemens ECAT EXACT HR-47 tomograph (CTI/Siemens Medical Systems, Knoxville, TN Inc.). The PET camera was calibrated by a phantom containing a $^{68}Ge/^{68}Ga$ solution with known radioactivity. A 15-min transmission scan was performed before the first emission scan and was used for photon attenuation correction of the emission recordings. Dynamic PET recording was acquired in a 3D acquisition mode. The tracer [^{15}O]-water was given as a 5-s intravenous injection of 500 MBq, followed by dynamic PET recordings for 5 min (20×3 s, 10×6 s, 6×10 s, and 6×20 s). Data were reconstructed using 2D iterative reconstruction (FORE OSEM). Each frame in the resulting dynamic PET image consisted of $128 \times 128 \times 47$ voxels of $0.7 \times 0.7 \times 3.1$ mm^3 with a central spatial resolution of 5 mm FWHM. During the dynamic PET scans, arterial blood (7 mL/min in total 35 mL removed from the pig) was continuously sampled and radioactivity concentrations were measured every 0.5 s by an automatic blood sampler (Allogg AB, Sweden) withdrawing 7 mL blood/min, i.e. 35 mL during the PET scan. Both dynamic PET data and arterial blood data were corrected for radioactive decay measured from the start of tracer administration.

Image analysis, kinetic modelling, and statistical analysis

A 15 mm (radius) circular formed region-of-interest (ROI) including the brain was defined in five adjacent transaxial slices of images of the mean radioactivity concentrations. The ROIs were combined to form one global volume-of-interest (VOI) containing a mixture of grey and white matter. Time courses of the radioactivity concentrations in this VOI were generated. The CBF was estimated from the dynamic [^{15}O]-water PET scans. The analytical solution of the model was fitted to data in order to estimate kinetic parameters. By denoting the tissue activity concentration as *M(t)*, and the arterial blood activity concentration as $C_i(t)$, the model predicts

$$M(t) = K_1 e^{-k_2 t} \otimes C_i(t) + V_0 C_i(t), \quad (1)$$

where ⊗ denotes a convolution integral. The model has three parameters: the clearance into the cell, K_1 (mL blood/min/mL brain tissue), the reverse rate constant k_2 (per min), and a vascular volume V_0 (mL blood/mL brain tissue). K_1 is assumed to be equal to CBF for freely diffusible substances such as [^{15}O]-water. In practice, the blood–brain barrier limits the passage of tracer from blood to cell. This effect causes CBF to be slightly underestimated by this equation as described by the Renkin–Crone relation [17, 18]. For each data set, CBF was estimated as K_1 by non-linear least-squares regression [19] of the one-tissue compartment model to the measured dynamic PET data. Each PET data point was weighted in proportion to the frame duration.

Statistics

Data were examined for outliers and skewness, and tested for normality using the Shapiro–Wilk method with *P* values less than 0.05 considered significant. For normally-distributed variables, we calculated the Pearson correlation coefficient r, and the *P* value between CBF and the monitored parameters. Spearman rank order correlation method was used for variables that are not normally distributed. Correction for multiple comparisons was made using the Benjamini–Hochberg step-up procedure [20] with the critical value for false discovery rate (FDR) set to $\alpha = 0.05$.

Step-wise regression with forward selection was used to test for the inclusion of best monitoring variable with threshold values for *F*-to-enter = 4.0 (minimum incremental *F* value to enter the model) and for *F*-to-leave = 3.9 (maximum incremental *F* value to remove from the model). The selection started without monitoring variables in the model. Then, we tested the inclusion of each monitoring variable that was not in the model, adding to the model the monitoring variable with the largest *F*-to-enter statistic provided that it is above the threshold. Then, it is tested to see if any variables already included have fallen below *F*-to-leave threshold. This process is repeated until no monitoring variables have *F*-statistics on the wrong side of the threshold.

Results

CBF was calculated in 37 pigs that were PET scanned between 79 and 314 min after onset of anaesthesia. The physiological monitoring variables are shown in Table 1.

Table 1 Estimated cerebral blood flow and measured physiological variables expressed both as mean and median

	Mean	Std dev	Median	Range	N
CBF (mL/mL/min)	0.54	0.16	0.51	0.15–0.91	37
pH	7.44	0.04	7.44	7.35–7.52	28
$PaCO_2$ (kPa)	6.3	0.7	6.2	5.0–7.9	28
PaO_2 (kPa)	18	5	16	10.7–29.0	27
HCT (%)	30	3	30	24.3–35.9	26
HR (min^{-1})	115	25	116	53–160	21
SBP (mmHg)	114	14	110	86–142	23
DBP (mmHg)	76	17	70	51–118	23
GLC (mmol/L)	4.9	1.4	4.8	2.3–8.1	26
TEMP (°C)	37.7	1.3	37.9	34.8–39.9	23
TIME (min)	115	68	127	79–314	37

CBF cerebral blood flow, *$PaCO_2$* arterial carbondioxide tension, *PaO_2* arterial oxygen tension, *HCT* haematocrit, *HR* heart rate, *SBP* systolic blood pressure, *DBP* diastolic blood pressure, *GLC* blood glucose, *TEMP* body temperature, *TIME* duration of anaesthesia, *N* number of observations

For all parameters, mean values were within the porcine reference intervals [21].

CBF and all nine monitored physiological variables passed the test for normality. The correlations and *P* values are shown in Table 2. CBF was associated with high $PaCO_2$, low blood pH, high HR, and high TEMP, whereas no associations were noted between CBF and PaO_2, HCT, SBP, DBP and GLC. However, no correlations were significant on 5% level when correcting for multiple comparisons. Thus, we screened the monitoring variables for their contribution to the prediction of CBF. Step-wise regression with forward selection was made to identify the monitoring parameters the best predicted CBF resulted in a linear combination of $PaCO_2$ (P = 0.025) and TEMP (P = 0.029). No other monitoring parameters added significantly to the prediction of CBF (Fig. 1).

Finally, we examined if time after onset of anaesthesia (TIME) affected the physiological condition of the pigs by comparing TIME to all other measures. TIME did not have clear outliers and was not highly skewed but did not pass the test for normality. We therefore used Spearman's method to test for correlations. The correlation coefficients for the relationship between TIME and CBF, and TIME and the nine monitoring variables are shown in Table 2. HR, TEMP and PaO_2 were significantly correlated to TIME after correcting for multiple comparisons.

Discussion

The mean CBF (0.54 mL/mL/min) was comparable with our previous study in pigs [6]. However, the variation in CBFs was high, even though standard conditions were

Table 2 Correlation coefficients between estimated cerebral blood flow and monitoring parameters

	pH	$PaCO_2$	PaO_2	HCT	HR	SBP	DBP	TEMP	GLC	TIME
CBF	- 0.35 0.064 28	0.45 0.016 28	- 0.22 0.28 27	0.22 0.29 26	0.49 0.024 21	0.06 0.80 23	- 0.07 0.76 23	0.41 0.052 23	0.13 0.53 26	0.26 0.11 37
pH	–	- 0.82 0.000 28	0.065 0.75 27	- 0.014 0.95 26	- 0.16 0.48 21	- 0.043 0.85 23	- 0.089 0.69 23	- 0.23 0.29 23	0.13 0.54 24	0.01 0.96 28
$PaCO_2$	–	–	- 0.11 0.59 27	0.30 0.14 26	0.24 0.31 21	0.27 0.21 23	0.21 0.33 23	0.34 0.12 23	- 0.13 0.56 24	0.10 0.62 28
PaO_2	–	–	–	- 0.23 0.28 25	- 0.60 0.004 21	0.40 0.059 23	0.26 0.23 23	0.035 0.87 23	- 0.24 0.27 23	**- 0.46** **0.015*** **27**
HCT	–	–	–	–	0.45 0.046 20	0.18 0.43 22	0.18 0.43 22	0.22 0.33 22	0.21 0.34 22	0.27 0.18 26
HR	–	–	–	–	–	0.022 0.92 21	0.039 0.87 21	0.33 0.14 21	0.21 0.40 18	**0.73** **0.000*** **21**
SBP	–	–	–	–	–	–	0.58 0.004 23	0.27 0.22 23	0.25 0.28 20	0.048 0.83 23
DBP	–	–	–	–	–	–	–	0.019 0.93 23	0.094 0.69 20	- 0.23 0.28 23
TEMP	–	–	–	–	–	–	–	–	0.19 0.42 20	**0.53** **0.010*** **23**
GLC	–	–	–	–	–	–	–	–	–	0.44 0.02 26

In white background. correlation coefficients between CBF and the measured monitoring variables. Each entry contains the correlation coefficient r (Pearsons), the P value, and the number of data. Positive correlation coefficients tend to increase together, whereas inverse relationships are observed with negative correlation. In grey background, correlation coefficients between TIME and all other parameters. Each entry contains the correlation coefficient p (Spearman's), the P value, and the number of data. HR, TEMP and PaO_2 were significantly correlated to TIME after correcting for multiple comparisons. Significant correlations are shown in bold and marked with *

used and the pigs were of the same sex, and had comparable age and body weight.

Out of nine monitored variables, we found significant correlations between CBF and $PaCO_2$, blood pH, HR, and TEMP. However, after correction for multiple comparisons with the Benjamini–Hochberg step-up procedure, none of these monitorering variables differed significantly. The reason could be that we compared many parameters where some are highly correlated, redundant or even extraneous. Instead, the step-wise regression could identify $PaCO_2$ and TEMP as the monitoring parameters that best predicted CBF. Thus, $PaCO_2$ and body temperature were important predictors of CBF that should be observed and controlled. The importance of $PaCO_2$ concentrations to predict CBF is in agreement with earlier studies in pigs [6, 22] and the fact that CO_2 is

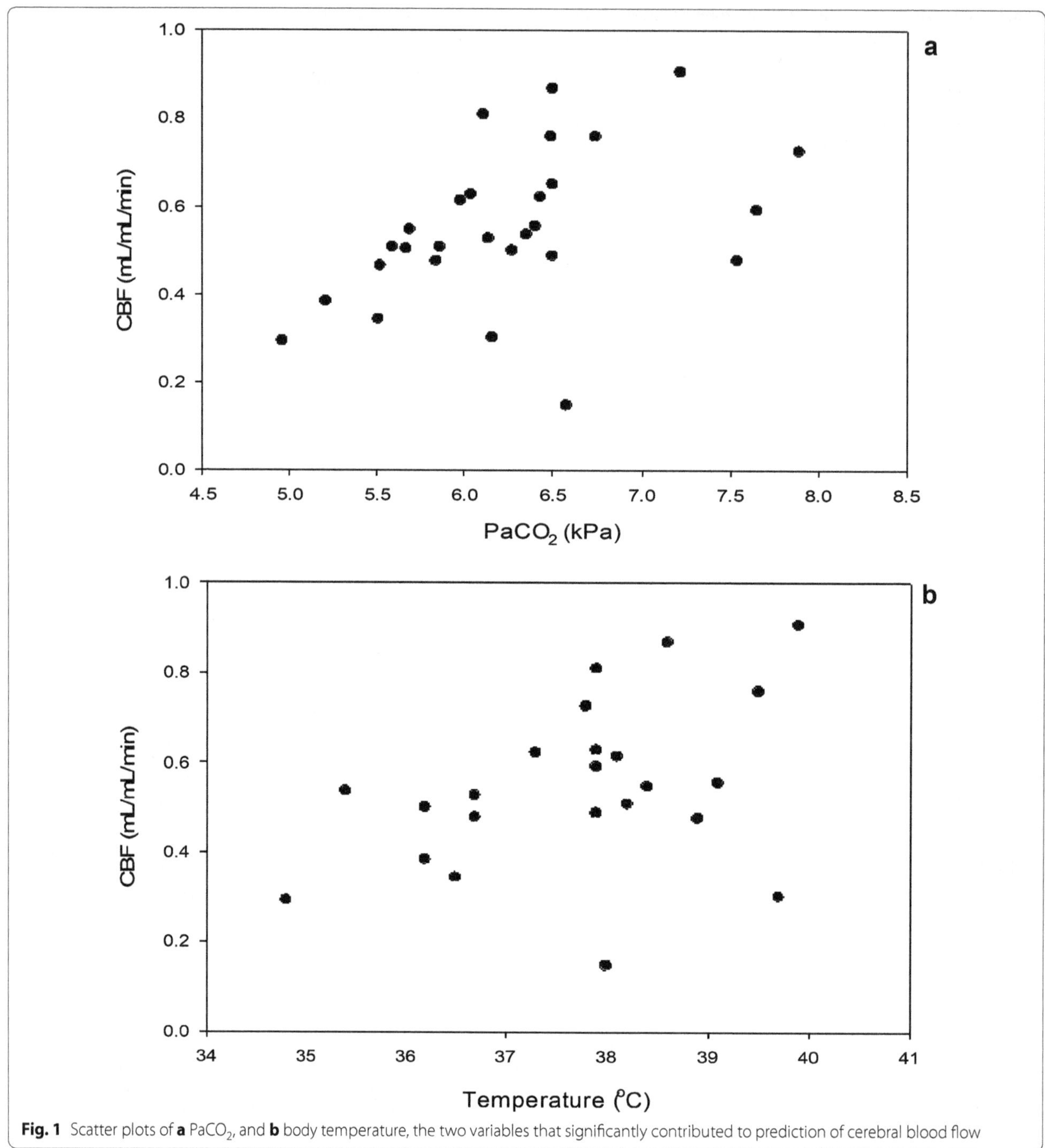

Fig. 1 Scatter plots of **a** $PaCO_2$, and **b** body temperature, the two variables that significantly contributed to prediction of cerebral blood flow

a strong vasodilator in the brain. $PaCO_2$ can be corrected by changing the minute volume of the respirator. We have recently shown that End-Tidal CO_2 ($ETCO_2$) can replace measurements of $PaCO_2$ when there is no access to arterial blood samples in pigs, and it is therefore possible to monitor CO_2-concentrations non-invasively [23]. The body temperature varied between slight hypothermia and normothermia. The importance of monitoring body temperature supports a previous pig study showing low CBF during severe hypothermia (body temperature < 37 °C) [24]. This effect underscores the importance of temperature monitoring and stabilization in pig brain studies. Hypothermia can be prevented by placing the pig on an electric blanket with thermostatic feedback to the temperature monitor during PET imaging procedures [25].

We found no correlations between CBF and PaO_2, HCT, HR, SBP, DBP and GLC. It is well-known that PaO_2 levels over 50 mmHg have no effect on CBF, while lower levels increase CBF [26]. HCT is the main determinant of blood viscosity, and in humans, higher HCT results in decreased CBF [27]. However, we found no such correlation between CBF and HCT in this study. Neither the HR, systolic nor the diastolic blood pressure was correlated to CBF. This can be explained by cerebral autoregulation which maintains a constant CBF in the mean blood pressure interval 65–140 mmHg and for variations in HR. Changes in blood pressure produce changes in cerebrovascular resistance, and this contributes to the maintenance of a constant CBF. However, a previous study reported that in ketamine anaesthetized pigs with a mean blood pressure of 102 mmHg, a 40% reduction in blood pressure (to 60 mmHg) reduced CBF with 15%, while a 43% increase in blood pressure (to 140 mmHg) increased CBF with 12% [28].

During this study some of the [^{15}O]-water PET scans were delayed due to technical reasons, which caused variation of the duration of anesthesia from 79 to 314 min. Therefore, we decided to investigate if duration of anaesthesia was correlated with monitorering variables and CBF. We found that TIME was correlated with HR, TEMP and PaO_2, but not with the other six monitorering variables and CBF. The correlation between TIME and HR can be explained by decreasing cardiac vagal activity known from dog studies (similar studies have not yet been performed in pigs) [29]. The correlation between TEMP and TIME can be explained by the fact that many pigs are slightly hypothermic shortly after anaesthesia, but body temperature is normalized by the feedback system connected to the warming blanket.

Ketamine and midazolam were used for the pre-medication and anaesthesia induction in all pigs. Isoflurane and N_2O were used to maintain anaesthesia. While ketamine and midazolam do not seem to affect CBF, isoflurane increases CBF [30–32]. In a previous study, CBF did not increase during hypercapnia in dogs anaesthetized with 2.8% isoflurane, whereas CBF increased during 1.4% isoflurane anaesthesia [33]. In our study, the pigs were anaesthetized with a vaporisor setting of 2% isoflurane and O_2/N_2O (1:2) and our results indicate that in pigs, cerebral autoregulation is maintained during anaesthesia maintained with 2% isoflurane. Also N_2O may affect CBF, as a study performed in healthy humans has shown that 30 and 60% N_2O increase CBF compared with pure oxygen [34].

It is a limitation on the study that we have only measured global CBF, and we cannot exclude the possibility of local heterogeneities in the CBF. It is therefore possible that correlations exist between monitoring variables and specific areas of the brain not seen in the global CBF. Due to the observational nature of our study, we cannot make any conclusions about the causal relationship of the variables included. Also, several of the observed physiological variables are individually correlated which further limits conclusions about causality. Future studies should therefore aim at investigating the effects of the individual physiological variables on CBF in an interventional study, as has already been done with $PaCO_2$ [6]. Until then the conclusions are drawn with caution.

Conclusions

The results indicate that monitoring of $PaCO_2$ and body temperature are crucial for maintaining stable levels of CBF and thus optimizing PET imaging of molecular mechanisms in the brain of pigs in vivo. The two variables should as far as possible be kept constant during PET scans of the pig brains. Furthermore, the duration of anaesthesia should be kept constant.

Authors' contributions

AKOA and OLM designed the study. AKOA collected the data. AKOA, MS and OLM performed the analyses and interpreted data together with NEZ. AKOA wrote the main manuscript text. All authors read and approved the final manuscript.

Author details

[1] Department of Nuclear Medicine and PET Centre, Faculty of Health, Aarhus University Hospital, Noerrebrogade 44, 10C, 8000 Aarhus C, Denmark.
[2] Department of Clinical Biochemistry, Faculty of Health, Copenhagen University Hospital Rigshospitalet, Blegdamsvej 9, 2100 Copenhagen, Denmark.

Acknowledgements

We thank the animal staff on Paaskehøjgaard and laboratory technicians at Aarhus PET Center for help in carrying out the PET studies. In addition, thanks to Michele Gammeltoft for proofreading in English.

Competing interests

The authors declare that they have no competing interests.

Funding

External funding was not used for this study.

References

1. Danielsen E, Smith DF, Poulsen PH, Østergaard L, Gee AD, Ishizu K, et al. Positron emission tomography of living brain in minipigs and domestic pigs. Scand J Lab Anim Sci. 1998;25(suppl 1):127–35.
2. Bender D, Olsen AK, Marthi MK, Smith DF, Cumming P. PET evaluation of the uptake of N-11C-methyl CP-643,051, an NK1 receptor antagonist, in the living porcine brain. Nucl Med Biol. 2004;31:699–704.
3. Andersen F, Watanabe H, Bjarkam C, Danielsen EH, Cumming P, DaNeX Study Group. Pig brain stereotaxic standard space: mapping of cerebral blood flow normative values and effect of MPTP-lesioning. Brain Res Bull. 2005;66:17–29.

4. Lind NM, Olsen AK, Moustgaard A, Jensen SB, Jakobsen S, Hansen AK, et al. Mapping the amphetamine–evoked dopamine release in the brain of the Göttingen minipig. Brain Res Bull. 2005;65:1–9.
5. Alstrup AKO, Smith DF. PET neuroimaging in pigs. Scand J Lab Anim Sci. 2012;1:1–21.
6. Olsen AK, Keiding S, Munk OL. Effect of hypercapnia on cerebral blood flow and blood volume in pigs studied by PET. Comp Med. 2006;56:416–20.
7. Watanabe H, Sakoh M, Andersen F, Rodell A, Sørensen JC, Østergaard L, Mouridsen K, Cumming P. Statistical mapping of effects of middle cerebral artery occlusion (MCAO) on blood flow and oxygen consumption in porcine brain. J Neurosci Methods. 2007;160:109–15.
8. Neto PR, Olsen AK, Gjedde A, Watanabe H, Cumming P. MDMA-evoked changes in cerebral blood flow in living porcine brain: correlation with hyperthermia. Synapse. 2004;53:214–21.
9. Ettrup KS, Sørensen JC, Rodell A, Alstrup AKO, Bjarkam CR. Hypothalamic deep brain stimulation influences autonomic and limbic circuitry involved in the regulation of aggression and cardiocerebrovascular control in the Göttingen minipig. Stereot Funct Neurosurg. 2012;90:281–91.
10. Hassoun W, Cavorsin ML, Ginovart N, Zimmer L, Gualda V, Bonnefoi F, Leviel V. PET study of the [11C] raclopride binding in the striatum of the awake cat: effects of anaesthetics and role of cerebral blood flow. Eur J Nucl Med. 2003;30:141–8.
11. Alstrup AKO, Landau AM, Holden JE, Jakobsen S, Schacht AC, Audrain H, et al. Effects of anesthesia and species on the uptake or binding of radioligands in vivo in the Göttingen minipig. Biomed Res Int. 2013. https://doi.org/10.1155/2013/808713.
12. Kuschinsky W, Wahl M. Local chemical and neurogenic regulation of cerebral vascular resistance. Physiol Rev. 1978;58:656–89.
13. Siesjo BK. Cerebral circulation and metabolism. J Neurosurg. 1984;60:883–908.
14. Ettrup KS, Glud AN, Orlowski D, Fitting LM, Meier K, Sørensen JC, et al. Basic surgical techniques in the Göttingen minipig: intubation, bladder catheterization, femoral vessel catheterization, and transcardial perfusion. J Vis Exp. 2011;52:e2652.
15. Olsen AK. Short-term effects of storage time and temperature on pH, pCO_2, and pO_2 in porcine arterial blood. Scand J Lab Anim Sci. 2003;4:197–201.
16. Toussaint P-J, Meyer E. A linear solution for calculation of K1 and k2 maps using the two-compartment CBF model. In: Gjedde A, Hansen SB, Knudsen GM, Paulson OB, editors. Physiological imaging of the brain with PET. Cambridge: Academic Press; 2001. p. 97–102.
17. Crone C. The permeability of capillaries in various organs as determined by the use of the 'indicator diffusion' method. Acta Physiol Scand. 1963;58:292–305.
18. Renkin EM. Exchangeability of tissue potassium in skeletal muscle. Am J Physiol. 1959;197:1211–5.
19. Marquardt DW. An algorithm for least-squares estimation of nonlinear parameters. J Soc Ind Appl Math. 1963;11:431–41.
20. Benjamini Y, Hochberg Y. Controlling the false discovery rate: a practical and powerful approach to multiple testing. J Royal Stat Soc. 1995;B57:289–300.
21. Bollen PJA, Hansen AK, Alstrup AKO. The laboratory swine. 2nd ed. Boca Raton: CRC Press LLC; 2010.
22. Poulsen PH, Smith DF, Østergaard L, Danielsen EH, Gee A, Hansen SB, et al. In vivo estimation of cerebral blood flow, oxygen consumption and glucose metabolism in the pig by [^{15}O] water injection, [^{15}O] oxygen inhalation and dual injections of [18F] fluorodeoxyglucose. J Neurosci Meth. 1997;77:199–209.
23. Alstrup AKO. End-tidal carbon dioxide ($ETCO_2$) can replace methods for measuring partial pressure of carbon dioxide (PCO_2) in pigs. Lab Anim Sci Prof. 2017:33–4 (in press).
24. Ehrlich MP, McCullough JN, Zhang N, Weisz DJ, Juvonen T, Bodian CA, Griepp RB. Effect of hypothermia on cerebral blood flow and metabolism in the pig. Ann Thorac Surg. 2002;73:191–7.
25. Alstrup AKO, Winterdahl M. Imaging techniques in large animals. Scand J Lab Anim Sci. 2009;36:55–66.
26. Bor-Seng-Shu E, Kita WS, Figueiredo EG, Paiva WS, Fonoff ET, Teixeira MJ, Panerai RB. Cerebral hemodynamics: concepts of clinical importance. Arq de Neuro Psiquiat. 2012;70:352–6.
27. Kirkness CJ. Cerebral blood flow monitoring in clinical practice. AACN. 2005;16:476–87.
28. Schmidt A, Ryding E, Åkeson J. Racemic ketamine does not abolish cerebrovascular autoregulation in the pig. Acta Anaesthesiol Scand. 2003;47:569–75.
29. Picker O, Scheeren TWL, Arndt JO. Inhalation anaesthetics increase heart rate by decreasing cardiac vagal activity in dogs. Br J Anaesth. 2001;87:748–54. https://doi.org/10.1093/bja/87.5.748.
30. De Cosmo G, Cancelli I, Adduci A, Merlino G, Aceto P, Valente M. Changes in hemodynamics during isoflurane and propofol anesthesia: a comparison study. Neurol Res. 2005;27:433–5.
31. Li CX, Patel S, Wang DJ, Zhang X. Effect of high dose isoflurane on cerebral blood flow in macaque monkeys. Magn Reson Imag. 2014;32:956–60.
32. Holmström A, Akeson J. Cerebral blood flow at 0.5 and 1.0 minimal alveolar concentrations of desflurane or sevoflurane compared with isoflurane in normoventilated pigs. J Neurosurg Anesthesiol. 2003;15:90–7.
33. McPherson RW, Traystman RJ. Effects of isoflurane on cerebral autoregulation in dogs. Anesthesiol. 1988;69:493–9.
34. Field LM, Dorrance DE, Krzeminska EK, Barsoum LZ. Effect of nitrous oxide on cerebral blood flow in normal humans. Br J Anaesth. 1993;70:154–9.

C-reactive protein, glucose and iron concentrations are significantly altered in dogs undergoing open ovariohysterectomy or ovariectomy

Elena Regine Moldal[1*], Mads Jens Kjelgaard-Hansen[2], Marijke Elisabeth Peeters[3], Ane Nødtvedt[4] and Jolle Kirpensteijn[5]

Abstract

Background: There are relatively few studies about the canine surgical stress response, a sequence of events orchestrated by the body in response to a surgical trauma which is sometimes, as shown in human surgery, deleterious to the patient. There is a need to identify objective markers to quantify this response in order to estimate tissue trauma and use the markers as potential early indicators of surgical complications. The study objective was to investigate the surgical stress response, measured by C-reactive protein (CRP), glucose and iron serum concentrations, to gonadectomy in female dogs, and to compare the response to ovariohysterectomy (OHE) with the response to ovariectomy (OVE). A randomized clinical trial was performed on a sample of 42 female dogs, which were divided into two groups: one group underwent OHE, the other OVE.

Results: Blood samples were collected immediately before surgery (T0), and at 1 (T1), 6 (T6), and 24 (T24) h after surgery, and serum frozen and stored at − 80 °C for later analysis. Upon thawing, the serum samples were subjected to measurement of CRP, glucose and iron concentration. Seventeen dogs in the OHE group and 19 dogs in the OVE group were included in the statistical analysis. There was a significant increase in glucose concentration at all time points compared with T0, and an increase of CRP at T6 and T24. Iron concentration was significantly decreased at T6 and T24. Differences between the two groups could not be detected for any of the three variables.

Conclusions: The study showed that both OHE and OVE induce a moderate surgical stress response in female dogs, measured by CRP, glucose and iron. A difference between the surgical techniques could not be detected for any of the variables, and hence; with regards to the parameters studied recommendations of one procedure over the other cannot be made and preferred technique remains the surgeon's choice.

Keywords: C-reactive protein, Glucose, Iron, Ovariectomy, Ovariohysterectomy, Surgery, Surgical stress response

*Correspondence: elena.moldal@nmbu.no
[1] Department of Companion Animal Clinical Sciences, Faculty of Veterinary Medicine and Biosciences, Norwegian University of Life Sciences, Oslo, Norway
Full list of author information is available at the end of the article

Background

The stress response to surgery involves an array of physiological events in the body, including endocrinological, immunological, and hematological alterations leading to a catabolic state [1, 2]. Even though these functions are beneficial in the acute survival situation, this response may in fact have negative effects on homeostasis and tissue healing [3].

The surgical stress response is believed to be proportional with the degree of tissue injury caused by the procedure [4, 5]. It is therefore important to choose surgical procedures that minimize the negative impact of surgery on the body. Complications after elective surgery in dogs and cats are not uncommon and have been reported to include hemorrhage, surgical site inflammation or infection, and increased attention to the surgical site [6, 7]. Female dogs are commonly neutered, most often by open ovariohysterectomy (OHE) or ovariectomy (OVE). Several authors argue that OVE should be the preferred method because of the belief that it is faster, safer, less invasive, and associated with fewer postoperative complications [8–10]. Open OHE in dogs has previously been shown to induce a significant, but short-lived neuroendocrine stress response [11]. Two previous studies by the authors comparing OVE and OHE failed to show differences between the two methods with regards to pain scores, time expenditure, and wound characteristics, as well as difference in the hemostatic stress response to surgery [12, 13]. However, one recent study identified significant differences in postoperative C-reactive protein (CRP) concentrations in three groups of dogs subjected to vasectomy, open OHE, or laparoscopic OHE [14]. CRP is an acute phase protein and a sensitive marker of inflammation [15–17], and can be used to quantify the inflammatory response to different surgical procedures in dogs [14]. Glucose is another biomarker commonly used to measure the stress response to surgery. A study comparing dogs subjected to open OHE with dogs subjected to the laparoscopic counterpart identified prolonged increases in glucose concentration in the open OHE group during the postoperative period [18]. Glucose is also an independent risk factor for postoperative wound infections in humans [19]. Hypoferremia is commonly seen after surgically induced inflammation in humans and is related to the extent of surgery [20]; however, information about iron concentration after surgery in dogs is scarce.

The aims of this study were to measure CRP, iron and glucose serum concentration as markers of the surgical stress response in dogs, and to test whether they differed between two commonly applied methods for surgical neutering, of which one—OVE—has been claimed to be less traumatic by some authors [8–10]. The hypothesis tested was: Surgery will cause significant increases of serum CRP and glucose and a decrease in serum iron-concentrations postoperatively, but to a lesser degree in the OVE compared to the OHE group.

Methods

The study was approved by the Ethics and Research Committee of the Department of Clinical Sciences of Companion Animals, Faculty of Veterinary Medicine, University of Utrecht (DCSCA), the Netherlands. It was performed as a prospective randomized clinical trial at the DCSCA between June 2006 and June 2007. Serum was stored at − 80 °C for a maximum of 4 years, and later transported to the University of Copenhagen on dry ice before analysis at the Central Laboratory, Department of Veterinary Clinical Sciences, University of Copenhagen, Denmark, in November 2010. The laboratory analysis was performed double blind in one analytical run, in random order, and unblinding did not take place until after statistical analysis of the data. Only the surgeon (MEP) knew what procedure was performed.

Study population

A total of 42 client-owned healthy intact bitches admitted to the DCSCA for elective neutering were prospectively entered into the study. Of these, 12 bitches were mongrels and 30 were pure-bred. Oral consent was obtained from the owners before the dogs underwent a thorough clinical examination to ensure that they were healthy. Only dogs assigned to ASA category 1 (normal, healthy animals) [21] were eligible for participation in the study, and all dogs went through their last estrus at least 6 weeks prior to presentation. Each dog was given a body condition score (BCS) at admission, with a score of 1 being emaciated and 5 being obese. The dogs were numbered consecutively at admission. Dogs were block randomized into one of two treatment groups, OVE or OHE, after induction of anesthesia [12].

Anesthesia, surgery, and analgesia

An intravenous (IV) catheter was inserted in the cephalic vein. The dogs were given a premedication of 1 mg/m^2 medetomidine intravenously (Domitor, Pfizer Animal Health, USA, 1 mg/mL) and 4 mg/kg carprofen IV (Rimadyl, Pfizer Animal Health, USA, 50 mg/mL) and anesthesia was induced with 1–2 mg/kg propofol IV (PropoVet, Abbott Laboratories, UK, 10 mg/mL) to effect. The dogs were then intubated and anesthesia was maintained with isoflurane (Isoflo, Abbott Laboratories, UK) in oxygen and air. Intermittent positive pressure ventilation (IPPV) was applied to ensure normocapnea and the volume was regulated to keep end-tidal CO_2 at normal levels (4.5–5 kPa). All dogs were given 10 mL/

kg/h Ringer's lactate IV (Stereofundin, Iso; B, Germany) at maintenance rate throughout the course of anesthesia and surgery. Intraoperative monitoring consisted of electrocardiogram (ECG), capnography, body temperature, and oxygen and vapor concentrations. In surgeries that lasted for more than one h, an additional dose corresponding to half of the original administered dose of medetomidine was administered IV. After surgery this was antagonized with 2.5 μg/m^2 atipamezole intramuscularly (IM) (Antisedan, Pfizer Animal Health, USA, 5 mg/mL) [12].

All surgeries were performed by one experienced ECVS Diplomate (MEP) with the help of an assistant, using a standardized surgical protocol for both procedures. Both OVE and OHE were carried out as open surgical procedures. The OVE dogs had their ovaries removed through a smaller incision than the OHE dogs, which additionally had their uterus removed [12].

All dogs were hospitalized for 24–32 h postoperatively. 10 μg/kg buprenorphine (Buprecare, Animalcare Ltd, UK, 0.3 mg/mL) was administered IV approximately 40 m before injecting atipamezole and then given subcutaneously (SC) every 6 h during the next 24 h. The rescue analgesia protocol consisted of administration of a higher dose of buprenorphine 20 μg/kg SC to animals showing pain scores > 15 on a modified version of the Short Form (SF) of the Glasgow Composite Measure Pain Scale [22]. Treatment at home consisted of 2 mg/kg carprofen orally every 12 h for an additional 2 days after discharge [12].

Blood sampling

Immediately after anesthetic induction an IV jugular catheter was inserted and secured in place. Just before the skin incision (T0) and just before closure of the abdominal incision (T1), and also at 6 h after T0 (T6), blood samples were collected from this catheter after discarding the first 5 mL of blood. The jugular catheter was then removed, and the 24-h blood sample (T24) was taken by direct venipuncture of the contralateral jugular vein. For all samples, a total of 11 mL blood was collected in one serum tube and two 3.2% citrate tubes, in that order. For T0, 10 additional mL blood was collected in heparin and EDTA for biochemistry and hematology, to confirm the animal's health before enrolment in the project. The following variables were analyzed: BUN (blood urea nitrogen), serum creatinine, alkaline phosphatase, bile acids, total plasma calcium, phosphorus, sodium, potassium, hematocrit, total leucocytes, and platelets.

All serum tubes were left in room temperature and centrifuged after 1 h at 4 °C at 1006*g* for 10 min before the serum was separated and placed directly in a − 80 °C freezer for later analysis at the Department of Veterinary Clinical Sciences.

Other

Hemostasis parameters and other variables including blood loss, surgical time, surgical wound characteristics, pain scores, and wound assessment scores were recorded and published in other studies [12, 13].

CRP

CRP levels were analyzed using a turbidimetric immunoassay (High Linearity CRP, Randox Laboratories Ltd., Crumlin, UK) performed on Advia 1800 Chemistry System (Siemens, Germany). Independently purified canine CRP was applied as calibrator (cat#8101, Life Diagnostics, West Chester, PA, USA) and control (TP-810CON, Tridelta, Kildare, Ireland). For complete assay performance, please see validation conducted by the laboratory performing the measurements [23, 24]. Automated reflex dilution was applied when measurement exceeded linear range, resulting in effective working range up to 600 mg/L. No prozone effect were observed up to 900 mg/L.

Glucose

Glucose was measured with the reagent Glucose Hexokinase/Glucose oxidase, including assay calibrator provided by manufacturer (Siemens, Germany) performed on the Advia 1800 Chemistry System. Imprecision was below 2%.

Iron

Iron was measured by using the reagent Iron RGT KT D/S, including calibrator provided by manufacturer (Siemens, Germany) on the Advia 1800 Chemistry System. Imprecision was below 2%.

Statistical analysis

Two dogs were excluded from the study, one because it was under treatment with phenobarbital for epilepsy, the other because of unexpected complications during surgery which lengthened the procedure but were not associated with the procedure per se. Also, because four serum samples were stored in a different freezer for a period of time, one sample from the OVE group and three samples from the OHE group were discarded. Thus, results from 36 dogs, 17 in the OHE group and 19 in the OVE group, were included in the statistical analysis. All statistical analyses were performed using the statistical software package Stata version 11 (Statacorp, College Station, USA). Three separate regression analyses were performed; one for each of the outcome variables CRP, glucose and serum iron concentrations. The explanatory variables were treatment group (OVE or OHE) and time [0 (=baseline), 1, 6, 24 h] in all models. Variables were initially evaluated for correlations between time points. Observations within each dog through time were not independent of each other. Therefore linear mixed regression models, including random effects for dog, were applied to detect differences between the treatment groups and between time points for each of the outcome variables. The overall effect of the categorical variable time was tested using likelihood ratio (LR) tests. The level of statistical significance was set to $P < 0.05$. The assumption of normally distributed residuals was assessed using normal quantile plots at the dog level.

Results

The mean age of participating dogs in the sample was 3.4 years, range 6 months to 10 years, and the mean weight 25 kg, range 12–36 kg. The groups did not differ with regards to age, body weight, body condition score, and surgical time [12]. Preoperative biochemical and hematological profiles in the dogs were within the reference intervals of the DCSCA. None of the dogs had pain scores > 15 and thus, rescue analgesia was not indicated in any of the animals.

CRP, glucose and iron

Mean and standard deviation for CRP, glucose and iron serum concentrations by time and group are presented in Table 1. The baseline (T0) values did not differ significantly between the groups for any of the three variables. Based on the observed correlations, an exchangeable correlation structure between time points was assumed for glucose and CRP, and a first-order autoregressive for iron concentration. The reported effects of treatment group and time are based on output from the three regression models for CRP, glucose and iron (Model output

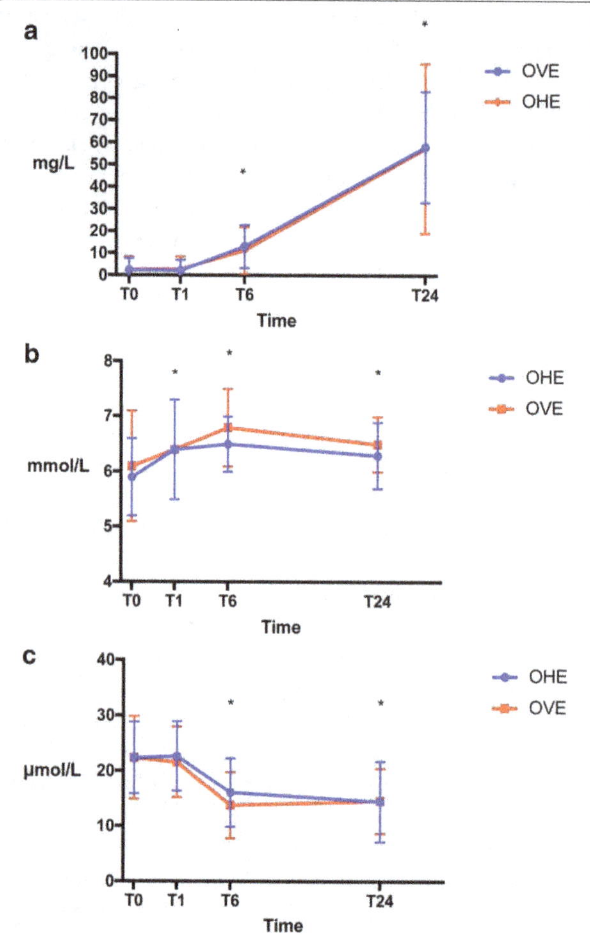

Fig. 1 Mean CRP (**a**), glucose (**b**), and iron (**c**) concentrations for the OHE and OVE group at each time point T0, T1, T6 and T24. There was no difference between groups for any of the parameters but the statistically significant changes from T0 are marked with asterisks

Table 1 Mean and standard deviation (SD) of CRP, glucose, and iron serum concentrations for dogs in the OHE and OVE group

Variable	Time	OHE mean	SD	OVE mean	SD	Reference interval
CRP (mg/L)	0	2.7	5.7	2.5	5.3	0.4–15.9
	1	2.9	5.7	2.3	4.8	
	6	11.4	10.7	13.2	9.8	
	24	57.6	38.4	58.3	25.0	
Glucose (mmol/L)	0	5.9	0.7	6.1	1.0	3.9–6.6
	1	6.4	0.9	6.4	0.9	
	6	6.5	0.5	6.8	0.7	
	24	6.3	0.6	6.5	0.5	
Iron (µmol/L)	0	22.4	6.5	22.4	7.5	5.4–32.2
	1	22.7	6.3	21.6	6.4	
	6	16.1	6.2	13.8	6.0	
	24	14.5	7.3	14.6	5.9	

available from the first author by request). CRP (Fig. 1a) was increased at T6 and T24 ($P < 0.001$) for both groups. There was no significant difference in CRP between groups ($P = 0.92$). The glucose concentration (Fig. 1b) was higher than baseline (T0) at all time points (LR test of group; $P = 0.004$), but no difference between groups was detected ($P = 0.27$). Iron concentration (Fig. 1c) was decreased at T6 and T24 compared to baseline ($P < 0.001$ for both), with no difference between groups ($P = 0.68$). Residuals were approximately normally distributed for all three models when assessed at the dog-level using normal quantile plots. The random dog-effect was highly significant for all three variables.

Discussion

Both OHE and OVE induced significant postoperative changes in CRP, glucose and iron concentrations. The hypothesis that OVE would cause a less marked stress response could however not be supported, which corroborates the authors' two previous studies comparing OVE and OHE [12, 13]. The detection of increased CRP after surgery is in accordance with previous human and canine studies [14–17, 25–28]. Increased glucose concentration perioperatively has also been registered in both species [11, 18, 19, 29].

Decreased iron concentration has been reported both after soft tissue and orthopedic surgery in humans [20, 30], and the magnitude of this decrease differs with surgical invasiveness [20]. Information about iron concentration in dogs after surgery is scarce, but unpublished observations by the authors indicate decreased concentrations after both skin-, abdominal- and orthopedic surgery compared with pre-operative values in dogs.

CRP is a major acute phase protein in dogs and the results expectedly indicate that a moderate inflammatory response occurs after both OVE and OHE. CRP has been shown to be a sensitive marker of inflammation and further has the ability to distinguish inflammatory states as a result of neoplasia, immune-mediated disease, surgery, and infections [14, 31–35]. It has been argued that CRP should be part of routine diagnostic testing because of its higher sensitivity than WBC [36, 37]. CRP can increase up to 95 times as a result of surgery [26], and this increase is related to the degree of tissue injury in dogs [14, 26]. Thus, CRP can be used to reflect the degree of surgical trauma [14]. In our study CRP increased approximately 20-fold from T0 to T24. There was no difference between groups. OHE has previously been shown to cause moderately elevated CRP in dogs [16, 26]; however, to a lesser degree than more invasive surgery like orthopedic surgery [26]. In a study of humans, a smaller elevation of CRP was detected after laparoscopic hysterectomy compared to the open abdominal procedure [38], and the same phenomenon has been identified in dogs [14]. The results from the current study serve to indicate that tissue trauma, as measured by CRP, is comparable for open OVE and OHE.

The glucose concentration significantly increased at T1 and T6, but slightly decreased again at T24; however, the difference from T0 to T24 was still statistically significant. There was no difference between the two groups. Blood glucose concentration is a useful measure of surgical stress in dogs [18], and has been identified as an independent risk factor for infection after surgery in humans [19, 29]. Hyperglycemia has deleterious effects on macrophage and neutrophil function [39], and this may explain why human patients suffering from diabetes mellitus are twice as likely to develop a post-operative infection compared to normoglycemic individuals [40, 41]. The pathophysiology behind postoperative hyperglycemia is partly induction of a hyperglycemic response by cortisol and growth hormone and partly insulin resistance and inhibition of insulin secretion, all induced by the neuroendocrine and metabolic stress response to surgery [5]. Glucose concentration has also been shown to have predictive value on the outcome in critically ill human patients [42]. In a study by Benson et al. [11], glucose was found to be elevated after anesthesia and surgery (OHE) in dogs. The increasing glucose concentration up to T6 corroborates a previous study on OHE in dogs [18]. In a study by Hardie et al. [43], 50% of dogs with sepsis that developed high glucose concentrations postoperatively died, whereas mortality in the group with normal glucose concentration was 14%. The difference was, however, not statistically significant ($P = 0.08$) [43]. The link between high glucose concentration and morbidity is not completely understood, but it has been suggested that the responsiveness of leukocytes stimulated with inflammatory mediators is inversely correlated with indices of in vivo glycemic control in humans [39]. As a minor study limitation it should be noted that time of postoperative feeding is not available for the dogs in the study. Also, because the postoperative glucose concentration was in the upper end of, and not outside, the reference interval for dogs in our study, a clinical relevance is considered unlikely. Nevertheless, it seems that OHE and OVE induce increased glucose concentration to a comparable extent.

The iron concentration decreased to a similar degree in both groups after surgery, at T6 and T24. An anemic state that resembles anemia of chronic disease commonly occurs in humans after surgery [20, 30], and can take up to 6 weeks to normalize [30]. This was previously believed to be purely due to blood loss; however, iron supplementation after orthopedic surgery has no major effect on erythropoiesis [44, 45]. Research in mice indicates that hypoferremia is mediated by interleukin 6 (IL-6) because it induces synthesis of the iron regulatory hormone hepcidin, an acute phase protein in humans [46, 47]. Transferrin, an iron binding transporter protein, is also a negative acute phase protein in dogs [31]. There are great similarities between dogs and humans in iron metabolism [48], and the mechanisms triggered postoperatively are likely to be similar as well. The iron concentration decreased to a similar extent in both groups.

It should be noted that several factors may influence the surgical stress response. Stress caused by hospitalization is commonly seen in dogs and may exacerbate the endocrine responses to surgery [18]. Care must be taken to avoid stress in surgical patients in order to minimize the catabolic events mediated by the stress response. This can in part be done with sedative and anesthetic drugs. In this study, medetomidine was used for premedication. Medetomidine has been shown to obtund the surgical stress response by preventing the catecholamine response induced by OHE [11], and could therefore have affected the glucose concentration to some degree. There is no evidence in the literature to say that medetomidine has an anti-inflammatory effect, and hence, an influence on CRP and iron concentration is considered unlikely. One could argue that the use of non-steroidal anti-inflammatory drugs (NSAIDs) such as carprofen would limit the inflammatory response to surgery; however, it is believed that NSAIDs do not directly block the production of IL-6 [49], which is proposed to be the main inducer of CRP [26, 50]. Also, it has previously been shown that CRP and iron as inflammatory markers are not affected by NSAID administration in humans [51], and neither meloxicam nor carprofen administration caused lower postoperative concentrations of CRP in a study of OHE in dogs [28]. Also, since carprofen administration would impact the two groups to a similar extent, we consider it a minor limitation to the study. The effects of stress and administration of anesthetic and analgesic drugs are also assumed to be similar for both groups, but it cannot be excluded that the drugs have masked the surgical stress response and hence masked a potential small difference between groups. A previous study has shown higher CRP concentrations after canine OHE performed by inexperienced surgeons [27]; however, since we used the same, experienced surgeon for all procedures, this is not relevant for the current study. The dogs were only followed for 24 h, and a follow-up to assess wound healing or inflammatory complications was not carried out. In humans, increased perioperative concentrations of glucose and CRP have been described as risk factors for postoperative infections [19, 52]. A study with longer follow-up of the animals with regards to complications resulting from surgery would have been of value.

The results from the current study show that open OVE and OHE provoke a moderate surgical stress response, as measured by CRP, glucose and iron concentration, of similar magnitude, likely because the two methods are too similar in surgical invasiveness to detect subtle differences. Laparascopic techniques may confer advantages over OHE and OVE in limiting inflammation and pain in the postoperative period [14, 18, 53–55].

Conclusions

The study showed that OHE and OVE induce a surgical stress response with postoperative increases in glucose concentration and CRP, and a decrease in iron concentration. No significant difference between the OHE and OVE group could be detected with regards to the parameters measured, and a recommendation of one procedure over the other can therefore not be made based on the findings of this study.

Abbreviations

CRP: C-reactive protein; DCSCA: The Department of Clinical Sciences of Companion Animals, Faculty of Veterinary Medicine, University of Utrecht; IL-6: interleukin 6; NSAIDs: non-steroidal anti-inflammatory drugs; OHE: ovariohysterectomy; OVE: ovariectomy.

Authors' contributions

ERM collected data, stored samples, and participated in the laboratory analyses. She was involved in statistical analysis of the data and responsible for manuscript preparation. MKH was responsible for the choice of laboratory variables. He performed the laboratory analyses and interpreted them, and was a major contributor in writing the manuscript. MEP was responsible for the design of the study and the acquisition of patients. She performed all surgeries and was a major contributor in writing the manuscript. AN performed the statistical analyses and was responsible for the interpretation of these. She wrote the statistics section of the manuscript and contributed to other aspects of manuscript preparation. JK was responsible for the study design and the acquisition of patients, as well as sample collection, handling, and interpretation of results. He was a major contributor in writing the manuscript. All authors read and approved the final manuscript.

Author details

[1] Department of Companion Animal Clinical Sciences, Faculty of Veterinary Medicine and Biosciences, Norwegian University of Life Sciences, Oslo, Norway. [2] Department of Veterinary Clinical Sciences, Faculty of Health and Medical Sciences, University of Copenhagen, Copenhagen, Denmark. [3] Department of Clinical Sciences of Companion Animals, Faculty of Veterinary Medicine, University of Utrecht, Utrecht, The Netherlands. [4] Department of Production Animal Clinical Sciences, Faculty of Veterinary Medicine and Biosciences, Norwegian University of Life Sciences, Oslo, Norway. [5] Hill's Pet Nutrition Inc, Topeka, KS, USA.

Acknowledgements

The authors wish to thank Professor Thomas Eriksen for valuable input during data collection, analysis, and manuscript preparation.

Competing interests

The authors declare that they have no competing interests.

Funding
The study was financed by the Research and Ethics Committee at the former Norwegian School of Veterinary Science.

References

1. Kehlet H, Wilmore DW. Multimodal strategies to improve surgical outcome. Am J Surg. 2002;183:630–41.
2. Kehlet H. Manipulation of the metabolic response in clinical practice. World J Surg. 2000;24:690–5.
3. Roizen MF. Should we all have a sympathectomy at birth? Or at least preoperatively? Anesthesiol Heart. 1988;68:482–4.
4. Kehlet H. The modifying effect of general and regional anesthesia on the endocrine–metabolic response to surgery. Reg Anesth Pain Med. 1982;7:4.
5. Desborough JP. The stress response to trauma and surgery. Br J Anaesth. 2000;85:109–17.
6. Burrow R, Batchelor D, Cripps P. Complications observed during and after ovariohysterectomy of 142 bitches at a veterinary teaching hospital. Vet Rec. 2005;157:829–33.
7. Pollari FL, Bonnett BN. Evaluation of postoperative complications following elective surgeries of dogs and cats at private practices using computer records. Can Vet J. 1996;37:672–8.
8. Okkens AC, Kooistra HS, Nickel RF. Comparison of long-term effects of ovariectomy versus ovariohysterectomy in bitches. J Reprod Fertil Suppl. 1997;51:227–31.
9. Okkens AC, vd Gaag I, Biewenga WJ, Rothuizen J, Voorhout G. Urological complications following ovariohysterectomy in dogs. Tijdschr Diergeneeskd. 1981;106:1189–98 **(in Dutch)**.
10. Van Goethem B, Schaefers-Okkens A, Kirpensteijn J. Making a rational choice between ovariectomy and ovariohysterectomy in the dog: a discussion of the benefits of either technique. Vet Surg. 2006;35:136–43.
11. Benson GJ, Grubb TL, Neff-Davis C, Olson WA, Thurmon JC, Lindner DL, et al. Perioperative stress response in the dog: effect of pre-emptive administration of medetomidine. Vet Surg. 2000;29:85–91.
12. Peeters ME, Kirpensteijn J. Comparison of surgical variables and short-term postoperative complications in healthy dogs undergoing ovariohysterectomy or ovariectomy. J Am Vet Med Assoc. 2011;238:189–94.
13. Moldal ER, Kristensen AT, Peeters ME, Nodtvedt A, Kirpensteijn J. Hemostatic response to surgical neutering via ovariectomy and ovariohysterectomy in dogs. Am J Vet Res. 2012;73:1469–76.
14. Kjelgaard-Hansen M, Strom H, Mikkelsen LF, Eriksen T, Jensen AL, Luntang-Jensen M. Canine serum C-reactive protein as a quantitative marker of the inflammatory stimulus of aseptic elective soft tissue surgery. Vet Clin Pathol. 2013;42:342–5.
15. Stahl WM. Acute phase protein response to tissue injury. Crit Care Med. 1987;15:545.
16. Hayashi S, Jinbo T, Iguchi K, Shimizu M, Shimada T, Nomura M. A comparison of the concentrations of C-reactive protein and α1-acid glycoprotein in the serum of young and adult dogs with acute inflammation. Vet Res Commun. 2001;25:117–20.
17. Baigrie RJ, Lamont PM, Kwiatkowski D, Dallman MJ, Morris PJ. Systemic cytokine response after major surgery. Br J Surg. 1992;79:757–60.
18. Devitt CM, Cox RE, Hailey JJ. Duration, complications, stress, and pain of open ovariohysterectomy versus a simple method of laparoscopic-assisted ovariohysterectomy in dogs. J Am Vet Med Assoc. 2005;227:921–7.
19. Vriesendorp TM, Morélis QJ, DeVries JH, Legemate DA, Hoekstra JBL. Early post-operative glucose levels are an independent risk factor for infection after peripheral vascular surgery. A retrospective study. Eur J Vasc Endovasc Surg. 2004;28:520–5.
20. van Iperen CE, Kraaijenhagen RJ, Biesma DH, Beguin Y, Marx JJM, van de Wiel A. Iron metabolism and erythropoiesis after surgery. Br J Surg. 1998;85:41–5.
21. American Society of Anesthesiologists. New classification of physical status. Anesthesiology. 1963;24:111.
22. Holton L, Reid J, Scott EM, Pawson P, Nolan A. Development of a behaviour-based scale to measure acute pain in dogs. Vet Rec. 2001;148:525–31.
23. Kjelgaard-Hansen M, Jensen AL, Kristensen AT. Evaluation of a commercially available human C-reactive protein (CRP) turbidometric immunoassay for determination of canine serum CRP concentration. Vet Clin Pathol. 2003;32:81–7.
24. Kjelgaard-Hansen M. Comments on measurement of C-reactive protein in dogs. Vet Clin Pathol. 2010;39:402–3.
25. McMahon AJ, O'Dwyer PJ, Cruikshank AM, McMillan DC, O'Reilly DSJ, Lowe GDO, et al. Comparison of metabolic responses to laparoscopic and minilaparotomy cholecystectomy. Br J Surg. 1993;80:1255–8.
26. Yamamoto S, Shida T, Miyaji S, Santsuka H, Fujise H, Mukawa K, et al. Changes in serum C-reactive protein levels in dogs with various disorders and surgical traumas. Vet Res Commun. 1993;17:85–93.
27. Michelsen J, Heller J, Wills F, Noble GK. Effect of surgeon experience on postoperative plasma cortisol and C-reactive protein concentrations after ovariohysterectomy in the dog: a randomised trial. Aust Vet J. 2012;90:474–8.
28. Kum C, Voyvoda H, Sekkin S, Karademir U, Tarimcilar T. Effects of carprofen and meloxicam on C-reactive protein, ceruloplasmin, and fibrinogen concentrations in dogs underdoing ovariohysterectomy. Am J Vet Res. 2013;74:1267–73.
29. Gandhi GY, Nuttall GA, Abel MD, Mullany CJ, Schaff HV, Williams BA, et al. Intraoperative hyperglycemia and perioperative outcomes in cardiac surgery patients. In: Mayo Clin Proc. 2005;80:862–6.
30. Biesma DH, Wiel AVD, Beguin Y, Kraaijenhagen J, Marx JJM. Post-operative erythropoiesis is limited by the inflammatory effect of surgery on iron metabolism. Eur J Clin Invest. 1995;25:383–9.
31. Ceron JJ, Eckersall PD, Martinez-Subiela S. Acute phase proteins in dogs and cats: current knowledge and future perspectives. Vet Clin Pathol. 2005;34:85–99.
32. Conner JG, Eckersall PD, Ferguson J, Douglas TA. Acute phase response in the dog following surgical trauma. Res Vet Sci. 1988;45:107–10.
33. Mischke R, Waterston M, Eckersall PD. Changes in C-reactive protein and haptoglobin in dogs with lymphatic neoplasia. Vet J. 2007;174:188–92.
34. Fransson BA, Karlstam E, Bergstrom A, Lagerstedt AS, Park JS, Evans MA, et al. C-reactive protein in the differentiation of pyometra from cystic endometrial hyperplasia/mucometra in dogs. J Am Anim Hosp Assoc. 2004;40:391–9.
35. Griebsch C, Arndt G, Raila J, Schweigert FJ, Kohn B. C-reactive protein concentration in dogs with primary immune-mediated hemolytic anemia. Vet Clin Pathol. 2009;38:421–5.
36. Nakamura M, Takahashi M, Ohno K, Koshino A, Nakashima K, Setoguchi A, et al. C-reactive protein concentration in dogs with various diseases. J Vet Med Sci. 2008;70:127–31.
37. Otabe K, Ito T, Sugimoto T, Yamamoto S. C-reactive protein (CRP) measurement in canine serum following experimentally-induced acute gastric mucosal injury. Lab Anim. 2000;34:434–8.
38. Ribeiro SC, Ribeiro RM, Santos NC, Pinotti JA. A randomized study of total abdominal, vaginal and laparoscopic hysterectomy. Int J Gynecol Obstet. 2003;83:37–43.
39. McManus LM, Bloodworth RC, Prihoda TJ, Blodgett JL, Pinckard RN. Agonist-dependent failure of neutrophil function in diabetes correlates with extent of hyperglycemia. J Leukoc Biol. 2001;70:395–404.
40. Van den Berghe G, Wouters P, Weekers F, Verwaest C, Bruyninckx F, Shetz M, et al. Intensive insulin therapy in critically ill patients. N Engl J Med. 2001;345:1359–67.
41. Shah BR, Hux JE. Quantifying the risk of infectious diseases for people with diabetes. Diabetes Care. 2003;26:510–3.
42. Finney SJ, Zekveld C, Elia A, Evans T. Glucose control and mortality in critically ill patients. JAMA J Am Med Assoc. 2003;290:2041–7.
43. Hardie EM, Rawlings CA, George JW. Plasma-glucose concentrations in cats and cats before and after surgery: comparison of healthy animals and animals with sepsis. Am J Vet Res. 1985;46:1700–4.
44. Zauber NP, Zauber AG, Gordon FJ, Tillis AC, Leeds HC, Berman E, et al. Iron supplementation after femoral head replacement for patients with normal iron stores. J Am Med Assoc. 1992;267:525–7.
45. Weatherall M, Maling TJ. Oral iron therapy for anaemia after orthopaedic surgery: randomized clinical trial. ANZ J Surg. 2004;74:1049–51.
46. Nemeth E, Valore EV, Territo M, Schiller G, Lichtenstein A, Ganz T. Hepcidin, a putative mediator of anemia of inflammation, is a type II acute-phase protein. Blood. 2003;101:2461–3.

47. Nemeth E, Rivera S, Gabayan V, Keller C, Taudorf S, Pedersen BK, et al. IL-6 mediates hypoferremia of inflammation by inducing the synthesis of the iron regulatory hormone hepcidin. J Clin Invest. 2004;113:1271–6.
48. Finch CA, Hegsted M, Kinney TD, Thomas ED, Rath CE, Haskins D, et al. Iron metabolism: the pathophysiology of iron storage. Blood. 1950;5:983–1008.
49. Borer LR, Peel JE, Seewald W, Schawalder P, Spreng DE. Effect of carprofen, etodolac, meloxicam, or butorphanol in dogs with induced acute synovitis. Am J Vet Res. 2003;64:1429–37.
50. Eckersall PD, Conner JG. Bovine and canine acute phase proteins. Vet Res Commun. 1988;12:169–78.
51. Hulton NR, Johnson DJ, Wilmore DW. Limited effects of prostaglandin inhibitors in *Escherichia coli* sepsis. Surgery. 1985;98:291–7.
52. Fransen EJ, Maessen JG, Elenbaas TWO, van Aarnhem EEHL, van Dieijen-Visser MP. Increased preoperative C-reactive protein plasma levels as a risk factor for postoperative infections. Ann Thorac Surg. 1999;67:134–8.
53. Hancock RB, Lanz OI, Waldron DR, Duncan RB, Broadstone RV, Hendrix PK. Comparison of postoperative pain after ovariohysterectomy by harmonic scalpel-assisted laparoscopy compared with median celiotomy and ligation in dogs. Vet Surg. 2005;34:273–82.
54. Davidson EB, Moll HD, Payton ME. Comparison of laparoscopic ovariohysterectomy and ovariohysterectomy in dogs. Vet Surg. 2004;33:62–9.
55. Culp WTN, Mayhew PD, Brown DC. The effect of laparoscopic versus open ovariectomy on postsurgical activity in small dogs. Vet Surg. 2009;38:811–7.

22

Antimicrobial resistance among pathogenic bacteria from mink (*Neovison vison*) in Denmark

Nanett Kvist Nikolaisen, Desireé Corvera Kløve Lassen, Mariann Chriél, Gitte Larsen, Vibeke Frøkjær Jensen and Karl Pedersen*

Abstract

Background: For proper treatment of bacterial infections in mink, knowledge of the causative agents and their antimicrobial susceptibility patterns is crucial. The used antimicrobials are in general not registered for mink, i.e. most usage is "off-label". In this study, we report the patterns of antimicrobial resistance among pathogenic bacteria isolated from Danish mink during the period 2014–2016. The aim of this investigation was to provide data on antimicrobial resistance and consumption, to serve as background knowledge for new veterinary guidelines for prudent and optimal antimicrobial usage in mink.

Results: A total number of 308 *Escherichia coli* isolates, 41 *Pseudomonas aeruginosa*, 36 *Streptococcus canis*, 30 *Streptococcus dysgalactiae*, 55 *Staphylococcus delphini*, 9 *Staphylococcus aureus*, and 20 *Staphylococcus schleiferi* were included in this study. Among *E. coli*, resistance was observed more frequently among the hemolytic isolates than among the non-hemolytic ones. The highest frequency of resistance was found to ampicillin, 82.3% and 48.0% of the hemolytic of the non-hemolytic isolates, respectively. The majority of the *P. aeruginosa* isolates were only sensitive to ciprofloxacin and gentamicin. Among the *Staphylococcus* spp., the highest occurrence of resistance was found for tetracycline. Regarding the nine *S. aureus*, one isolate was resistant to cefoxitin indicating it was a methicillin-resistant *Staphylococcus aureus*. Both β-hemolytic *Streptococcus* species showed high levels of resistance to tetracycline and erythromycin. The antimicrobial consumption increased significantly during 2007–2012, and fluctuated at a high level during 2012–2016, except for a temporary drop in 2013–2014. The majority of the prescribed antimicrobials were aminopenicillins followed by tetracyclines and macrolides.

Conclusions: The study showed that antimicrobial resistance was common in most pathogenic bacteria from mink, in particular hemolytic *E. coli*. There is a need of guidelines for prudent use of antimicrobials for mink.

Keywords: Antimicrobial consumption, Antimicrobial resistance, *Escherichia coli*, Mink, *Neovison vison*, *Pseudomonas aeruginosa*, *Staphylococcus delphini*, *Streptococcus canis*

Background

The Danish production of mink (*Neovison vison*) skins was over 17 million annually (2013–2016). In 2016, this corresponded to 30% of the world production of 55.7 million skins [1]. In the Danish mink production, a range of bacterial species are causing a wide variety of infectious diseases. Among the most important ones are *Escherichia coli* (causing e.g. enteritis, pneumonia, and septicemia), *Streptococcus canis* and *Streptococcus dysgalactiae* (e.g. pneumonia, wound infections, and mastitis), various staphylococci such as *Staphylococcus delphini*, *Staphylococcus aureus*, and *Staphylococcus schleiferi* (e.g. wound infections, dermatitis, pleuritis, pneumonia, and mastitis) and *Pseudomonas aeruginosa* (e.g. hemorrhagic pneumonia) [2]. Antimicrobials are prescribed for treatment of these infections, but the usage of antimicrobial

*Correspondence: kape@vet.dtu.dk
National Veterinary Institute, Technical University of Denmark, Kemitorvet, Anker Engelundsvej 1, 2800 Lyngby, Denmark

drugs may lead to the selection for resistance [3, 4]. Therefore, it is important to follow the development of resistance over time for the major bacterial pathogens. The consumption of antimicrobials for mink in Denmark increased over several years up to 2012 [5, 6]. Rising public focus on animal welfare may have contributed to the increase in 2011–2012 [6]. On the other hand, rising focus on antimicrobial consumption in the mink production may have contributed to the significant decrease in 2013 and 2014 [5, 6].

At present, only one antimicrobial product containing oxytetracycline is registered specifically for use in mink on the Danish market. Therefore, most antimicrobial use is "off-label" and dosages are extrapolated from other animal species, for which the products are registered, while knowledge on absorption and plasma concentrations in mink are sparse.

Here we present the results of the surveillance of antimicrobial resistance among pathogenic bacteria isolated from mink submitted for diagnostic at the National Veterinary Laboratory in a 3-year period, 2014–2016, and compare the results with previous data. The reported findings of antimicrobial resistance levels are discussed in relation to patterns in antimicrobial prescription for mink.

Methods

Bacterial isolates and culture conditions

Bacterial isolates were obtained from clinical samples from carcasses submitted to the National Veterinary Institute, DTU, during the period 2014–2016. The isolates were considered causative agents in infections that had led to the submission of the animals for laboratory examination. They had been recovered from pathological material by conventional culture methods and identified by matrix-associated laser desorption/ionization—time of flight mass spectrometry (MALDI-TOF MS). Mass spectra were obtained using an Autoflex Speed instrument (Bruker Daltonics, Bremen, Germany) calibrated with the Bruker *Escherichia coli* Bacterial Test Standard for Mass Spectrometry. Isolates were analysed with the MALDI Biotyper RTC 3.1 software using a BDAL database of library spectra (Bruker Daltonics). Only one isolate was included from each submission. They originated from many farms (n = 284 out of approx. 1400 Danish mink farms) and were assumed to be representative for Danish mink farms.

The *E. coli* isolates (n = 308) consisted of 158 hemolytic and 150 non-hemolytic isolates. They were derived from samples of liver, lung, mammary gland, feces, intestine, spleen, or uterus. The *S. canis* (n = 36) and *S. dysgalactiae* (n = 30) isolates were derived from mammary gland, liver, lung, paw, skin, or thoracic cavity. The staphylococci included in this investigation were primarily of the species *S. delphini* (n = 55) and a few of *S. aureus* (n = 9) or *S. schleiferi* (n = 20). They were derived from lung, liver, urine, skin, uterus, nose, or kidney. Isolates of *P. aeruginosa* (n = 41) were mainly isolated from the lung, except a few deriving from the spleen, liver, or thoracic cavity; all *P. aeruginosa* isolates were found in association with outbreaks of hemorrhagic pneumonia.

Antimicrobial susceptibility testing

The minimal inhibitory concentration (MIC) of different antimicrobial agents was determined by the broth dilution susceptibility testing method using a semiautomatic system (SensiTitre, Trek Diagnostic Systems Ltd., UK) according to recommendations by the Clinical Laboratory Standards Institute [7]. The susceptibility test-panels and their test ranges are presented in Tables 1, 2, 3, 4, 5, 6 and 7. In the test result for *P. aeruginosa,* only apramycin, ciprofloxacin, colistin, gentamicin, spectinomycin, and streptomycin were reported due to intrinsic resistance towards the remaining antimicrobials [8, 9] (Table 3).

MIC values were interpreted using clinical breakpoints when available [see Additional file 1]. Since there are no approved breakpoints for mink pathogens, these interpretations must be regarded cautiously. Test ranges were as stated by Pedersen et al. [10]. Resistance percentages were calculated from isolates with MIC values above the breakpoint for resistance. In this study, the resistance level for each antimicrobial was considered low when <10% of the isolates were above the resistance breakpoint and considered high when resistance levels were >40%. Comparison between resistance levels in hemolytic and non-hemolytic *E. coli* was performed by using a Fisher's exact test [11]. Results were considered significant when $P < 0.05$.

Consumption of antimicrobial agents

Data on antimicrobial consumption in mink from 2007 to 2016 were extracted from the national veterinary prescription database, VetStat [12, 13]. VetStat data are considered to cover more than 99% of the total prescribed amounts of antimicrobials for veterinary use [14]. This study included all records on sales of antimicrobial drug for systemic use when (1) prescribed for mink, and/or (2) prescribed to mink farms with no other animal species recorded on the farm. The temporal developments in antimicrobial consumption were presented as annual kg active compound together with the trend in number of breeding females as a measure of population size.

To enable comparison of individual classes of antimicrobials, the consumption was measured in Defined Animal Doses. To adjust for fluctuations in population size,

Table 1 MIC distributions and occurrence of resistance of hemolytic *Escherichia coli* (n = 158) isolates from Danish mink (2014–2016)

	Distribution (n) of MICs (µg/ml)																		
	0.015	0.031	0.063	0.125	0.25	0.5	1	2	4	8	16	32	64	128	256	512	1024	2048	%R
Amox + clav								12	23	110	11	2							1.3
Ampicillin							2	17	8		1		130						82.3
Apramycin									110	42	5		1						0.6
Cefotaxime				154	1				1	2									1.9
Ceftiofur						156			1		1								0.6
Chloramphenicol								4	96	50		3	2	3					5.1
Ciprofloxacin	106	50			1		1												0
Colistin							150	7				1							0.6
Florfenicol								8	122	24				4					2.5
Gentamicin						52	93	8		1		4							2.5
Nalidixic acid									155				1	2					1.9
Neomycin								128	25		2		3						3.2
Spectinomycin											113	12	7	6	9	11			16.5
Streptomycin										53	14	7	16	20	48				57.6
Sulphamethoxazole													69					89	56.3
Tetracycline								69	2		1	2	84						55.1
Trimethoprim							93	1					64						40.5

Vertical lines indicate breakpoints for resistance (see breakpoint table in Additional file 1 A). White fields indicate test range for each antimicrobial. Values greater than the test range represent MIC values greater than the highest concentration in the range. MICs equal to or lower than the lowest concentration, are given as the lowest concentration in the test range

R resistance, *n* number of isolates, *amox + clav* amoxicillin with clavulanic acid (1:2)

Table 2 MIC distributions and occurrence of resistance of non-hemolytic *Escherichia coli* (n = 150) isolates from Danish mink (2014–2016)

	Distribution (n) of MICs (µg/ml)																		
	0.015	0.031	0.063	0.125	0.25	0.5	1	2	4	8	16	32	64	128	256	512	1024	2048	%R
Amox + clav								21	52	64	12	1							0.7
Ampicillin							2	29	42	5			72						48.0
Apramycin									103	43	4								0
Cefotaxime				146	3					1									0.7
Ceftiofur						147	2				1								0.7
Chloramphenicol								6	61	74	2	2		5					4.7
Ciprofloxacin	83	53	3		2	2		1		6									4.0
Colistin							144	6											0
Florfenicol								8	93	47	1			1					1.3
Gentamicin						52	88	9		1									0
Nalidixic acid									138	3				9					6.0
Neomycin								123	18	2	1	1	5						4.7
Spectinomycin											107	21		3	5	14			14.7
Streptomycin										86	12	5	2	11	34				34.7
Sulphamethoxazole													97					53	35.3
Tetracycline								98	10				42						28.0
Trimethoprim							114						36						24.0

Vertical lines indicate breakpoints for resistance (see breakpoint table in Additional file 1 A). White fields indicate test range for each antimicrobial. Values greater than the test range represent MIC values greater than the highest concentration in the range. MICs equal to or lower than the lowest concentration, are given as the lowest concentration in the test range

R resistance, *n* number of isolates, *amox + clav* amoxicillin with clavulanic acid (1:2)

an estimated treatment proportion (TP) per year was calculated as;

$$TP = \sum \frac{\text{active compound}}{\text{DADD kg} * (\text{animal biomass} * \text{days})}$$

where DADDkg (mg/kg) is the number of defined daily dosage for treatment of one kg biomass, defined on product level as the recommended average daily dose, according to the principles described previously by Jensen et al.

Table 3 MIC distributions and occurrence of resistance of *Pseudomonas aeruginosa* (n = 41) isolates from Danish mink (2014–2016)

	Distribution (n) of MICs (μg/ml)																		%R
	0.015	0.031	0.063	0.125	0.25	0.5	1	2	4	8	16	32	64	128	256	512	1024	2048	
Apramycin									31	10									-
Ciprofloxacin			1	21	13	5	1												0
Colistin							14	20	6	1									17
Gentamicin						4	26	11											0
Spectinomycin													1	5	16	19			-
Streptomycin										2	6	26	7						-

Vertical lines indicate breakpoints for resistance when available (see breakpoint table in Additional file 1 A). White fields indicate test range for each antimicrobial. Values greater than the test range represent MIC values greater than the highest concentration in the range. MICs equal to or lower than the lowest concentration, are given as the lowest concentration in the test range

R resistance, *n* number of isolates

Table 4 MIC distributions and occurrence of resistance of *Streptococcus canis* (n = 36) isolates from Danish mink (2014–2016)

	Distribution (n) of MICs (μg/ml)															%R
	0.063	0.125	0.25	0.5	1	2	4	8	16	32	64	128	256	512	1024	
Cefoxitin					24	11	1									-
Chloramphenicol						15	21									0
Ciprofloxacin				16	20											0
Erythromycin			17				1			18						53
Forfenicol					15	21										0
Gentamicin				1	1	14	19	1								-
Penicillin	34		2													6
Spectinomycin									21	3			1	11		-
Streptomycin								3	14	2	1	16				-
Sulphamethoxazole										9	13	3			11	-
Tetracycline							1	1			34					97
Tiamulin			21	2					1	2	10					-
TMP+Sulpha			36													0
Trimethoprim				29	4	3										0

Vertical lines indicate breakpoints for resistance when available (see breakpoint table in Additional file 1 B). White fields indicate test range for each antimicrobial. Values greater than the test range represent MIC values greater than the highest concentration in the range. MICs equal to or lower than the lowest concentration, are given as the lowest concentration in the test range

R resistance, *n* number of isolates, *TMP + Sulpha* trimethoprim with sulphamethoxazole (1:19)

[5]; active compound was the annual antimicrobial use summarized on 4th or 5th ATCvet level [15]; the live animal biomass was estimated from number of breeding females registered at Kopenhagen Fur, and data on litter size and growth, as described by Jensen et al. [5]. A TP of 10 DADD/1000 biomass × days corresponds to 1% of the population biomass being treated on an average day.

Results

Resistance occurrence

In the hemolytic *E. coli* isolates, the highest occurrence of resistance was recorded for ampicillin (82.3%). Additionally, high resistance levels were found for streptomycin, sulphonamides, tetracyclines, and trimethoprim (>40%) (Table 1). For these compounds as well as spectinomycin, resistant isolates were recorded from any sampling site. For other tested antimicrobials, resistance levels were low.

Among the hemolytic *E. coli*, 45 different phenotypic resistance profiles were recorded. Only 19 of 158 isolates were sensitive to all 17 tested antimicrobials. Multiresistance, i.e. being resistant to three or more compounds, was recorded in 60% of all the isolates. The most common phenotypes were resistant to ampicillin-streptomycin-sulphonamide-tetracycline/trimethoprim (see Additional file 2). Mono-resistance was recorded in 10% of the isolates. Resistance for up to 10 compounds was recorded.

Table 5 MIC distributions and occurrence of resistance of *Streptococcus dysgalactiae* (n = 30) isolates from Danish mink (2014–2016)

	Distribution (n) of MICs (μg/ml)															
	0.063	0.125	0.25	0.5	1	2	4	8	16	32	64	128	256	512	1024	%R
Cefoxitin				1	24	5										-
Chloramphenicol						5	24	1								0
Ciprofloxacin			1	19	10											0
Erythromycin			12	1						17						57
Forfenicol					5	24	1									0
Gentamicin					3	15	11	1								-
Penicillin	30															0
Spectinomycin									16	4				10		-
Streptomycin							1	4	7	1	1	16				-
Sulphamethoxazole										17	4	3	2	1	3	-
Tetracycline				1	1	1	2			6	19					83
Tiamulin			15	1							14					-
TMP+Sulpha			30													0
Trimethoprim				18	11	1										0

Vertical lines indicate breakpoints for resistance when available (see breakpoint table in Additional file 1 B). White fields indicate test range for each antimicrobial. Values greater than the test range represent MIC values greater than the highest concentration in the range. MICs equal to or lower than the lowest concentration, are given as the lowest concentration in the test range

Table 6 MIC distributions and occurrence of resistance of *Staphylococcus delphini* (n = 55) isolates from Danish mink (2014–2016)

	Distribution (n) of MICs (μg/ml)															
	0.063	0.125	0.25	0.5	1	2	4	8	16	32	64	128	256	512	1024	%R
Cefoxitin				33	20	1	1									0
Chloramphenicol						1	24	29	1							0
Ciprofloxacin		30	22	2	1											0
Erythromycin			17	25	1		1			11						20
Forfenicol					2	32	21									0
Gentamicin			54	1												0
Penicillin	18	11	15	2	3	3	2	1								47
Spectinomycin										21	30			4		7
Streptomycin							45	7		1	2					5
Sulphamethoxazole										47	5	3				0
Tetracycline				25	2					3	25					51
Tiamulin			53	1	1											0
TMP+Sulpha			54							1						2
Trimethoprim				2	10	24	17	1			1					2

Vertical lines indicate breakpoints for resistance (see breakpoint table in Additional file 1 B). White fields indicate test range for each antimicrobial. Values greater than the test range represent MIC values greater than the highest concentration in the range. MICs equal to or lower than the lowest concentration, are given as the lowest concentration in the test range

R resistance, *n* number of isolates, *TMP + Sulpha* trimethoprim with sulphamethoxazole (1:19)

Resistance among the non-hemolytic *E. coli* isolates was also highest for ampicillin (48%), followed by streptomycin, sulphonamide, and trimethoprim (>25%) (Table 2). For these antimicrobials and tetracycline, resistant isolates were observed for all kind of samples. For other tested antimicrobials, resistance was at low levels.

The hemolytic and non-hemolytic *E. coli* isolates showed similar resistance patterns, e.g. both showed the highest level of resistance to ampicillin. However, higher levels of resistance were in general observed among the hemolytic isolates than among the non-hemolytic isolates (Tables 1, 2). The differences were statistically

Table 7 MIC distributions and occurrence of resistance of *Staphylococcus schleiferi* (n = 20) isolates from Danish mink (2014–2016)

	Distribution (n) of MICs (μg/ml)														
	0.063	0.125	0.25	0.5	1	2	4	8	16	32	64	128	256	512	%R
Cefoxitin				17	2		1								0
Chloramphenicol							17	3							0
Ciprofloxacin		8	12												0
Erythromycin			19							1					5
Forfenicol						18	2								0
Gentamicin			17	3											0
Penicillin	18		1						1						10
Spectinomycin										13	6			1	5
Streptomycin							13	7							0
Sulphamethoxazole										11	8	1			0
Tetracycline				9						1	10				55
Tiamulin			14	5	1										0
TMP+Sulpha			19	1											0
Trimethoprim					2	16	2								0

Vertical lines indicate breakpoints for resistance (see breakpoint table in Additional file 1 B). White fields indicate test range for each antimicrobial. Values greater than the test range represent MIC values greater than the highest concentration in the range. MICs equal to or lower than the lowest concentration, are given as the lowest concentration in the test range

significant for ciprofloxacin (P < 0.03) and highly significant (P < 0.001) for ampicillin, streptomycin, sulphonamide, tetracycline and trimethoprim. Only for ciprofloxacin the resistance levels were higher in the non-hemolytic isolates (4%) than in the hemolytic isolates (1%) (Tables 1, 2).

All the 41 *P. aeruginosa* isolates were sensitive to ciprofloxacin and gentamicin. Colistin resistance was found in 17% of the isolates. All isolates were susceptible to apramycin in a concentration below 16 μg/mL (Table 3).

The two species of beta-hemolytic streptococci tested in this study, presented similar resistance patterns (Tables 4, 5). The majority of the 36 *S. canis* isolates and the 30 *S. dysgalactiae* isolates were resistant to tetracycline (97% and 83%, respectively). Additionally, high levels of resistance to erythromycin were found in both streptococci species with more than 40% of the isolates (Tables 4, 5). As all the isolates of *S. dysgalactiae* were sensitive to penicillin, and two of the *S. canis* isolates were resistant.

The two staphylococcus species tested in this study, presented similar resistance patterns except for penicillin (Tables 6, 7). Among the 55 *S. delphini* isolates the highest occurrence of resistance were found for tetracycline (51%), penicillin (47%) and erythromycin (20%) (Table 6). Among the 20 *S. schleiferi* isolates about half of the isolates were resistant to tetracyclines, but only two isolates were resistant penicillin (Table 7).

Only nine *S. aureus* isolates were available for testing. They were susceptible to the majority of the tested antimicrobials, while five of the isolates were resistant to penicillin and four to tetracyclines. One of the isolates was resistant to cefoxitin, suggesting that this *S. aureus* isolate was a methicillin-resistant *S. aureus* (MRSA).

Antimicrobial consumption

The overall antimicrobial consumption in the mink production measured in kg active compound, increased by 130% from 2007 to 2012, followed by a slight temporary decrease, most pronounced in 2014 (Fig. 1). From 2010 there has been an increase in number of breeding females, which may explain for some of the increase in usage (Fig. 1). Taking into account the changes in population size, the antimicrobial consumption increased by 109%, from 23 DADD/(1000 biomass × days) in 2007 to 48 DADD/(1000 biomass × days) in 2012 (Fig. 2). In 2014, the antimicrobial consumption decreased to around 30 DADD/(1000 biomass × days), and since increasing towards 40 DADD/(1000 biomass × days) in 2016. The rise during the period 2007–2012 was mainly related to the use of aminopenicillins (mainly amoxicillin), tetracyclines and macrolides, which are by far the most frequently used antimicrobials in the mink production (Fig. 2). Lincomycin in combination with spectinomycin has been commonly used, but it has been decreasing the past years. Cephalosporins and fluoroquinolones comprised less than 0.01% of the antimicrobial consumption in Danish mink during 2007–2012; amphenicols (florfenicol) comprised 0.06% and colistin comprised 0.2% of the consumption.

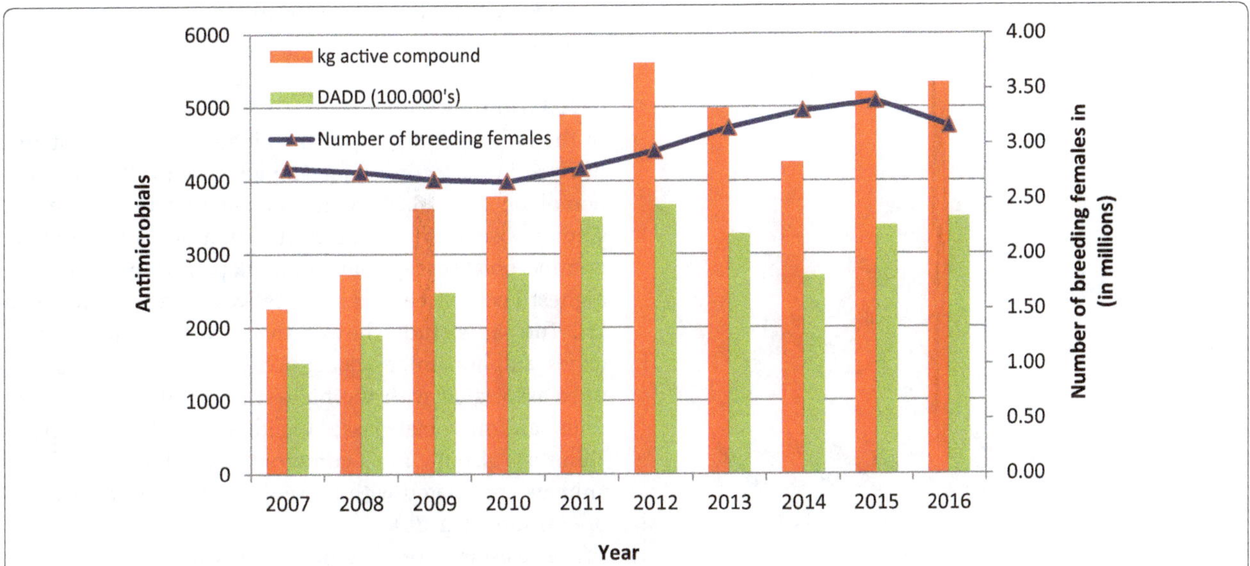

Fig. 1 Antimicrobial prescriptions in Danish mink production (2007–2016). The prescription of antimicrobials given in kg active compound and DADD per year, and the curve indicating number of breeding females (in millions). DADD: defined animal daily dose is the assumed average maintenance dose needed to treat one kg animal

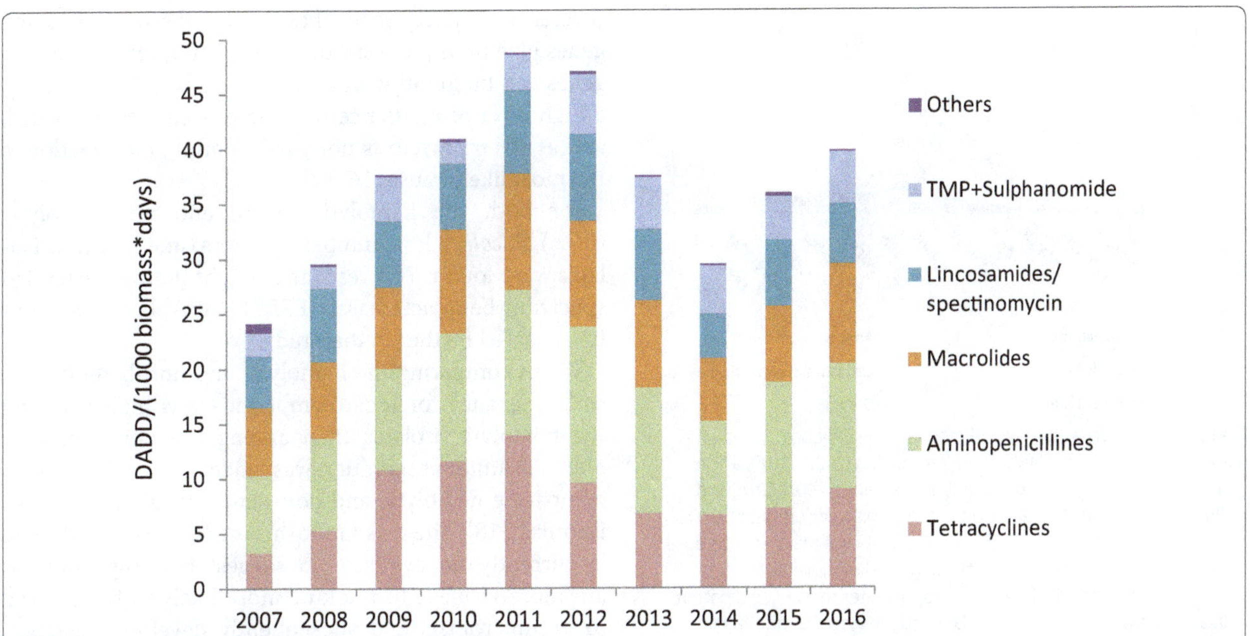

Fig. 2 Antimicrobial prescriptions in the Danish mink production (2007–2016) by antimicrobial class. *DADD* defined animal daily dose is the assumed average maintenance dose needed to treat one kg animal. Others: Pleuromutilins, amphenicols, aminoglycosides, cephalosporins, colistin, fluoroquinolones, penicillin. TMP + sulphonamide: trimethoprim with sulphonamide

The seasonal pattern shows a dramatic peak in antimicrobial consumption in May (Fig. 3a). This is true for all antimicrobial classes, but most pronounced for the most used antimicrobials; aminopenicillins, macrolides, lincosamides with spectinomycin, and tetracyclines (Fig. 3a). The prescription of tetracycline also increases into the autumn (June–October), when the kits are growing and the biomass is significantly higher (Fig. 3b). In contrast, during the period from pelting (November–December) until the whelping

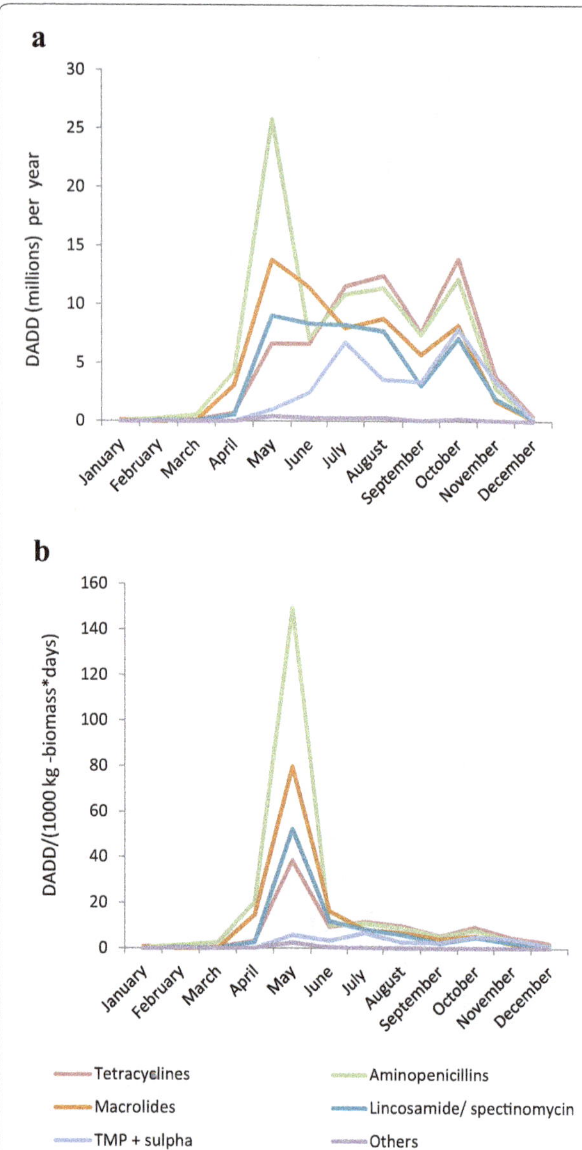

Fig. 3 Seasonal patterns in antimicrobial prescriptions by antimicrobial class in the Danish mink production (2007–2016). **a** The graph is a monthly average from the time period 2007–2016, and illustrates the seasonal pattern in antimicrobial consumption. *DADD* defined animal daily dose is the assumed average maintenance dose needed to treat one kg animal. **b** The graph is a monthly average from the time period 2007–2016, and illustrates the seasonal pattern in antimicrobial consumption relative to the size of Danish mink production (monthly average, 2007–2016). DADD/(1000 kg – biomass * day) = number of DADD's used within a given period per tonnes live biomass multiplied by number of days at risk within the time period (month), the unit describes the prescribed antimicrobials relative to the biomass on the farm, i.e. the decrease during autumn as the kits grow and the biomass increases. Others: Pleuromutilins, amphenicols, aminoglycosides, cephalosporins, colistin, fluoroquinolones, penicillin. TMP + sulpha: trimethoprim with sulphonamide

season (May), the prescription of antimicrobial was very low (Fig. 3b).

Discussion

In the present study, by far the highest level of resistance in *E. coli* was recorded for ampicillin, with 82.3% of the hemolytic and 48.0% of the non-hemolytic isolates. A similar observation was reflected in a previous study on antimicrobial susceptibility in mink pathogens, where the highest occurrence of resistance was found to ampicillin [2]. The same study showed that streptomycin, tetracyclines, sulphonamides, spectinomycin, and trimethoprim were associated with the highest levels of resistance [2]. These antimicrobial classes together with the aminopenicillins are also the most commonly used, but much fewer animals are treated with these drugs compared to aminopenicillins (Fig. 3b).

The resistance profiles of *E. coli,* with more than 50% of the isolates being resistant to sulphonamide and streptomycin, which are not commonly used in Danish mink, might be related to usage and/or to co-selection [16]. The potential of *E. coli* to transfer resistance plasmids and thereby spread antimicrobial resistance is well known; several resistance genes have been discovered, some genes give multiple resistances, and numerous resistance genes can be found within one isolate [17]. In this study, a high level of resistance to streptomycin was recorded, and as streptomycin is not used in mink, co-selection is the most likely cause [16, 17].

For both the hemolytic (1.9%) and non-hemolytic (0.7%) *E. coli,* a low number of cefotaxime resistant isolates were found. This resistance might indicate extended spectrum beta-lactamases (ESBL) status, but it was not investigated further in this study.

When comparing the hemolytic and non-hemolytic *E. coli,* resistance for most compounds was higher among the hemolytic isolates than among the non-hemolytic ones. A similar observation was made in a previous study, comparing hemolytic and non-hemolytic *E. coli* in Danish mink [18]. The reason for this is not known, and there is currently no evidence to suggest that these strains are more virulent to mink or more likely to be exposed to antimicrobials and subsequently develop resistance. However, this needs to be further investigated. In pigs, the hemolytic *E. coli* O149 is the most important pathogen in weaning diarrhea, and hemolysis is thought to be involved in the pathogenesis, although other toxins than hemolysin are known to be important [19].

In mink, *P. aeruginosa* is causative of hemorrhagic pneumonia, and this bacterium is well recognized because of its intrinsic resistance to most antimicrobials [8, 9]. High susceptibility was found to ciprofloxacin, colistin, and gentamicin. The few colistin-resistant strains found in this study might belong to the Gaussian distribution of the susceptible wild types (Table 3). In a previous study, all *P. aeruginosa* isolates were found susceptible to gentamicin and colistin [2].

In this study, both group G (*S. canis*) and group C (*S. dysgalactiae*) streptococci were investigated. In the two streptococcus species, high resistance levels to tetracycline were found; *S. canis*: 97% and *S. dysgalactiae*: 83%. High levels of resistance to tetracycline were also found in a previous study [2]. Resistance to macrolides, represented by erythromycin was high in data from 2008 [2] and this pattern was also found in the present study with more than 50% of the isolates being resistant in both species (Tables 4, 5). Whether the high levels of resistance to macrolides and tetracycline reflects the similarly high consumption of these compounds (Fig. 2) is uncertain. The tiamulin and spectinomycin MIC distributions showed a distinct division into two groups in both species. This might indicate the grouping of susceptible wild type and a resistant population (Tables 4, 5). Penicillin resistance was low in the streptococci despite high consumption of aminopenicillins; this is a pattern known also from other species, e.g. humans and cattle [20]. In this study, two *S. canis* isolates had a MIC value of 0.25 μg/mL to penicillin while the other isolates had MIC values $\leq$0.063 μg/mL. This needs to be further investigated.

The taxonomy of staphylococci has changed so that isolates from mink that were previously identified as *S. intermedius* are now considered to belong to the species *S. delphini*. Thus, the isolates reported by Pedersen et al. [2] as *S. intermedius* were likely all *S. delphini*. Among *S. delphini*, far the highest level of resistance was found to tetracycline (51%). A similar pattern was observed in 2008 [2], as high levels of resistant isolates were found to tetracycline, penicillin and erythromycin.

One of the *S. aureus* isolates was resistant to cefoxitin. This observation subsequently prompted an investigation of occurrence of MRSA in mink, and it has become evident that MRSA is widespread on Danish mink farms. The majority of the isolates are livestock-associated MRSA CC398, and belonging to spa-types t034 and t011, which are also most prevalent in pigs [21].

In general, the occurrence of resistance towards cephalosporins and fluoroquinolones is very low in bacterial isolates from Danish mink, most likely due to the very low consumption of the compounds both in Danish mink and other production animals in Denmark (Fig. 2) [20].

There was a marked increase in antimicrobial prescription in May (Fig. 3a). The reason is probably that that mink kits are born around early May, and the antimicrobials are mainly for treatment of pre–weaning mink diarrhea. In the peri-weaning period May–July, the prescription of aminopenicillins was 27% higher than macrolides and 75% higher compared to the use of tetracyclines. In contrast, tetracyclines were used 10% more than aminopenicillins and 65% more than macrolides in autumn. Thus aminopenicillins are in general used to treat pre- and post-weaning animals in the spring, whereas tetracyclines are used mainly in the almost full-grown animals in the autumn. Consequently, more animals can be treated with the given amount of aminopenicillins in the spring, than the tetracycline in the autumn. This explains the difference between Fig. 3a, b.

Conclusions

For *E. coli*, high levels of resistance were recorded, especially among hemolytic isolates, to the most used compounds ampicillin and tetracyclines. High resistance levels to streptomycin and sulphonamides were recorded, probably due to co-resistance. The most commonly used antimicrobials are also reflected in the resistance patterns of Gram positive bacteria. The antimicrobial consumption data displays an overall decrease from 2011 to 2014, and then a gradual increase in 2015 and 2016.

There is a need for guidelines regarding treatment and susceptibility of relevant pathogens in Danish mink for veterinarians and farmers to optimize (and minimize) the use of antimicrobial compounds.

Authors' contributions

NKN and DCKL collected resistance data and drafted the manuscript. MC recovered resistance data from LIMS databases. GL was responsible for collecting bacterial isolates for sensitivity testing. VFJ provided descriptive analyses on antimicrobial usage from VetStat. KP validated resistance data and completed the manuscript. All authors contributed to the manuscript. All authors read and approved the final manuscript.

Acknowledgements

This investigation was supported by grants from the Pelsdyravlerfonden, 2014–2016. The skilled technical assistance from Mrs. Susanne M Ranebro and Pia T Hansen is gratefully acknowledged.

Competing interests

The authors declare that they have no competing interests.

Funding

This investigation was supported by a grant from The Fur Animal Levy Fund and the Danish Veterinary and Food Administration.

References

1. Kopenhagen Fur: Historical data. http://www.kopenhagenfur.com/da/minkavl/historisk-data/verdensproduktion-i-minkskind. Accessed 28 Feb 2017.
2. Pedersen K, Hammer AS, Sørensen CM, Heuer OE. Usage of antimicrobials and occurrence of antimicrobial resistance among bacteria from mink. Vet Microbiol. 2008;133:115–22.

3. Aarestrup FM, Seyfarth AM, Emborg H-D, Pedersen K, Hendriksen RS, Bager F. Effect of abolishment of the use of antimicrobial agents for growth promotion on occurrence of antimicrobial resistance in fecal enterococci from food animals in Denmark. Antimicrob Agents Chemother. 2001;45:2054. doi:10.1128/AAC.45.7.2054-2059.2001.
4. Garcia-Miguera L, Hendriksen RS, Fraile L, Aarestrup FM. Antimicrobial resistance of zoonotic and commensal bacteria in Europe: the missing link between consumption and resistance in veterinary medicine. Vet Microbiol. 2014;170:1–9.
5. Jensen VF, Sommer HM, Struve T, Clausen J, Chriél M. Factors associated with usage of antimicrobials in commercial mink (*Neovison vison*) production in Denmark. Prev Vet Med. 2016. doi:10.1016/j.prevetmed.2016.01.023.
6. Anononymous. DANMAP 2014—Use of antimicrobial agents and occurrence of antimicrobial resistance in bacteria from food and humans in Denmark. Copenhagen, Denmark. ISSN 1600-2032. 2015.
7. Clinical and Laboratory Standards Institute. Performance standards for antimicrobial disk and dilution susceptibility test for bacteria isolated from animals; Approved standard, 4th ed. CLSI document VET01-A4, CLSI, Wayne, Pennsylvania, USA, 2013.
8. Clinical Lab Standards Institute—CLSI: Intrinsic Resistance, M100 S27:2017. http://em100.edaptivedocs.info/GetDoc.aspx?doc=CLSI%20M100%20S27:2017&scope=user. Accessed 28 Feb 2017.
9. The European Committee on antimicrobial susceptibility testing—EUCAST: expert rules and intrinsic resistance 27 Sep 2016. http://www.eucast.org/expert_rules_and_intrinsic_resistance/ Accessed 28 Feb 2017.
10. Pedersen K, Pedersen K, Jensen H, Finster K, Jensen VF, Heuer OE. Occurrence of antimicrobial resistance in bacteria from diagnostic samples from dogs. J Antimicrob Chemother. 2007;60:775–81. doi:10.1093/jac/dkm269.
11. Social science statistics: statistical test calculators, http://www.socscistatistics.com/tests/Default.aspx. Accessed 2 Mar 2017.
12. Stege H, Bager F, Jacobsen E, Thougaard A. VETSTAT-the Danish system for surveillance of the veterinary use of drugs for production animals. Prev Vet Med. 2003;57:105–15.
13. Anonymous. VetStat. The Danish Veterinary and Food Administration. http://www.foedevarestyrelsen.dk/Leksikon/Sider/VetStat.aspxx. Accessed Mar 2017.
14. Anonymous. DANMAP 2001—use of antimicrobial agents and occurrence of antimicrobial resistance in bacteria from food and humans in Denmark. Copenhagen, Denmark. ISSN 1600-2032. 2002.
15. WHO Collaborating Centre for Drug Statistics Methodology. New ATC/DDDs and alterations from the October 2015 meeting. http://www.whocc.no/news/new_atc_ddds_and_alterations_from_the_october_2015_meeting. Accessed 10 Apr 2016.
16. Tadesse DA, Zhao S, Tong E, Ayers S, Singh A, Bartholomew MJ, McDermott PF. Antimicrobial drug resistance in *Escherichia coli* from humans and food animals, United States, 1950–2002. Emerg Infect Dis. 2012;18:741–9.
17. Guerral B, Junker E, Schroeter A, Malorny B, Lehmann S, Helmuth R. Phenotypic and genotypic characterization of antimicrobial resistance in German *Escherichia coli* isolates from cattle, swine and poultry. J Antimicrob Chemother. 2003;52:489–92. doi:10.1093/jac/dkg362.
18. Vulfson L, Pedersen K, Chriel M, Frydendahl K, Andersen Holmen T, Madsen M, Dietz HH. Serogroups and antimicrobial susceptibility among *Escherichia coli* isolated from farmed mink (*Mustela vison Schreiber*) in Denmark. Vet Microbiol. 2001;79:143–53.
19. Fairbrother JM, Gyles CL. Colibacillosis. In: Zimmerman JJ, Karriker LA, Ramirez A, Schwartz KJ, Stevenson GW, editors. Diseases of Swine. 10th ed. Hoboken: Wiley; 2012. p. 723–47.
20. Anononymous. DANMAP 2015—use of antimicrobial agents and occurrence of antimicrobial resistance in bacteria from food and humans in Denmark, ISSN 1600-2032. 2016.
21. Hansen JE, Larsen AR, Skov RL, Chriél M, Larsen G, Angen Ø, Larsen J, Lassen DCK, Pedersen K. Livestock-associated methicillin-resistant *Staphylococcus aureus* is widespread in farmed mink (*Neovison vison*). Vet Microbiol. 2017;207:44–9.
22. Clinical Lab Standards Institute (CLSI): Bacterial breakpoint data from M100 S27:2017. http://em100.edaptivedocs.info/GetDoc.aspx?doc=CLSI%20M100%20S27:2017&scope=user. Accessed 28 Feb 2017.
23. Clinical Lab Standards Institute (CLSI): Bacterial breakpoint data from VET01S ED3:2015. http://vet01s.edaptivedocs.info/GetDoc.aspx?doc=CLSI%20VET01S%20ED3:2015&scope=user. Accessed 28 Feb 2017.
24. European Committee on Antimicrobial Susceptibility Testing, EUCAST: Data from the EUCAST clinical breakpoints—bacteria (v 7.0, 2017-01-01). http://www.eucast.org/clinical_breakpoints/. Accessed 28 Feb 2017.
25. European Committee on Antimicrobial Susceptibility Testing, EUCAST: epidemiological cut-off values (ECOFFs), antimicrobial wild type distributions of microorganism. https://mic.eucast.org/Eucast2/SearchController/search.jsp?action=init. Accessed 29 May 2017.

23

The use of phoxim and bendiocarb for control of fleas in farmed mink (*Mustela vison*)

Kim Søholt Larsen[1*], Martin Sciuto[2] and Jan Dahl[3]

Abstract

Background: Fleas (*Ceratophyllus sciurorum*) are common on farmed mink in Denmark. When present, the fleas have a negative impact on the health of the farmed mink and are of nuisance for farm staff. Severe infestations of fleas cause anemia, poor growth and may result in death of mink kits. Changed behavior of the dams is also observed. Further it has been demonstrated that the fleas are vectors of Aleutian disease virus. Flea control is based on use of a few insecticides and resistance has been reported against permethrin. There is thus a need for new flea control products. In this blinded, randomized clinical trial according to GCP standard, phoxim spray and bendiocarb powder for flea control on mink farms were investigated.

Results: Both the phoxim spray solution and bendiocarb powder were found to be efficient for the control of *C. sciurorum* fleas on farmed mink. Phoxim treatments reduced the number of fleas by 98.4% and the bendiocarb treatments reduced the number of fleas by 99.0% in the mink nest boxes when compared to counts in controls. No clinical signs were observed post treatment.

Conclusions: The study demonstrated that phoxim sprayed on the animals and the use of bendiocarb powder in the nest box material were highly efficient for the control of the *C. sciurorum* fleas on farmed mink. Both products were safe to use at the recommended dose rate. Both compounds are recommended to be integrated in a new farm management plan suggested here.

Keywords: Bendiocarb, Farmed mink, Fleas, Phoxim

Background

Mink farmers are often confronted with flea infestations in mink (*Mustela vison*) and the need of an adequate treatment [1, 2]. The squirrel flea, *Ceratophyllus sciurorum*, is the most common pest on farmed mink in Denmark and several other countries [3]. Severe flea infestations may cause anemia, poor growth and may result in death of the very young mink kits. Furthermore, the flea infested dams may become restless and thus often leave the nest boxes. This is associated with poor care of the kits, starvation and subsequently death. Skin and fur can also be damaged when the mink reacts to the fleas by scratching and biting [4]. A flea problem is typically detected when observing fleas on the mink, finding increased numbers of anemic or dead newborn kits or when the farm personnel is being bitten by fleas. The squirrel flea has also been demonstrated to be the vector of pathogenic organisms, e.g., Aleutian mink disease virus [5]. Control of the squirrel fleas on mink farms is thus of vital importance for the health of the mink.

The squirrel flea is almost only present on the host while blood feeding. After the blood meal they leave their host and are then found in the host's surrounding, typically in the straw material of the nest box. It is also in the nest box material that the fleas lay their eggs and where the development from egg to adult flea takes place [4].

Only two insecticides are at present registered for flea control in mink farms in Denmark, namely diflubenzuron

*Correspondence: kim@kslinnovation.dk
[1] KSL Innovation ApS, Ramløsevej 25, 3200 Helsinge, Denmark

and permethrin. Both products are talc powder formulated and are spread/dusted in the straw material in the nest box of the mink. These treatments are made preventively but permethrin is also used when fleas are observed on the farms. Failure of controlling the fleas using permethrin has been experienced on farms not only in Denmark [1, 6], but also in other countries [4]. The reduced efficacy observed in Denmark seems to be due to the presence of permethrin resistance [6] but poor management practice on the farms is also part of the flea problem [7]. There is thus a need for finding new well tolerated insecticides for squirrel flea control on farmed mink.

The purpose of this study was to evaluate the efficacy of phoxim and bendiocarb formulations for flea control on farmed mink.

Methods

Trial design

Phoxim was applied as a 0.1% phoxim aqueous dilution spray (1.9 mL per 100 cm^2 body surface) (Sebacil® Vet., Bayer) and bendiocarb as a 1.25% bendiocarb powder (4 g per nest box) (Ficam® D, Bayer) on an established flea infestation. Two control groups (water spray or talc powder without any insecticide, respectively) were included. Each nest box in the treated and the control groups was regarded as a separate unit as the migration of fleas between nest boxes is very limited or does not occur at all. Each cage in the study with one mink was separated from the next by an empty cage. The trial was blinded, by separation of study roles: the dispenser was not involved in any clinical examination throughout the study and the staff counting flea numbers was unaware of the treatment minks had received.

Farms and animals

The study was designed as a field study and two commercial standard mink farms were selected. Both farms were located in Jutland, Denmark and both farms had a record of squirrel flea problems for several years. The chains of cages were placed under a roof and with a pathway between the chains. Each cage consisted of a wooden nest box (0.075 m^2) and a wire netting box (0.27 m^2). All nest boxes were newly packed with barley straw. Below the straw a folded newspaper was placed to avoid material from falling out of the nest box. Food for the mink was applied on the top of the wire netting boxes. The mink used were 160 barren female mink, 1 or 2 years of age. The animals were of different breeds. One unit with 80 mink on each farm was used. The mink were split randomly into two treatment groups. Forty mink were included in the treatment groups (20 mink in each group) and 40 were acting as controls (again 20 mink in each group). The animals were inspected daily by the farm personal during the trial period. Further, a veterinarian also inspected all animals prior to treatment and at the end of the study. Clinical visual inspection of the animal in the wire netting box was performed with special emphasis on the hair and skin prior to the treatment and at the end of the study 7 days later.

Treatments

The aim of the treatments was either controlling the fleas on the mink or the fleas in the nest box material. The first product tested was 50% w/v phoxim (Sebacil® Vet.) administered as a 0.1% phoxim aqueous dilution sprayed once. Considering the body surface of minks to be similar to those of ferrets (ferrets with a body weight of 0.75 kg and 1.0 kg do have a body surface area of 0.082 m^2 and 0.099 m^2, respectively [8, 9]), the topical spray-dosing of the mink were conducted according to Table 1.

The 0.1% phoxim water-based solution was sprayed on the mink. The second product used was 1.25% w/w bendiocarb powder (Ficam® D), which was applied to the straw material in the nest box at a dose of 4 g. Twenty-five millilitre of water and 4 g of talc powder were used as control references for the phoxim and bendiocarb treatments, respectively. The treatments were performed the day after 50 *C. sciurorum* fleas were placed in each of the nest boxes. The effect of the treatments was measured as the number of fleas found in the material of each nest box 1 week after the treatments.

Table 1 Dosing table for 0.1% phoxim aqueous dilution sprayed on the body surface of mink

Calculation of body surface area (BSA)			Application volume for animals in the body weight range of	
BW in gram	BSA in m^2	Target volume (mL)	Weight range (g)	IVP (mL)
750	0.082	15.7	750–999	19
1000	0.099	19.1	1000–1249	22
1250	0.115	22.1	1250–1499	25
1500	0.130	25.0	1500–1749	28
1750	0.144	27.7	1750–1999	30
2000	0.158	30.3	2000–2249	33
2250	0.171	32.8	2250–2499	35
2500	0.183	35.1	2500–2749	37

The target volume was calculated based on a recommended dose of 25 mL per adult animal of 1.5 kg body weight. Body surface area (BSA) in $m^2 = K \times$ [body weight (BW) in grams$^{2/3}$] $\times 10^{-4}$, K = constant of 9.94 for ferrets

Experimental infestation

The barren female mink were transferred to cages with new straw bedding material. No fleas were thus present in the nest boxes before the artificial infestation. All nest boxes were then artificially infested with 50 adult fleas (*C. sciurorum*) on the day before treatment. The fleas used for this study were collected from the same farm where the mink were originating. This was done to prevent any possible transmission of pathogenic organisms between farms. The fleas for each nest box were kept in separate tubes for up to 24 h before the day of use.

Parasite counting

On study day 7 all material in the nest boxes was transferred into large plastic bags for counting of live fleas within 72 h after collection. Each bag was given a unique code number. The staff performing the flea counting (entomologists) was blinded by means of the coded bags. Counting of fleas was done by looking through the material from each of the nest boxes and counting all adult live fleas found in the material.

Statistical analyses

Data for both trials were analysed in a loglinear model with treatment group and farm as explanatory variables (PROC GENMOD, SAS Institute, NC, USA). The interaction between farm and treatment was evaluated. Effects are reported per farm, and if the interaction between farm and treatment was non-significant, an overall effect was calculated. Initially a Poisson distribution was assumed, but if the model fit, evaluated as a high Pearson Chi square, indicated a low fit of the model, a negative binomial distribution was assumed. Finally, if overdispersion was still present after this, a post hoc adjustment of P-values and confidence intervals was calculated, using the P-scale option in PROC GENMOD (SAS Institute) (adjusting P-values and confidence-intervals by the Pearson Chi square statistics divided by degrees of freedom).

Results are presented as percentage reduction in each treatment-group, compared to the respective control-group.

Thus, the efficacy of the two compounds included in this study was evaluated on their ability to control fleas present in the mink nesting material compared to untreated controls.

Results

Three bags with nest material could not be used for flea counting: One sample from one farm had lost the cage code label during the collection process and two samples from the other farm were excluded due to incorrect numbering in the registration process. These three nest boxes were excluded in this study and data from flea counts in 157 nest boxes are thus included in this study.

No animals experienced health problems, no animals received additional medical treatment and no nest material was removed from the nest boxes. No changes in normal behaviour were observed as well as no side effects were observed during the study period.

Phoxim treatment

Due to overdispersion (scaled Pearson Chi square = 4.73), the Poisson-model was discarded and a negative binomial distribution was assumed. This improved model fit considerably better, but some overdispersion was still present (scaled Pearson Chi square = 1.44). Confidence intervals and P-values were adjusted using the P-scale-option.

Initially an interaction between farm and treatment-effect was examined, giving a non-significant P-value of 0.34. Results are presented as results per farm and in a combined analysis (Table 2).

Bendiocarb treatment

Due to overdispersion (scaled Pearson Chi square = 4.41), the Poisson-model was discarded, and negative binomial distribution was assumed. This improved model fit considerably better, but some overdispersion was still present (scaled Pearson Chi square = 1.41). Confidence intervals and P-values were adjusted using the P-scale-option.

Initially an interaction between farm and treatment-effect was examined, giving a non-significant P-value of 0.08.

Using 0.1% phoxim the reduction in farm 1 was 98.8% and in farm 2, 97.9% with an overall reduction of 98.4% (Tables 3, 4). Use of 4 g of 1.25% bendiocarb in the mink

Table 2 Statistics for the phoxim treatment group

Farm number	Number of nests		Nests with fleas		Average number of fleas[a]		Average number of fleas in positive nests[a]	
	1	2	1	2	1	2	1	2
Treatment	20	20	4	5	0.3 (0.1–0.8)	0.4 (0.2–1.0)	1.5 (0.5–4.1)	1.6 (0.7–3.8)
Control	20	20	20	20	24.8 (18.8–32.7)	18.9 (14.2–25.0)	24.8 (18.8–32.7)	18.9 (14.2–25.0)

[a] Assuming a negative binomial distribution

nest boxes, reduced the number of fleas by 98.2% in farm 1 and 99.7% in farm 2. Overall the reduction was 99.0% (Table 5).

Discussion

In the present study the bendiocarb and phoxim containing products were found to control the fleas and to be easy to apply. Phoxim has already been tested for flea control on farmed mink [10]. However, another treatment strategy was used, i.e. using spontaneously infested nest boxes, two treatments of insecticide regime and a dosage not related to the weight of the mink. Due to this, a direct comparison with the present study is not possible.

The number of fleas collected in the untreated control nest boxes after 7 days showed a reduction in the number of fleas of approximately 50% in the control group. A likely explanation would be that some of the fleas infesting the mink are removed by oral grooming. It is known that farmed mink perform oral grooming [11, 12] but the effect of this grooming on the flea population has not been demonstrated. Removal of fleas (*Ctenocephalides felis*) by oral grooming has been observed in, e.g., cats. Here, by grooming, the cats removed between 4.1 and 17.6% of the fleas daily [13]. It was also demonstrated that cats with fleas groomed twice the rate of the flea free cats [14]. Another explanation for the reduced number of fleas could be that the fleas are simply leaving the nest boxes. However, no fleas were observed outside the nest boxes containing the flea hosts when *C. sciurorum* fleas were reared in captivity [15].

This spontaneous reduction of the number of fleas did not affect the validity of the trial as the number of fleas persisting in the control group was sufficient for a meaningful calculation of efficacy. The numbers meet requirements given by the relevant EMEA guideline.

Based on the present results from the phoxim and bendiocarb treatments, these compounds are suitable for flea control. As mink farmers perform management routines on the farm on a yearly basis related to the synchronous life cycle of the mink, a flea management plan could be included in these routines. In a management plan, the mink farmer can treat the fleas efficiently by simple hygiene measures (removing the straw in the nest boxes) in combination with a repeated chemical control (treating the mink and/or the nest boxes with a flea control product, respectively). In this flea management plan the phoxim spraying should be done at specific times of the year when the animals are moved in traps between the cages anyway. The bendiocarb powdering of the nest box material should then be done when the animals are moved to newly packed nest boxes. Both types of products may be used for flea control when the mated bitches are placed in newly packed nest boxes in mid-April; at the end of June/early July when the kittens are moved to newly packed nest boxes and in the autumn when the animals for breeding are selected and gathered). In early March when the farmer is preparing for the mating the phoxim treatment is the most preferred. It should be

Table 3 Farm specific flea reductions in phoxim treatment group compared to its control and combined effect

	Farm 1	P-value	Farm 2	P-value	Combined	P-value
Reduction	98.8% (96.7%–99.6%)	< 0.0001	97.9% (94.6%–99.2%)	< 0.0001	98.4% (96.8%–99.2%)	< 0.0001

Table 4 Statistics for the bendiocarb treatment group

Farm number	Number of nests		Nests with fleas		Average number of fleas[a]		Average number of fleas in positive nests[a]	
	1	2	1	2	1	2	1	2
Treatment	19	19	2	1	0.3 (0.01–0.7)	0.06 (0.01–0.44)	2.5 (0.8–7.6)	1 (0.1–9.2)
Control	20	19	18	18	14.7 (10.2–20.9)	18.4 (12.8–26.5)	16.3 (12.7–20.8)	19.4 (15.3–24.7)

[a] Assuming a negative binomial distribution

Table 5 Farm specific flea reductions in bendiocarb treatment group compared to its control and combined effect

	Farm 1	P-value	Farm 2	P-value	Combined	P-value
Reduction	98.2% (94.0%–99.5%)	< 0.0001	99.7% (98.2%–99.9%)	< 0.0001	99.0% (97.3%–99.7%)	< 0.0001

noted that the latter two flea control products should not be used at the same animal or nest box and that there is a need for the treatment chosen to be repeated after 1 month.

Conclusions

The treatment of a 0.1% aqueous phoxim dilution sprayed on the animals or with 4 grams of the 1.25% bendiocarb dusted in the next box material was highly efficient in reducing the number of fleas applied to the nesting materials experimentally before treatment. It is suggested that these compounds are implemented in a yearly flea management plan on mink farms.

Authors' contributions

KSL planned and performed the study, was the contact person for the mink farmers and was the major contributor in writing the manuscript. MS assisted the in-field data collection and contributed further to the manuscript. JD did the statistical evaluations of the study. All authors read and approved the final manuscript.

Author details

[1] KSL Innovation ApS, Ramløsevej 25, 3200 Helsinge, Denmark. [2] KSL Consulting ApS, Lejrvej 17, 1, 3500 Værløse, Denmark. [3] Jan Dahl Consult, Østrupvej 89, 4350 Ugerløse, Denmark.

Acknowledgements

The authors thank the mink farmers and their staff for providing the opportunity to work on the farms and their help in handling the mink.

Competing interests

The study was conducted independently of any involvement from the producer of the compounds, Bayer Animal Health, Germany and Bayer A/S, Denmark.

Funding

This study was funded by Bayer Animal Health, Germany and Bayer A/S, Denmark.

References

1. Knorr M, Rasmussen AM, Larsen KS. An interview study regarding pest problems on Danish mink farms. Annual report 2014. Aarhus N: Kopenhagen Fur; 2015. p. 175–82. https://issuu.com/kopenhagenfur/docs/fagli g___rsberetning_2014/129.
2. Larsen KS. Flea and flea control—a questionnaire. Dansk Pelsdyravl. 1992;1:19–20 **(in Danish)**.
3. Larsen KS. Fleas and farmed mink. Norw J Agri Sci. 1992;9:420–5.
4. Larsen KS. A study of the squirrel flea, *Ceratophyllus sciurorum sciurorum*, related to its occurrence on farmed mink. Ph.D. thesis, University of Aarhus; 1995.
5. Lazov CM, Jensen TH, Larsen KS, Hansen MS, Chriél M, Larsen LE, Struve T, Hjulsager CK. Transmission of Aleutian Mink Disease Virus with fleas. Annual report 2015. Aarhus N: Kopenhagen Fur; 2016. p. 91–4. https://issuu.com/kopenhagenfur/docs/faglig___rsberetning_2015_revideret.
6. Larsen KS. Resistance demonstrated in fleas from Danish mink farms. Dansk Pelsdyravl. 2016;4:50. http://ipaper.ipapercms.dk/KopenhagenFur/DanskPelsdyravlApril2016/?page=50 **(in Danish)**.
7. Larsen KS. Why do I have fleas on the farm?. Dansk Pelsdyravl. 2015;5:34–5. http://ipaper.ipapercms.dk/KopenhagenFur/DanskPelsdyravlJuni2015/?page=34 **(in Danish)**.
8. Jones KL, Granger LA, Kearney MT, da Cunha AF, Cutler DC, Shapiro ME, Tully TN, Shiomitsu K. Evaluation of a ferret-specific formula for determining body surface area to improve chemotherapeutic dosing. Am J Vet Res. 2015;76(2):142–8.
9. The Merck Veterinary Manual, weight to body surface area conversion, http://www.merckvetmanual.com/mvm/appendixes/reference_guide s/weight_to_body_surface_area_conversion.html, last full review Oct 2015.
10. Larsen KS, Siggurdsson H, Mencke N. Efficacy of imidacloprid, imidacloprid/permethrin and phoxim for flea control in the Mustelidae (ferret, mink). Parasitol Res. 2005;97(Suppl 1):S107–12. https://doi.org/10.1007/s00436-005-1453-0.
11. Malmkvist J, Hansen SW. Why do farm mink chew? NJF Report No. 116. NJF Seminar No. 280, Helsingfors, Finland; 1997. p. 211–6.
12. Malmkvist J, Sørensen DD, Larsen T, Palme R, Hansen SW. Weaning and separation stress: maternal motivation decreases with litter age and litter size in farmed mink. Appl Anim Beh Sci. 2016;181:152–9.
13. Hinkle NC, Koeler PG, Patterson RS. Host grooming efficacy for relation of cat flea (Siphonaptera: Pulicidae) populations. J Med Entomol. 1998;35:266–9.
14. Eckstein RA, Hart BL. Grooming and control of fleas in cats. Appl Anim Behav Sci. 2000;68:141–50.
15. Larsen KS. Laboratory rearing of the squirrel flea *Ceratophyllus sciurorum sciurorum* with notes on its biology. Ent Exp et Appl. 1995;76:241–5.

24

Changes in the faecal bile acid profile in dogs fed dry food vs high content of beef

Kristin Marie Valand Herstad[1*], Helene Thorsen Rønning[2], Anne Marie Bakke[3], Lars Moe[1] and Ellen Skancke[1]

Abstract

Background: Dogs are fed various diets, which also include components of animal origin. In humans, a high-fat/low-fibre diet is associated with higher faecal levels of bile acids, which can influence intestinal health. It is unknown how an animal-based diet high in fat and low in fibre influences the faecal bile acid levels and intestinal health in dogs. This study investigated the effects of high intake of minced beef on the faecal bile acid profile in healthy, adult, client-owned dogs (n = 8) in a 7-week trial. Dogs were initially adapted to the same commercial dry food. Thereafter, incremental substitution of the dry food by boiled minced beef over 3 weeks resulted in a diet in which 75% of each dog's total energy requirement was provided as minced beef during week 5. Dogs were subsequently reintroduced to the dry food for the last 2 weeks of the study. The total taurine and glycine-conjugated bile acids, the primary bile acids chenodeoxycholic acid and cholic acid, and the secondary bile acids lithocholic acid, deoxycholic acid (DCA) and ursodeoxycholic acid (UDCA) were analysed, using liquid chromatography–tandem mass spectrometry.

Results: The faecal quantities of DCA were significantly higher in dogs fed the high minced beef diet. These levels reversed when dogs were reintroduced to the dry food diet. The faecal levels of UDCA and taurine-conjugated bile acids had also increased in response to the beef diet, but this was only significant when compared to the last dry food period.

Conclusions: These results suggest that an animal-based diet with high-fat/low-fibre content can influence the faecal bile acids levels. The consequences of this for canine colonic health will require further investigation.

Keywords: Commercial dry food, Healthy client-owned dogs, Minced beef, Primary and secondary bile acids

Background

Bile acids (BA) are essential for digestion and absorption of dietary lipids and lipid-soluble vitamins in the small intestine in mammals as well as in other vertebrates [1]. Studies mainly performed in cell-lines from humans and laboratory animals describe that BA also function as signalling molecules by activating receptors in the gall bladder, intestine and accessory digestive organs. These receptors and their ligands are involved in the regulation of lipid and glucose homeostasis [2–4] and they are believed to modulate the immune response in the liver and intestine [5]. However, high levels of some of these BA are toxic for colonic cells [6–8], and their concentrations are therefore tightly regulated [9].

The primary BA, cholic acid (CA) and chenodeoxycholic acid (CDCA) are synthetized from cholesterol and conjugate with either glycine or taurine in the liver. The latter is the most common in dogs [10, 11]. Most conjugated BA (> 95%) are reabsorbed in the ileum [12] and are returned to the liver through the enterohepatic circulation. BA that escape absorption, are deconjugated and converted through 7 alpha-dehydroxylation to secondary BA by colonic bacteria. The secondary BA deoxycholic acid (DCA) and lithocholic acid (LCA) originate from CA and CDCA, respectively [13]. Ursodeoxycholic acid

*Correspondence: kristin.herstad@nmbu.no
[1] Department of Companion Animal Clinical Sciences, Faculty of Veterinary Medicine, Norwegian University of Life Sciences (NMBU), Oslo, Norway

(UDCA) is also produced by bacterial transformation from the primary BA CDCA [14].

Although dogs have adapted to a diet containing considerable amounts of carbohydrates through the domestication process, they were originally carnivores [15, 16]. In humans, a diet consisting of high content of animal derived protein and fat, and low content of carbohydrates, has been associated with increased faecal levels of BA, including DCA [8]. High levels of DCA may contribute to the formation and/or progression of colorectal tumours in humans [17] and mice [7, 18]. In contrast, UDCA is considered to have chemopreventative properties, and may counteract the effect of DCA, as demonstrated in human colon cancer cell lines [19, 20]. Colorectal tumours are rarely diagnosed in dogs [21, 22], yet they are considered more common in dogs than in other animal species [23]. Since similar molecular mechanisms have been described in the colorectal tumorigenesis in humans and dogs [24–26], and as dogs live in similar environments as humans, knowledge regarding how diet influences the faecal BA composition may be valuable for both dogs and humans.

Characterization of the pre- and postprandial serum concentrations of total BA aids in identifying impaired hepatic function and is useful in diagnosing portosystemic shunts (PSS) in dogs [27]. However, the various BA are rarely measured in faeces, and studies characterizing the canine faecal BA profile are sparse [28–30]. Furthermore, little is known about how a meat-based diet influences the levels of these BA.

The aim of this study was therefore to use liquid chromatography–tandem mass spectrometry (LC–MS/MS) to characterize the faecal BA profiles in healthy dogs before, during and after a diet with high content of boiled minced beef (MB).

Methods

The study protocol was reviewed and approved according to the guidelines of the ethics committee at the Faculty of Veterinary Medicine and Biosciences, Norwegian University of Life Sciences (NMBU) (Approval Number: 14/04723-23). All dog-owners gave a written informed consent before participation and were informed that they could leave the study at any time.

Animals, study design and diets

The study population consisted of a heterogeneous population of healthy client owned dogs (n = 11) of both gender and of various breeds and ages. They were included in a 7-week prospective dietary intervention study (Table 1). Three dogs did not complete the study due to loose faeces/diarrhoea (faecal score > 4.5, based on a five-point scale where grade 1 represents hard, dry faeces and grade 5 represents watery diarrhoea) [31]. Thus, eight dogs completed all the diet periods and were included in the present investigation. A detailed description of the study, the dogs and the diets have been described previously [32]. In brief, all the dogs were adapted to a commercial dry food diet for 2 weeks (CD1). Thereafter, each dogs received a mixture of boiled minced beef (MB) and CD diet for 3 weeks, where the MB was gradually increased in weekly increments at the expense of the CD diet. Water was added to the minced beef at a ratio of 3 parts MB:1 part water and simmered for 15 min or until the meat was completely cooked. The meat with any remaining water was mixed with the CD, cooled, and served. The amount of MB given each week was calculated to provide 25 (low minced beef, LMB), 50 (moderate minced beef, MMB) and 75 (high minced beef, HMB) percent of the dog's total energy requirement. Finally, all the dogs were reintroduced to the original CD diet in the last 2 weeks of the study (CD2). The energy requirement for each adult dog was estimated according to information provided by the owner concerning type and amount of diet fed prior to the study and/or the range of 350–500 kJ ME × $BW^{0.75}$ based on activity level, coat quality, body weight and body condition score [33]. The energy content in diets were kept constant for each dog throughout the study period. The calculated content of macronutrients for these diets were as follows: CD: 27.1/100 g dry matter (DM) proteins, 16.3/100 g DM lipids, 48.3/100 g DM nitrogen-free extract (NFE; carbohydrate-containing fraction) and 10.4/100 g DM fibre (non-starch polysaccharides); and HMB: 46.2/100 g DM proteins, 33.1/100 g DM lipids, 15.6/100 g DM NFE, and 3.4/100 g DM fibre. The detailed composition of the diets are found in Additional file 1.

The data presented herein are from faecal samples collected and analysed from each of the dogs during the

Table 1 Demographic overview of the eight client-owned dogs included in a 7-week dietary intervention study

Dog no.[a]	Breed	Gender Female F/ male M	Age (years)	Body weight (kg)
1	English Springer Spaniel	F	8	19.5
3	Small Munsterlander	F	6	21.5
4	Eurasier	F	1.5	17.7
5	Irish Setter	M	4	21.5
6	Mixed breed	M	5	14.7
7	English Setter	M	5	28
10	English Cocker Spaniel	F	8	10.3
11	German Shorthaired Pointer	F	3	19.9

[a] Dog no. 2, 8 and 9 did not complete all the diet periods

last 3 days from diet periods CD1 and HMB, and from the last 2 days from diet period CD2. All faecal samples analysed had normal faecal consistency. Samples were freeze-dried (Christ Alpha 1–4; SciQuip, Shropshire, UK) [34] and subsequently frozen and stored at − 80 °C prior to further processing.

Sample preparation

Liquid chromatography–tandem mass spectrometry (LC–MS/MS) was used to analyse faecal BA. These included CA, CDCA, DCA, LCA, UDCA, and glycine- and taurine conjugated forms of these BA. A detailed overview of the BA are found in Additional file 2. The method for extraction of BA was based on Hagio et al. [35] with the following modifications: A total of 100 µL of 0.1 µg/mL internal standard was added to each freeze-dried faecal sample of 100 mg. Centrifugation of samples were performed at 4 °C. The evaporation steps were performed at room temperature. The methanol extracts were purified with solid phase extraction using an Oasis HLB cartridge (Waters, Milford, MA, USA), following the generic Oasis HLB protocol. The eluates were evaporated to dryness at room temperature under a stream of air and the dry residues were reconstituted in 1 mL methanol/10 mM ammonium acetate (1 + 1). The extracts were filtered through 0.22 µm nylon spin filters (Spin-X, Costar, Corning Inc., Corning, NY, USA) for 3 min at 11,000×*g*. The filtered extracts were transferred to HPLC-vials and subsequently stored at − 20 °C until LC–MS/MS analysis.

Liquid chromatography–tandem mass spectrometry (LC–MS/MS)

The analysis was performed with an Agilent 1290 liquid chromatography system (Agilent Technologies, Waldbronn, Germany) coupled online with an Agilent G6490 triple quadrupole mass spectrometer (Agilent Technologies, Singapore) with a JetStream ESI ion source. The LC–MS/MS method described by Hagio et al. [35] was modified. The separation was done on a Waters Acquity BEH C18 column, 100 mm × 2.1 mm i.d. and 1.7 µm particles, with 10 mM ammonium acetate in water as mobile phase A and acetonitrile as mobile phase B (MPB). The flow rate was 0.4 mL/min and the column temperature 40 °C. The gradient started with 1 min 20% MBP, then went from 20 to 50% MPB in 9 min, then from 50 to 95% MBP in 0.1 min followed by 3 min in 95% MBP. The column was equilibrated in 20% MPB for 3 min before the next injection. Total analysis time was 15 min. The injection volume was 1 µL and the auto sampler temperature 4 °C.

All BA were ionized in negative mode and detected as their (M-H)—ions. The monitored ion transitions and compound specific parameters are given in Additional file 3a. All common MS/MS-parameters are provided in Additional file 3b.

Due to the ubiquitous presence of BA in faeces it was impossible to obtain a truly negative sample material. The method validation was therefore performed by spiking a pooled faecal sample with BA and subtracting the BA levels in the same sample without addition, to evaluate both linearity, precision and limit of detection. The precision study was done by spiking six samples at 100 µg/g. The linearity was evaluated from spiked samples at five levels; 0.1, 0.5, 1, 10 and 50 µg/g. Grade 1 water was used as negative control. The faecal BA concentrations were calculated relative to the spiked samples used to evaluate the precision. Therefore, this method is only semi-quantitative. The faecal BA concentrations are expressed in µg/g DM.

The precision at 100 µg/g was < 13% for all compounds. The limits of detection for all BA was 1 µg/g. Chromatograms of faecal BA from one dog (id 7), are shown in Additional file 4.

Statistical methods

Data were tested for normality using the Shapiro–Wilk normality. Non-parametric Wilcoxon signed-rank test was used to calculate statistical differences between the various BA between the diet periods (CD1 vs HMB and CD2 vs HMB) without correction for multiple comparison. The software Graph Pad, PRISM v.7 (CA, USA) was used. A two-dimensional Principal component analysis (PCA) plot was generated using PRIMER7 [36]. A P value below 0.05 was considered statistically significant.

Results

The secondary BA, DCA were significantly higher in the HMB samples compared with the levels in both CD1 and CD2 samples ($P = 0.05$ and 0.04, respectively). Higher quantities of UDCA were detected in the HMB samples compared with that of CD2 samples ($P = 0.02$), but this was not significant when compared to CD1 samples ($P > 0.1$, Fig. 1). Although the median values for the primary BA, CA and CDCA were higher in HMB samples, the differences were not statistically significant ($P > 0.1$, Fig. 1). However, the levels of taurine-conjugated BA were significantly higher in the HMB samples compared with the CD2 samples ($P = 0.02$), but not compared with CD1 samples ($P > 0.5$). Concentrations of glycine-conjugated BA were measured, but were below quantification limit in all dogs (Table 2).

As evaluated by a PCA plot, the majority of HMB samples are displayed along the first axis (PC1) and the

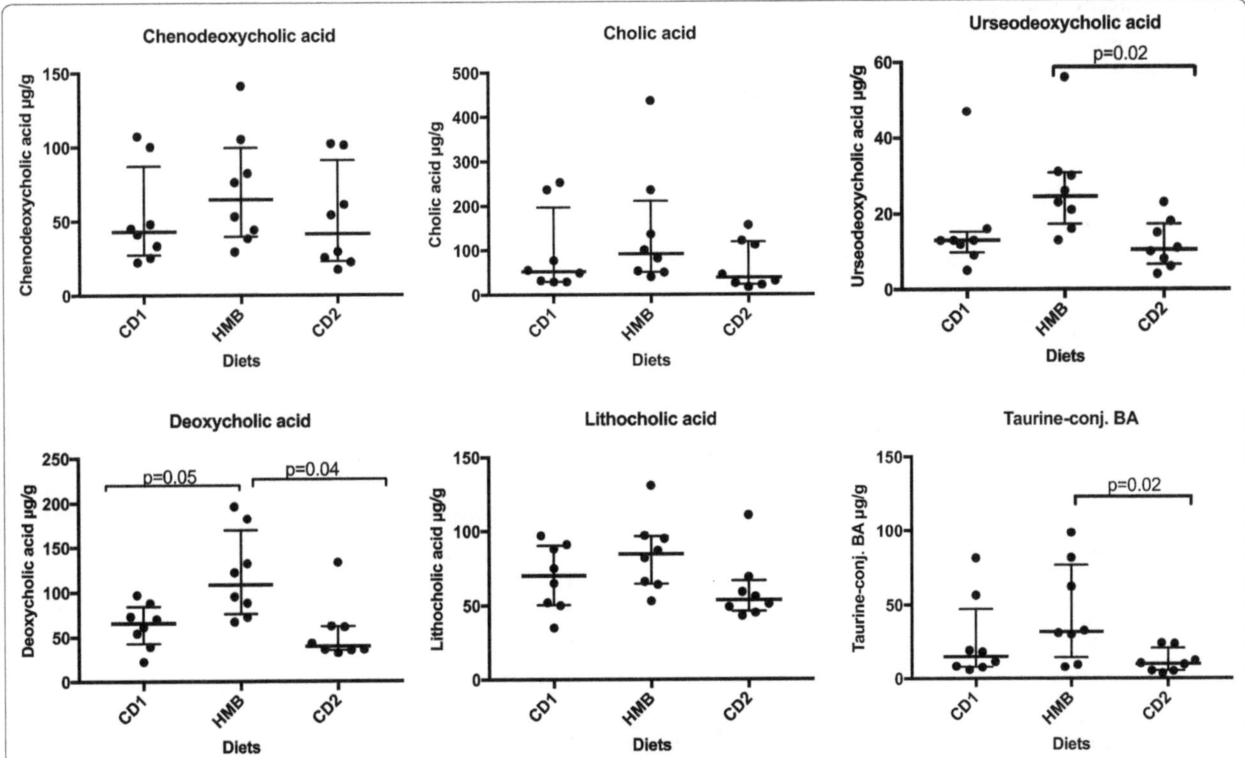

Fig. 1 Median concentrations with interquartile ranges of bile acids (BA) (µg/g faeces) in samples of eight dogs fed commercial dry food at the start and end of the study (CD1 and CD2) and high minced beef (HMB). Significant differences of faecal BA in diet periods CD1 vs HMB and CD2 vs HMB are indicated (Wilcoxon signed-rank test without correction for multiple comparison). *CD1* Commercial dry food given the first 2 weeks of the study, *CD2* commercial dry food given the last 2 weeks of the study, *HMB* high minced beef, *CA* cholic acid, *CDCA* chenodeoxycholic acid, *DCA* deoxycholic acid, *LCA* litocholic, *UDCA* ursodeoxycholic acid, Taurine-conj. BA (taurine-conjugated CA, CDCA, DCA, and LCA)

vectors (bile acids), particularly LCA, DCA and UDCA, are directed towards the HMB samples (Fig. 2).

The variability in breed, age and body size between both genders of dogs made it impossible to perform any statistical testing for any possible impact of these factors on the faecal BA composition.

Discussion

A diet shift from commercial dry food (CD) to high minced beef (HMB) and vice versa, during a 7-week dietary intervention study influenced faecal BA profiles in healthy client-owned dogs. Specifically, the secondary BA, DCA and UDCA increased in the HMB samples compared with the CD1 and/or CD2 samples, likely due to the presence of colonic bacteria with 7 alpha-dehydroxylating capabilities that transform primary BA to secondary BA. It is known that members within *Clostridium* and *Eubacterium* have this capability [13, 37]. We have previously reported, using the same study population, significantly higher relative abundances of an OTU in the family *Clostridiaceae* in the HMB samples [32]. This bacterial taxa was classified within a BLAST search to be *Clostridia hiranonis* with 97% identity. Interestingly, this species is capable of converting CA and CDCA into DCA and LCA, respectively [38]. Thus, the increased presence of this taxa may explain the higher faecal quantity of DCA in dogs fed HMB. The concomitant rise in the quantity of UDCA, rather than LCA, may indicate the possibility that increased bacterial transformation of CDCA to UDCA [14] is more likely to occur than bacterial transformation of CDCA to LCA in dogs. Moreover, the bacterial 7 beta-dehydroxylation of UDCA yield LCA [13, 39], but the low quantity of LCA may suggest that this process is not dominant in the intestine of dogs. However, since we used a semi-quantitative approach, these results needs to be validated in studies where the exact faecal quantities of BA are measured.

The apparent lack of glycine-conjugated BA in the faeces, yet detectable levels of taurine-conjugated BA, confirm that dogs primarily conjugate their bile acids with taurine rather than glycine [40–42]. Furthermore, the significantly higher taurine-conjugated BA levels measured in the faeces collected during the HMB period compared to the CD2 period suggest that the high lipid levels of the HMB diet can induce greater primary BA secretion. However, observed levels of primary BA, CA and

Table 2 Concentrations of faecal bile acids (µg/g)

Dog_id[a]	Diet	CA	CDCA	DCA	LCA	UDCA	G-DCA	G-LCA	T-CA	T-CDCA	T-DCA	T-LCA
1	CD1	32	41	54	52	13	1	1	3	1	1	0
	HMB	40	53	67	53	21	0	2	5	1	1	0
	CD2	112	61	36	43	8	4	2	2	1	1	0
3	CD1	55	45	73	65	16	2	1	5	2	2	0
	HMB	437	105	182	95	56	4	1	28	1	52	1
	CD2	122	102	62	59	23	0	2	4	1	1	0
4	CD1	49	48	97	97	13	5	1	19	7	41	14
	HMB	50	29	72	66	13	0	1	31	4	22	5
	CD2	26	25	43	56	11	0	1	11	2	7	4
5	CD1	29	25	61	75	12	2	1	5	2	8	3
	HMB	53	38	95	82	26	4	2	7	1	17	5
	CD2	22	22	36	49	10	2	1	1	0	2	1
6	CD1	29	22	39	50	9	2	1	2	1	5	3
	HMB	137	76	132	97	30	7	3	10	1	16	4
	CD2	17	17	32	45	6	6	2	2	1	5	2
7	CD1	77	33	22	35	5	8	1	2	1	3	2
	HMB	236	82	196	131	31	10	3	21	3	66	9
	CD2	31	29	35	51	4	5	2	3	1	4	2
10	CD1	253	107	88	88	13	8	2	8	2	7	2
	HMB	82	44	88	64	16	11	3	2	1	5	1
	CD2	157	101	133	111	18	18	3	7	2	11	4
11	CD1	237	100	70	91	47	0	1	29	7	15	6
	HMB	101	141	122	87	23	3	2	11	1	17	3
	CD2	45	54	61	69	15	5	2	3	1	6	2

The concentrations were determined semiquantitatively

CA cholic acid, *CDCA* chenodeoxycholic acid, *DCA* deoxycholic acid, *LCA* litocholic, *UDCA* ursodeoxycholic acid, glycine-conjugated DCA (G-DCA) and LCA (G-LCA), taurine-conjugated CA (T-CA), CDCA (T-CDCA), DCA (T-DCA), and LCA (T-LCA))

[a] Detailed demographics of these dogs are given in Table 1

CDCA were variable between dogs and not significantly increased in response to the HMB diet. The variable response between dogs in this study may be explained by differing BA metabolism, intestinal peristalsis, intestinal pH and/or gastrointestinal absorption of BA, as well as differences in the intestinal microbiota composition, which may result in different levels of secondary bile acid in response to diet in these individuals [1, 43].

The hydrophobicity of the BA influences their cytotoxic potential, ranking UDCA as the most hydrophilic and LCA as the most hydrophobic (BA hydrophobicity scale: UDCA < CA < CDCA < DCA < LCA) [44]. DCA has been shown to induce oxidative damage of DNA in vitro, which may result in abnormal cell proliferation of mutagenic, apoptosis-resistant cells [17, 45–47]. In contrast to the possible cytotoxic effects of DCA and LCA on colonic cells, UDCA is believed to have chemoprotective potential [19, 48]. A previous study of ten laboratory dogs described that oral treatment with UDCA resulted in lower ratio of secondary to primary BA [10]. Interestingly, the quantity of faecal UDCA in humans appear to be low in general [49], in contrast to the levels in dogs observed in this study. Whether dogs generally are adapted to having an intestinal microbiota that transform higher quantities of primary BA to UDCA compared to humans, also in response to a high-fat intake, merits further investigations.

In contrast to dietary fat, plant-fibre is thought to protect against colorectal cancer development in humans. Dietary fibres are fermented to short chain fatty acids (SCFA), which purportedly have anti-inflammatory and anti-carcinogenic properties [50]. One mode of action suggested is that the production of SCFA by bacterial fermentation of non-digestible carbohydrates reduces luminal pH and bacterial 7 alpha-dehydroxylase activity, and hence conversion of primary to the secondary BA, DCA and LCA is inhibited [51]. Fibres also bind to BA and thus facilitate their excretion [52]. Moreover, antioxidants in plants, such as beta-carotene and alpha-tocopherol may inhibit the detrimental effects of DCA on colonic cells [47]. In dogs, animal-fibres, such as collagen, has been suggested to have the same properties as plant-fibre [53],

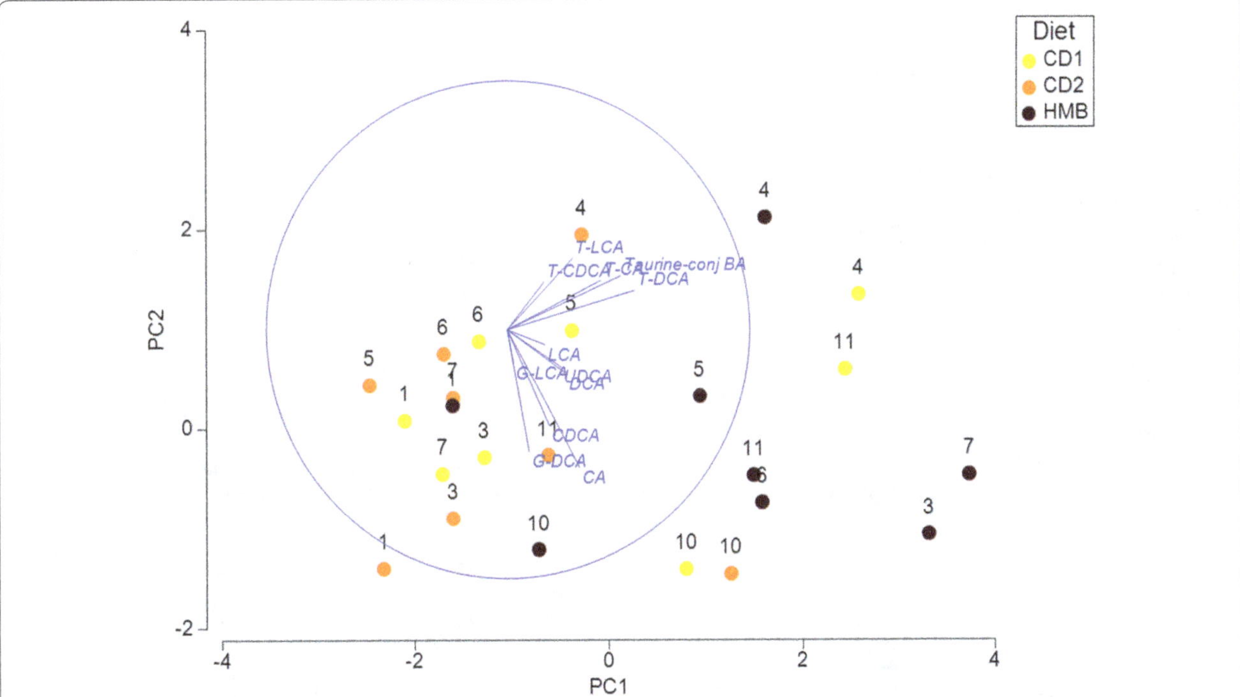

Fig. 2 A Principal component analysis (PCA) plot showing the relationship between samples. The data are displayed across the two main principal components (PC1 and PC2). Each point represents one sample and each colour represents diet period. Closer clustering between points indicate higher relative commonality with respect to bile acid composition in those samples. Concomitantly, larger distances between points indicate lower relative commonality of bile acid composition in those samples. The first axis, PC1 accounted for 55% of the variability and PC2 accounted for 20% of the variability. The directions of the vectors (blue lines) corresponding to BA, particularly LCA, UDCA and DCA are directed towards the HMB samples. *CD1* Commercial dry food given the first 2 weeks of the study, yellow points; *CD2* commercial dry food given the last 2 weeks of the study, orange points, *HMB* high minced beef, black points, *CA* cholic acid, *CDCA* chenodeoxycholic acid, *DCA* deoxycholic acid, *LCA* litocholic, *UDCA* ursodeoxycholic acid, Taurine-conj. BA (taurine-conjugated CA, CDCA, DCA, and LCA)

and thereby limit any potential toxic effects from secondary BA.

In humans, a diet with high content of protein and fat and low content of fibre, is associated with a higher risk of colorectal cancer [8, 54, 55]. Moreover, elevated serum and faecal levels of DCA have been observed in humans with colorectal adenoma and carcinoma compared with healthy controls [56, 57]. Dogs are fed various diets, which also include more animal-based diets preferred by some pet owners [58, 59]. Yet dogs rarely develop colorectal cancer [21, 60]. Given dogs' carnivorous origins, it may not be surprising to find metabolic differences between humans and dogs that can explain differences in the risks of developing chronic intestinal, associated digestive organ and systemic diseases. For instance, dogs' lipoprotein transportation of fat differs from that of humans [61], which may be the reason why atherosclerosis is not a major issue in dogs. Future studies should evaluate the faecal levels of BA, and particularly DCA and UDCA in dogs with colorectal cancer, non-tumour related colonic diseases, as well as healthy controls to gain an understanding of BA involvement in intestinal health in dogs.

The main limitation of this study was the small and heterogeneous sample size. Factors such as age, breed, body size/weight, gender, as well as previously fed diets may have influenced the faecal bile acid composition in our dogs. Previous studies have found that these aforementioned factors may influence the intestinal microbiota composition [62–65]. Whether the metabolites produced by the microbiota, including bile acids, also are influenced by these factors needs to be determined in future, adequately powered studies. Moreover, the influence of the individual dietary components, such as fat, starch, proteins, micronutrients, fibre, collagen etc., on the outcome was not tested. Although the discussion primarily focused on the influence of dietary fat, the presence and/or absence of other diet components most likely also influenced the faecal bile acid composition.

Conclusions

A diet shift from commercial dry food to one of high beef content and vice versa, resulted in changes in the faecal BA profiles of healthy client-owned dogs. A high-fat/low-fibre diet in humans results in accumulation of secondary BA in the colon, particularly DCA, which has cytotoxic effects on colonic cells. Interestingly, our results in dogs revealed that the increase in DCA was accompanied by an increase in UDCA, the latter believed to have a chemoprotective mode of action. Since dogs have evolved from carnivorous wolves, and therefore presumed tolerant of high protein, high fat diets, they may have a different metabolism of BA, or have protective mechanisms against potential harmful effects induced by secondary BA, in order to maintain colonic health. Further studies are needed to more specifically evaluate the role of BA in colonic diseases of dogs.

Abbreviations

BA: bile acids; CA: cholic acid; CD: commercial dry food; CDCA: chenodeoxycholic acid; DCA: deoxycholic acid; DM: dry matter; HMB: high minced beef; LC–MS/MS: liquid chromatography–tandem mass spectrometry; LMB: low minced beef; MB: minced beef; MMB: moderate minced beef; MPB: mobile phase B; NFE: nitrogen-free extract; OTU: operational taxonomic unit; PCA: principal component analysis; SCFA: short chain fatty acid; UDCA: ursodeoxycholic acid.

Authors' contributions

KH, ES and LM designed the study. KH performed sample collection. AMB calculated the rations for the different diet periods. KH performed laboratory work. HTR conducted the LC–MS/MS-analysis. KH performed the statistical analysis. KH wrote the manuscript, with contributions from all authors during manuscript preparation. All authors read and approved the final manuscript.

Author details

[1] Department of Companion Animal Clinical Sciences, Faculty of Veterinary Medicine, Norwegian University of Life Sciences (NMBU), Oslo, Norway. [2] Matriks AS, Forskningsparken, Gaustadallèen 21, 0349 Oslo, Norway. [3] Department of Basic Sciences and Aquatic Medicine, Faculty of Veterinary Medicine, Norwegian University of Life Sciences (NBMU), Oslo, Norway.

Acknowledgements

The authors thank Christina Steppeler for her excellent help with the preparation of samples used for the analysis of BAs and Professor Eystein Skjerve for valuable comments during the statistical analysis. We would also like to express our gratitude to the dog-owners and dogs participating in this study.

Competing interests

The authors declare that they have no competing interests.

Funding

The Felleskjøpet and the Astri and Birger Torsted Foundation provided financial support.

References

1. Hofmann AF, Hagey LR, Krasowski MD. Bile salts of vertebrates: structural variation and possible evolutionary significance. J Lipid Res. 2010;512:226–46.
2. Fiorucci S, Distrutti E. Bile acid-activated receptors, intestinal microbiota, and the treatment of metabolic disorders. Trends Mol Med. 2015;2111:702–14.
3. Makishima M, Okamoto AY, Repa JJ, Tu H, Learned RM, Luk A, et al. Identification of a nuclear receptor for bile acids. Science. 1999;2845418:1362–5.
4. Nguyen A, Bouscarel B. Bile acids and signal transduction: role in glucose homeostasis. Cell Signal. 2008;2012:2180–97.
5. Fiorucci S, Cipriani S, Mencarelli A, Renga B, Distrutti E, Baldelli F. Counter-regulatory role of bile acid activated receptors in immunity and inflammation. Curr Mol Med. 2010;106:579–95.
6. Bernstein H, Bernstein C, Payne CM, Dvorakova K, Garewal H. Bile acids as carcinogens in human gastrointestinal cancers. Mutat Res. 2005;5891:47–65.
7. Bernstein C, Holubec H, Bhattacharyya AK, Nguyen H, Payne CM, Zaitlin B, et al. Carcinogenicity of deoxycholate, a secondary bile acid. Arch Toxicol. 2011;858:863–71.
8. O'Keefe SJ, Li JV, Lahti L, Ou J, Carbonero F, Mohammed K, et al. Fat, fibre and cancer risk in African Americans and rural Africans. Nat Commun. 2015;6:6342.
9. Kim I, Ahn SH, Inagaki T, Choi M, Ito S, Guo GL, et al. Differential regulation of bile acid homeostasis by the farnesoid X receptor in liver and intestine. J Lipid Res. 2007;4812:2664–72.
10. Imamura M, Nakajima H, Takahashi H, Yamauchi H, Seo G. Bile acid metabolism, bacterial bowel flora and intestinal function following ileal pouch-anal anastomosis in dogs, with reference to the influence of administration of ursodeoxycholic acid. Tohoku J Exp Med. 2000;1902:103–17.
11. Zhang J, He K, Cai L, Chen YC, Yang Y, Shi Q, et al. Inhibition of bile salt transport by drugs associated with liver injury in primary hepatocytes from human, monkey, dog, rat, and mouse. Chem Biol Interact. 2016;255:45–54.
12. Borgstrom B, Lundh G, Hofmann A. The site of absorption of conjugated bile salts in man. Gastroenterology. 1968;544(Suppl):781–3.
13. Ridlon JM, Kang DJ, Hylemon PB. Bile salt biotransformations by human intestinal bacteria. J Lipid Res. 2006;472:241–59.
14. Hirano S, Masuda N, Oda H. In vitro transformation of chenodeoxycholic acid and ursodeoxycholic acid by human intestinal flora, with particular reference to the mutual conversion between the two bile acids. J Lipid Res. 1981;225:735–43.
15. Axelsson E, Ratnakumar A, Arendt ML, Maqbool K, Webster MT, Perloski M, et al. The genomic signature of dog domestication reveals adaptation to a starch-rich diet. Nature. 2013;4957441:360–4.
16. Dressman JB. Comparison of canine and human gastrointestinal physiology. Pharm Res. 1986;33:123–31.
17. Bernstein C, Bernstein H, Garewal H, Dinning P, Jabi R, Sampliner RE, et al. A bile acid-induced apoptosis assay for colon cancer risk and associated quality control studies. Cancer Res. 1999;5910:2353–7.
18. Cao H, Luo S, Xu M, Zhang Y, Song S, Wang S, et al. The secondary bile acid, deoxycholate accelerates intestinal adenoma-adenocarcinoma sequence in Apc (min/+) mice through enhancing Wnt signaling. Fam Cancer. 2014;134:563–71.
19. Akare S, Jean-Louis S, Chen W, Wood DJ, Powell AA, Martinez JD. Ursodeoxycholic acid modulates histone acetylation and induces differentiation and senescence. Int J Cancer. 2006;11912:2958–69.
20. Im E, Martinez JD. Ursodeoxycholic acid (UDCA) can inhibit deoxycholic acid (DCA)-induced apoptosis via modulation of EGFR/Raf-1/ERK signaling in human colon cancer cells. J Nutr. 2004;1342:483–6.
21. Schäffer E. Incidence and types of canine rectal carcinomas. J Small Anim Pract. 1968;9:491–6.
22. Valerius KD, Powers BE, McPherron MA, Hutchison JM, Mann FA, Withrow SJ. Adenomatous polyps and carcinoma in situ of the canine colon and rectum: 34 cases (1982–1994). J Am Anim Hosp Assoc. 1997;33:156–60.
23. Lingeman CH, Garner FM. Comparative study of intestinal adenocarcinomas of animals and man. J Natl Cancer Inst. 1972;482:325–46.

24. Tang J, Le S, Sun L, Yan X, Zhang M, Macleod J, et al. Copy number abnormalities in sporadic canine colorectal cancers. Genome Res. 2010;203:341–50.
25. Tang J, Li Y, Lyon K, Camps J, Dalton S, Ried T, et al. Cancer driver-passenger distinction via sporadic human and dog cancer comparison: a proof-of-principle study with colorectal cancer. Oncogene. 2014;337:814–22.
26. Youmans L, Taylor C, Shin E, Harrell A, Ellis AE, Seguin B, et al. Frequent alteration of the tumor suppressor gene APC in sporadic canine colorectal tumors. PLoS ONE. 2012. https://doi.org/10.1371/journal.pone.0050813.
27. Gerritzen-Bruning MJ, van den Ingh TS, Rothuizen J. Diagnostic value of fasting plasma ammonia and bile acid concentrations in the identification of portosystemic shunting in dogs. J Vet Intern Med. 2006;201:13–9.
28. Blake AB, Guard BC, Honneffer JB, Kumro FG, Kennedy OC, Lidbury JA, et al. Dogs with exocrine pancreatic insufficiency have dysbiosis and abnormal fecal lactate and bile acid concentrations. American College of Veterinary Internal Medicine (ACVIM) abstracts; Maryland, USA, 2017. J Vet Intern Med. 2017;31:1286.
29. Guard BC, Alexander C, Honneffer JB, Lidbury JA, Steiner JM, Swanson KS, et al. Effect of the bile acid sequestrand cholestyramine on fecal bile acid concentrations in healthy dogs. American College of Veterinary Internal Medicine (ACVIM) abstracts; Maryland, USA, 2017. J Vet Intern Med. 2017;31:1280.
30. Guard BC, Jonika MM, Honneffer JB, Lidbury JA, Steiner JM, Suchodolski JS. Development and analytical validation of an assay for the quantification of canine fecal bile acids. American College of Veterinary Internal Medicine (ACVIM) abstracts; Maryland, USA, 2017. J Vet Intern Med. 2017;31:1289.
31. Moxham G. Waltham feces scoring system- A tool for veterinarians and pet owners. How does your pet rate? Waltham®Focus. 2001;112:24–45.
32. Herstad KMV, Gajardo K, Bakke AM, Moe L, Ludvigsen J, Rudi K, et al. A diet change from dry food to beef induces reversible changes on the faecal microbiota in healthy, adult client-owned dogs. BMC Vet Res. 2017;131:147.
33. Thes M, Koeber N, Fritz J, Wendel F, Dillitzer N, Dobenecker B, et al. Metabolizable energy intake of client-owned adult dogs. J Anim Physiol Anim Nutr (Berl). 2016;1005:813–9.
34. Hartviksen M, Bakke AM, Vecino JG, Ringo E, Krogdahl A. Evaluation of the effect of commercially available plant and animal protein sources in diets for Atlantic salmon (*Salmo salar* L.): digestive and metabolic investigations. Fish Physiol Biochem. 2014;40:1621–37.
35. Hagio M, Matsumoto M, Fukushima M, Hara H, Ishizuka S. Improved analysis of bile acids in tissues and intestinal contents of rats using LC/ESI-MS. J Lipid Res. 2009;501:173–80.
36. Clarke KR, Gorley RN. PRIMER v7: user manual/tutorial. Plymouth: PRIMER-E; 2015. p. 296.
37. Doerner KC, Takamine F, LaVoie CP, Mallonee DH, Hylemon PB. Assessment of fecal bacteria with bile acid 7 alpha-dehydroxylating activity for the presence of bai-like genes. Appl Environ Microbiol. 1997;633:1185–8.
38. Kitahara M, Takamine F, Imamura T, Benno Y. *Clostridium hiranonis* sp. nov., a human intestinal bacterium with bile acid 7alpha-dehydroxylating activity. Int J Syst Evol Microbiol. 2001;51:39–44.
39. Ridlon JM, Harris SC, Bhowmik S, Kang DJ, Hylemon PB. Consequences of bile salt biotransformations by intestinal bacteria. Gut Microbes. 2016;71:22–39.
40. Nakayama F. Composition of gallstone and bile: species difference. J Lab Clin Med. 1969;734:623–30.
41. Wildgrube HJ, Stockhausen H, Petri J, Fussel U, Lauer H. Naturally occurring conjugated bile acids, measured by high-performance liquid chromatography, in human, dog, and rabbit bile. J Chromatogr. 1986;353:207–13.
42. Washizu T, Ikenaga H, Washizu M, Ishida T, Tomoda I, Kaneko JJ. Bile acid composition of dog and cat gall-bladder bile. Nihon Juigaku Zasshi. 1990;522:423–5.
43. Jones BV, Begley M, Hill C, Gahan CG, Marchesi JR. Functional and comparative metagenomic analysis of bile salt hydrolase activity in the human gut microbiome. Proc Natl Acad Sci USA. 2008;10536:13580–5.
44. Hofmann AF. Bile acids: the good, the bad, and the ugly. News Physiol Sci. 1999;14:24–9.
45. Booth LA, Gilmore IT, Bilton RF. Secondary bile acid induced DNA damage in HT29 cells: are free radicals involved? Free Radic Res. 1997;262:135–44.
46. Glinghammar B, Inoue H, Rafter JJ. Deoxycholic acid causes DNA damage in colonic cells with subsequent induction of caspases, COX-2 promoter activity and the transcription factors NF-kB and AP-1. Carcinogenesis. 2002;235:839–45.
47. Rosignoli P, Fabiani R, De Bartolomeo A, Fuccelli R, Pelli MA, Morozzi G. Genotoxic effect of bile acids on human normal and tumour colon cells and protection by dietary antioxidants and butyrate. Eur J Nutr. 2008;476:301–9.
48. Alberts DS, Martinez ME, Hess LM, Einspahr JG, Green SB, Bhattacharyya AK, et al. Phase III trial of ursodeoxycholic acid to prevent colorectal adenoma recurrence. J Natl Cancer Inst. 2005;9711:846–53.
49. Kakiyama G, Muto A, Takei H, Nittono H, Murai T, Kurosawa T, et al. A simple and accurate HPLC method for fecal bile acid profile in healthy and cirrhotic subjects: validation by GC–MS and LC–MS. J Lipid Res. 2014;555:978–90.
50. Macfarlane GT, Macfarlane S. Bacteria, colonic fermentation, and gastrointestinal health. J AOAC Int. 2012;951:50–60.
51. Bingham SA. Diet and colorectal cancer prevention. Biochem Soc Trans. 2000;282:12–6.
52. Kritchevsky D. Influence of dietary fiber on bile acid metabolism. Lipids. 1978;1312:982–5.
53. Depauw S, Hesta M, Whitehouse-Tedd K, Vanhaecke L, Verbrugghe A, Janssens GP. Animal fibre: the forgotten nutrient in strict carnivores? First insights in the cheetah. J Anim Physiol Anim Nutr (Berl). 2011;971:146–54.
54. Cross AJ, Ferrucci LM, Risch A, Graubard BI, Ward MH, Park Y, et al. A large prospective study of meat consumption and colorectal cancer risk: an investigation of potential mechanisms underlying this association. Cancer Res. 2010;706:2406–14.
55. Russell WR, Gratz SW, Duncan SH, Holtrop G, Ince J, Scobbie L, et al. High-protein, reduced-carbohydrate weight-loss diets promote metabolite profiles likely to be detrimental to colonic health. Am J Clin Nutr. 2011;935:1062–72.
56. Reddy BS, Wynder EL. Metabolic epidemiology of colon cancer. Fecal bile acids and neutral sterols in colon cancer patients and patients with adenomatous polyps. Cancer. 1977;396:2533–9.
57. Bayerdorffer E, Mannes GA, Ochsenkuhn T, Dirschedl P, Wiebecke B, Paumgartner G. Unconjugated secondary bile acids in the serum of patients with colorectal adenomas. Gut. 1995;362:268–73.
58. Freeman LM, Michel KE. Evaluation of raw food diets for dogs. J Am Vet Med Assoc. 2001;2185:705–9.
59. Laflamme DP, Abood SK, Fascetti AJ, Fleeman LM, Freeman LM, Michel KE, et al. Pet feeding practices of dog and cat owners in the United States and Australia. J Am Vet Med Assoc. 2008;2325:687–94.
60. Van der Gaag I. The histological appearance of large intestinal biopsies in dogs with clinical signs of large bowel disease. Can J Vet Res. 1988;521:75–82.
61. Bauer JE. Lipoprotein-mediated transport of dietary and synthesized lipids and lipid abnormalities of dogs and cats. J Am Vet Med Assoc. 2004;2245:668–75.
62. Benno Y, Nakao H, Uchida K, Mitsuoka T. Impact of the advances in age on the gastrointestinal microflora of beagle dogs. J Vet Med Sci. 1992;544:703–6.
63. Kim J, An JU, Kim W, Lee S, Cho S. Differences in the gut microbiota of dogs (*Canis lupus* familiaris) fed a natural diet or a commercial feed revealed by the Illumina MiSeq platform. Gut Pathog. 2017;9:68.
64. Li Q, Lauber CL, Czarnecki-Maulden G, Pan Y, Hannah SS. Effects of the dietary protein and carbohydrate ratio on gut microbiomes in dogs of different body conditions. MBio. 2017;8(1):e01703–16. https://doi.org/10.1128/mBio.01703-16.
65. Simpson JM, Martineau B, Jones WE, Ballam JM, Mackie RI. Characterization of fecal bacterial populations in canines: effects of age, breed and dietary fiber. Microb Ecol. 2002;442:186–97.

Measurement of single kidney glomerular filtration rate in dogs using dynamic contrast-enhanced magnetic resonance imaging and the Rutland-Patlak plot technique

Jan-Niklas Mehl[1*], Matthias Lüpke[1], Ann-Cathrin Brenner[1], Peter Dziallas[2], Patrick Wefstaedt[2] and Hermann Seifert[1]

Abstract

Background: Nephropathies are among the most common diseases in dogs. Regular examination of the kidney function plays an important role for an adequate treatment scheme. The determination of the glomerular filtration rate (GFR) is seen as the gold standard in assessing the kidney status. Most of the tests have the disadvantage that only the complete glomerular filtration rate of both kidneys can be assessed and not the single kidney glomerular filtration rate. Imaging examination techniques like dynamic contrast-enhanced magnetic resonance imaging have the potential to evaluate the single kidney GFR. There are studies in human medicine describing the determination of the single kidney GFR using this technique. To our knowledge there are no such studies for dogs.

Results: An exponential fit was found to describe the functional interrelation between signal intensity and contrast medium concentrations. The changes of contrast medium concentrations during the contrast medium bolus propagation were calculated. The extreme values of contrast medium concentrations in the kidneys were reached at nearly the same time in every individual dog (1st maximum aorta 8.5 s, 1st maximum in both kidneys after about 14.5 s; maximum concentration values varied between 17 and 125 µmol/mL in the aorta and between 4 and 15 µmol/mL in the kidneys). The glomerular filtration rate was calculated from the concentration changes of the contrast medium using a modified Rutland-Patlak plot technique. The GFR was 12.7 ± 2.9 mL/min m^2 BS for the left kidney and 12.0 ± 2.2 mL/min/m^2 BS for the right kidney. The mean values of the coefficient of determination of the regression lines were averagely 0.91 ± 0.08.

Conclusions: The propagation of contrast medium bolus could be depicted well. The contrast medium proceeded in a similar manner for every individual dog. Additionally, the evaluation of the single kidney function of the individual dogs is possible with this method. A standardized examination procedure would be recommended in order to minimize influencing parameters.

Keywords: Dog, Dynamic contrast-enhance MRI, Glomerular filtration rate, Kidney, Renal function, Rutland-Patlak plot

*Correspondence: jan.mehl@gmx.de
[1] Institute for General Radiology and Medical Physics, University of Veterinary Medicine Hannover, Foundation, Bischofsholer Damm 15, 30173 Hannover, Germany
Full list of author information is available at the end of the article

Background

In companion animal medicine, the importance of canine nephropathies should not be underestimated. The prevalence of chronic kidney disease (CKD) have been assessed to be up to 3.74% [1–4]. The progressive course of this disease requires a changing treatment scheme. Therefore, periodic control examinations are recommended for an adequate treatment [5]. Endogenous creatinine and blood urea nitrogen are used most frequently in clinical practise for evaluating the renal function but these are neither sensitive enough to reveal subclinical or border-line renal failure [6, 7], nor are they suitable for evaluating single kidney function [8, 9]. The measurement of the glomerular filtration rate (GFR) is classified as being the best single test for assessing kidney function [10]. Despite this, this tool is seldom used in veterinary medicine because of its high cost and effort [6]. It might also be a useful screening method for early monitoring the kidney function of dog breeds that are predisposed for nephropathies [6].

Inulin-clearance is reputed to be the gold standard for GFR measurement. However, this examination can only be performed under elaborate clinical conditions [11]. Creatinine [6, 7, 12, 13] and Gadolinium-1,4,7,10-tetraazacyclododecane-1,4,7,10-tetraacetic acid (Gd-DOTA) [8, 14] are seen as eligible markers for measuring GFR in humans and rats.

As stated in numerous studies in human medicine, functional magnetic resonance imaging (fMRI) is used to assess the GFR. The main advantage is the absence of ionising radiation. This fact should not be underestimated regarding repeated evaluations of the kidney status.

Nevertheless, MRI devices are still not widely distributed in veterinary clinics and high costs for this kind of examination have to be mentioned [15]. Additionally, limitations of renal fMRI examinations contribute to the lack of agreement on the quantification of the concentration of the contrast medium depending on signal intensity (SI) as well as a standardised protocol for the examination and analysis [16].

There is no consensus on a suitable model for the calculation of GFR either [17, 18]. Previous studies introduced or developed different models for GFR measurements including various amounts of compartments [18–23]. GFR was calculated in our study using a modified Rutland-Patlak plot (RPP) model. The model was used the first time by Hackstein et al. [19] to determine the GFR via fMRI measurements and describes a graphical solution of a simplified two-compartment model [19]. The main advantage of this model is its simplicity because it is just a two-compartment model and no other physiological parameters are needed for calculating the GFR [21].

The fMRI-data were analysed to answer the following questions: (1) Is it possible to evaluate the single-kidney functions in dogs using fMRI-bolus-tracking? and (2) How much influence do different evaluation parameters have on the calculation of the modified RPP?

Methods

Dogs

Eight healthy Beagle dogs (four males and four females) were included. They were kept as experimental animals at the Clinic for Small Animals at the University of Veterinary Medicine Hannover, Foundation, Germany. All procedures were approved by the animal welfare officer of the University of Veterinary Medicine Hannover, Foundation and the Lower Saxony State Office for Consumer Protection and Food Safety, Oldenburg, Germany (TV-No. 33.9-42502-04-08/1600).

The age of the dogs ranged from 4 to 11 years with a mean age of 8.5 years and a standard deviation of 2.9 years. The body weight (BW) of the dogs ranged from 14 kg to 22 kg with a mean BW of 17.5 kg and a standard deviation of 2.7 kg.

GFR measurement by the clearance of exogenously administered creatinine

To evaluate the kidneys' health status, the dogs' GFR was measured by determining the modified plasma-clearance of exogenously administered creatinine according to a test that has been evaluated previously [24, 25].

This method is accepted as a simple and accurate method [6, 24, 25] that can be reliably performed in clinical daily routine without special elaborate examination methods [7, 12, 13].

An exact calculated amount of 5% creatinine solution (LABOKLIN GmbH & Co.KG, 97688 Bad Kissingen, Germany) depending on the body surface (BS) of the dog was injected subcutaneously in every dog (2 g creatinine/m^2 BS). BS was calculated with the help of the BW.

$$BS[\mathrm{m}^2] = 0.1 \cdot BW\,[\mathrm{kg}]^{0.667}$$

According to the test specifications four blood samples were taken per dog. They were sent to an external laboratory (LABOKLIN GmbH & Co.KG) and analysed there.

Serial dilution

For analysing the fMRI measurements in vivo a functional correlation between SI and concentration of contrast medium had to be established. Therefore, a serial dilution of the contrast medium was made. 25 test tubes were filled with 0.9% NaCl and the contrast medium in concentrations from 0 to 80 mmol/L. All tubes were put into a water quench which was heated up to 38 °C and examined in MRI with the same settings as the fMRI measurements for the dogs (see Table 1—bolus track).

All MRI examinations were performed with a Philips Achieva 3 Tesla scanner.

Due to turbulence in the water, this measurement was read 4 times at intervals of 14, 106 and 127 min. The mean SIs of the different contrast medium concentrations were determined. The functional correlation between SI and concentration of contrast medium was calculated from 0 to 15 mmol/L (SI 0–1200) using the software Origin Pro® (OriginLab Corporation, Massachusetts, USA). As fit-functions a third-degree polynomial and an ascending exponential function were chosen.

MRI examination of the dogs

For preparing the anaesthesia and injecting the contrast medium all dogs were given a vein catheter either in the cephalic vein or the saphenous vein. An extension line type Heidelberger was attached to the vein catheter in order to administer the contrast medium manually during the examinations. The anaesthesia of all dogs was started with an injection of levomethadon [0.2 mg/kg intravenously (i.v.)], diazepam (1 mL/10 kg i.v.) and propofol (4–6 mg/kg i.v.). Hereafter, the dogs were intubated, and the anaesthesia was continued by inhalant anaesthesia (1–1.2% end-tidal expired isoflurane).

All dogs were in a supine position for the MRI-examinations and a body coil was used. The pre-settings for the fMRI sequence (bolus track) were chosen according to Table 1. The images of the sequence are created in a so called subtraction procedure. This means that the SIs of the third image in the sequence are taken as reference values and subtracted from all subsequent images. Every fMRI examination took about 15 min (see Additional file 1).

Bolus track

The contrast medium (Dotarem 0.5 mmol/mL; Querbet, 95943 RoissyCdGCedex, France) was injected as bolus at a dose of 0.1 mmol/kg (0.2 mL/kg). To insert the complete amount of contrast medium first 6 mL of 0.9% NaCl were poured into the extension line type Heidelberger. After that the contrast medium was injected and finally the extension line was rinsed with 15 mL of 0.9% NaCl.

Image analysis

In order to measure the SI changes of the functional MR-images, the sequences were loaded in the computer software ImageJ®. After that, manually drawn regions of interest (ROIs) were created once for all slices. The ROIs were put over both kidneys and cortices. Furthermore, a ROI was drawn over the aorta representing the vascular space. All ROIs were created within the boundaries of the tissues. Additionally, small rectangular ROIs were drawn closely to the left and right kidney as the aorta to establish a correction factor (Fig. 1). They were needed to calculate the concentrations of contrast medium in the organs.

First of all we compared the progression of SI changes in all the different ROIs of all dogs. The mean values of the SI-changes were measured until the end of MRI-examination and transferred to Excel® (Microsoft Corporation).

To convert the SIs of the different ROIs to concentrations of contrast medium in the ROIs the functional correlation of the serial dilution was used.

The slice thickness of the fMRI examinations was thicker than the volume of the relevant organs.

Therefore the complete kidney could be implied for the calculation of the GFR and not just a small part of the renal parenchym. Additionally an enlarged slice thickness leads to an improved signal to noise ratio.

Thus, SI in the voxels of the measured ROIs contained SI contributions of the organs and the residual tissues.

Therefore, the distortion caused by the residual tissue had to be corrected. In order to calculate the volume of the organs in the ROIs, the diameters of aorta, kidneys and cortices were measured in the T2-weighted images (Table 1). After that, the volume of the residual tissue was computed by subtracting the volumes of the organs. The real concentration c_{tissue} in the tissues could be calculated according to the following formula.

Table 1 MR sequence parameters

Parameter	Bolus track	Anatomical sequence
Sequence	T1-FFE = fast field echo = gradient echo sequence	T2 W-TSE_HR = Turbo-Spin-Echo
Repetition time (ms)	4.2628	1510.694
Echo time (ms)	1.281	100
Flip angle	40°	90°
Voxel size (mm)	1.74 × 1.74 × 45	0.73 × 0.73 × 5
Time between two slices (s)	0.58	
Slice thickness (mm)	45	5
Slice orientation	Dorsal	Transversal/dorsal

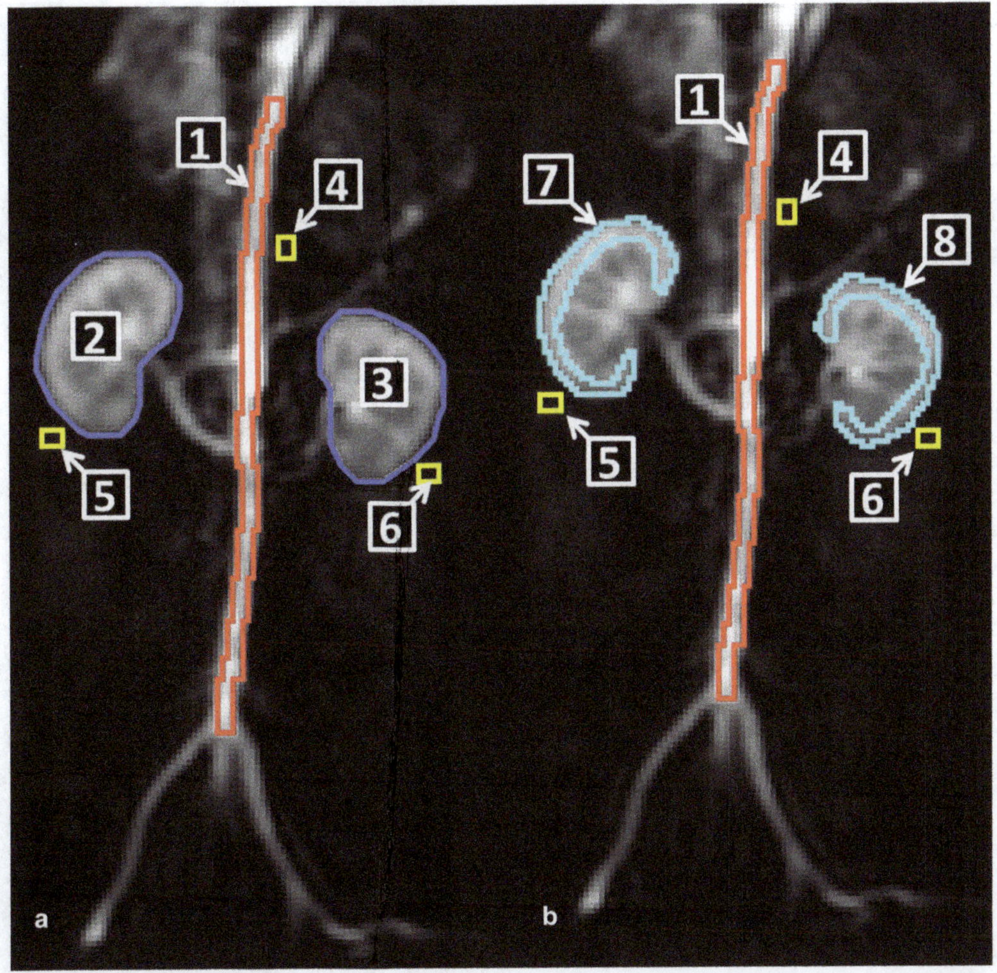

Fig. 1 Localisation of different ROIs for analysing the Bolus track sequence. The different numbers represent: 1 $ROI_{aorta\ all}$ (red), 2 $ROI_{right\ kidney}$ (blue), 3 $ROI_{left\ kidney}$ (blue), 4 $ROI_{correction\ aorta}$ (yellow), 5 $ROI_{correction\ right\ kidney}$ (yellow), 6 $ROI_{correction\ left\ kidney}$ (yellow), 7 $ROI_{right\ cortex}$ (cyan) and 8 $ROI_{left\ cortex}$ (cyan)

$$c_{tissue} = c_{Voxel} \times \frac{V_{Voxel}}{V_{tissue}} - c_{residual\ tissue} \times \frac{V_{residual\ tissue}}{V_{tissue}}$$

c_{Voxel} is the concentration of contrast medium in the complete voxel, V_{Voxel} is the volume of the voxel, V_{tissue} is the measured volume of the tissue in the voxel, $c_{residual\ tissue}$ is the concentration of the contrast medium in the residual space of the voxel, and $V_{residual\ tissue}$ is the volume of the residual tissue.

To eliminate the artefacts which were mainly caused by breathing movement a Savitzky–Golay filter [26] was used. The best results were found when the filter was put over 15 pictures (8.7 s).

For all dogs, the temporal changes of contrast medium concentrations were calculated and compared. Starting point for integration (t = 0 s) was the last image before a SI ascent caused by the arrival of the contrast bolus in the ROI_{aorta} could be measured.

Rutland-Patlak plot

In order to calculate the single kidney GFR a modified Rutland-Patlak plot (RPP) was computed using the previously calculated time-dependent changes of the contrast medium concentrations in the affected organs. As stated previously [20] the RPP had to be modified due to the delayed propagation of the contrast medium in the renal vessels compared to the aorta. To fulfil all requirements of the RPP-model [19], the course of the concentrations in the kidneys was shifted by a time span (Δt). Thus, the RPP-formula was modified by Δt. The final RPP-formula sets up a straight line equation. The y-value is plotted against the x-value to calculate the gradient $p.V_{vas}$ graphically. This enables the single kidney GFR to be calculated.

$$\underbrace{\frac{c_{kidney}(t+\Delta t)\cdot V_{kidney}}{c_{aorta}(t)}}_{y} = V_{vas} + p\cdot V_{vas}\cdot \underbrace{\frac{\int_0^t c_{aorta}(t')dt'}{c_{aorta}(t)}}_{x}$$

$$\Leftrightarrow y = b + m\cdot x$$

c_{kidney} is the concentration of contrast medium in the kidney, V_{kidney} is the volume of the kidney and c_{aorta} is the concentration in the aorta. V_{vas} is the volume of the vascular space and p is the constant of proportionality.

The time span between the first concentration maxima in the ROI_{aorta} and ROI_{kidney} was taken as Δt.

Due to the heterogeneous propagation of the contrast bolus in the different dogs the starting point for integration was set to the point of time when the second maximum concentration was reached in the aorta. The time interval of the RPPs was 60 s. The starting point also marked the first pair of the x-value and y-value that was plotted in the RPPs.

In order to calculate the glomerular filtration rate of a single kidney the gradient had to be multiplied by 60 and divided by the BS in order to state the results in mL/min/m^2 BS. To calculate the GFR of the plasma the results were multiplied by the factor [1 – hematocrit (hct)]. As the hct had not been measured during MRI-examination and all dogs were seen as clinically healthy, a typical hct of 0.47 was assumed according to the study of Bourgès-Abella who tried to establish reference values for Beagles, which were held under laboratory conditions [27].

Additionally, the influence of different sizes of ROI_{aorta} on the calculation of the GFR was determined. As displayed in Fig. 2 two more ROIs were drawn over the aorta in order to measure the influence of size and localisation of the ROIs in the vascular space. One rectangular ROI was drawn above the bifurcation of the arteria renalis dexter ($ROI_{a.renalis\ dexter}$) having the dimensions 3 voxels × 5 voxels; a second rectangular ROI ($ROI_{highest\ SI}$) of the same size was drawn over the point where the highest value of SI could be measured. A RPP was computed for these different ROIs.

Statistical analysis

For statistical analysis the computer software OriginPro® (OriginLab Corporation, Massachusetts, USA) was used. The different RPPs were compared using box-plots. Additionally, a t-test of paired samples was performed to compare the left and right kidney function.

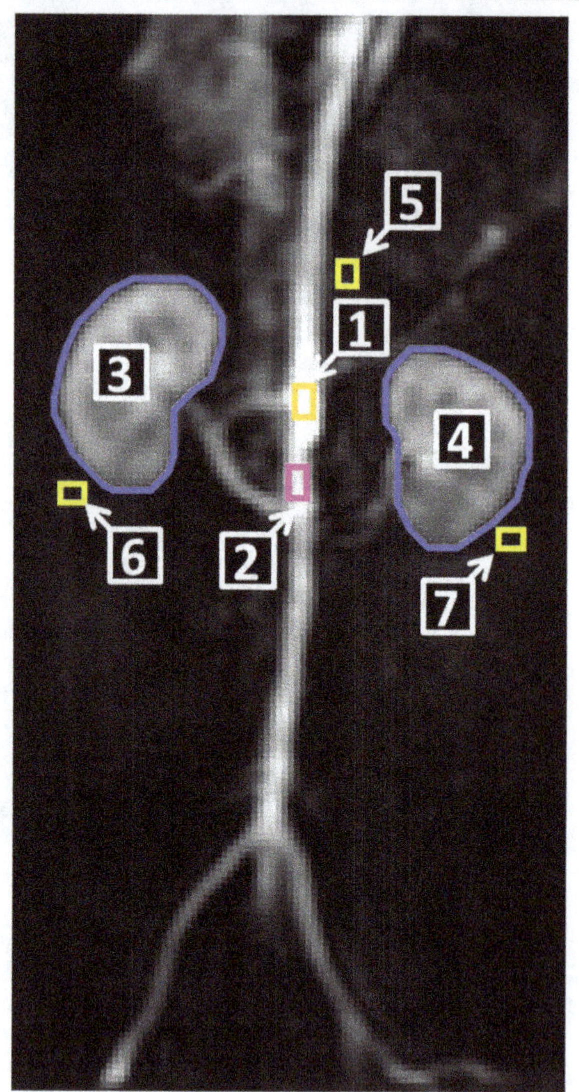

Fig. 2 Different ROIs drawn over the aorta to measure the influence of ROI placement. $ROI_{highest\ SI}$ (1; orange) $ROI_{a.renalis\ dexter}$ (2; magenta); $ROI_{kidneys}$ (3, 4; blue); $ROI_{correction\ aorta}$ (yellow; 5), $ROI_{correction\ right\ kidney}$ (yellow, 6), $ROI_{correction\ left\ kidney}$ (yellow, 7)

Results

Reference method

All concentrations of the dogs' endogenous serum-creatinine values were within the limits of the reference range as well as the results for the calculation of the "modified plasma-creatinine-clearance". In summary, all eight tested dogs could be judged healthy with regard to the kidney function according to the reference method.

Serial dilution

The measured values and the mean value of all four measurements can be seen in Fig. 3. The results of all four single measurements are displayed by different symbols and the mean value by a continuous line. At first SI rose with increasing concentration of contrast medium, then reached a maximum value and decreased again.

As demonstrated in Fig. 3 the correlation of SI and the concentration of the contrast medium was not linear. Although the SI exceeded 1200 for three dogs for a very short time, the fit function between SI and contrast medium was just computed in this range. The fitting in this range showed the best results for the lower concentrations and a pretty good approximation for the higher values.

The best results were found for an exponential ascent and a third degree polynomial. Comparing these two functions using the Akaike information criteria (AIC) [28] showed that the exponential ascent was with higher probability correct (4.8 times higher). The exponential fit curve is shown in Fig. 4 and described by the following equation:

$$c_{Gadolinium}[\text{mmol/L}] = a + b \cdot e^{x \cdot S[a.u.]}$$

"$c_{\text{Gadolinium}}$" is the concentration of Gadolinium-DOTA, "a" = − 1.933, "b" = 1.996, "x" = 0.001876 and "S" is the SI.

Image analysis

The time course and spatial extension of contrast medium could be seen very clearly through the whole bolus track sequence of every dog. For every ROI an unambiguous increase and decrease in SI could be measured.

With the determined equation all values for SI could be converted to definite concentrations in every ROI. As demonstrated in Fig. 5 smoothing the curves in the graphs helped to identify and interpret the extreme values of concentration of contrast medium and curve progression. The filter was set over 15 pictures all the time.

After corrections concerning the residual tissue had been performed the curve progression showed a pretty similar shape for each dog. As displayed in Fig. 6 the characteristic propagation of the contrast medium's concentration in $\text{ROI}_{\text{aorta all}}$ culminated in a first maximum value after the first increase. Afterwards, concentration decreased until a characteristically minimum value. Hereafter, the concentration of contrast medium increased again until a second lower maximum and after that it decreased continuously again. The second maximum was influenced mainly by the bolus of contrast medium that ran a second time through the aorta.

A similar curve propagation could also be monitored for the ROIs of both kidneys and cortexes: in comparison to $\text{ROI}_{\text{aorta all}}$ a timely individually slightly delayed increase in SI could be monitored for all eight dogs.

Although the curve propagation of all dogs was of a similar nature the extreme values were reached at

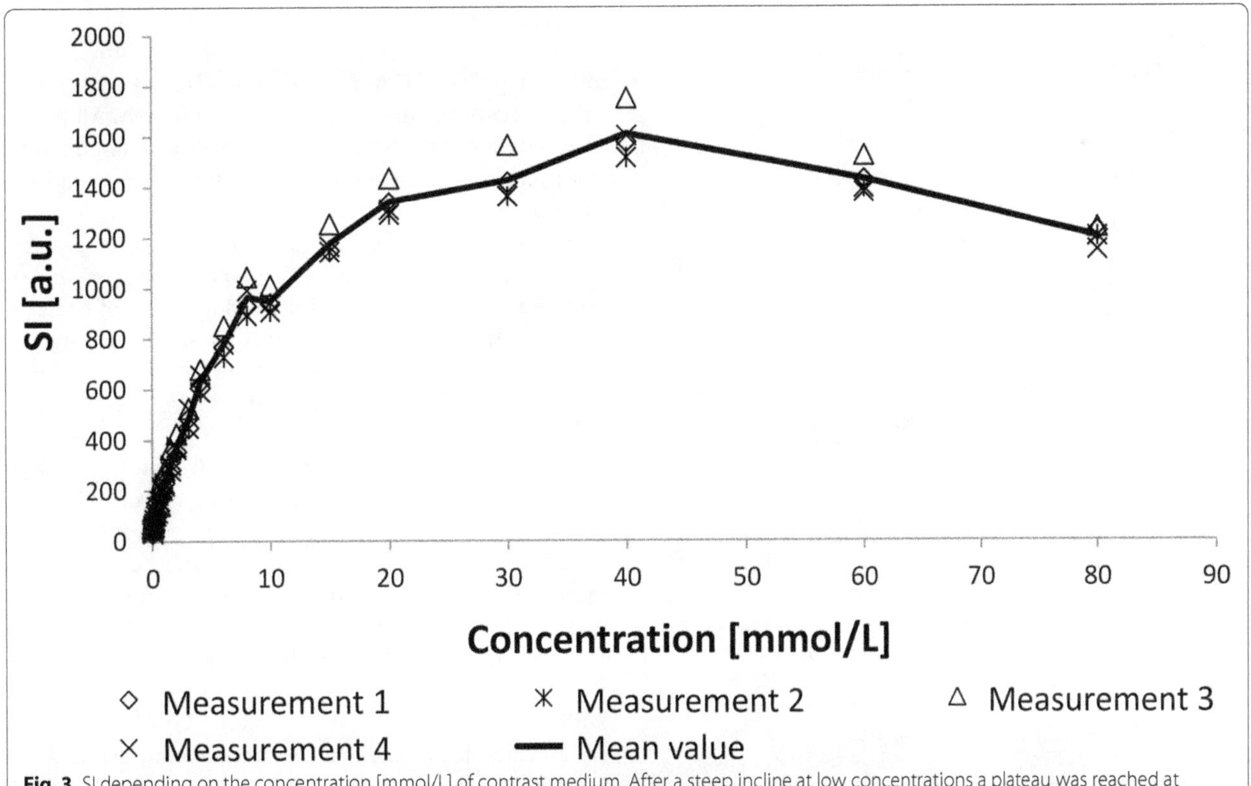

Fig. 3 SI depending on the concentration [mmol/L] of contrast medium. After a steep incline at low concentrations a plateau was reached at concentrations of about 40 mmol/L. The more the concentration increased a diminished SI could be observed due to T_2*-effects

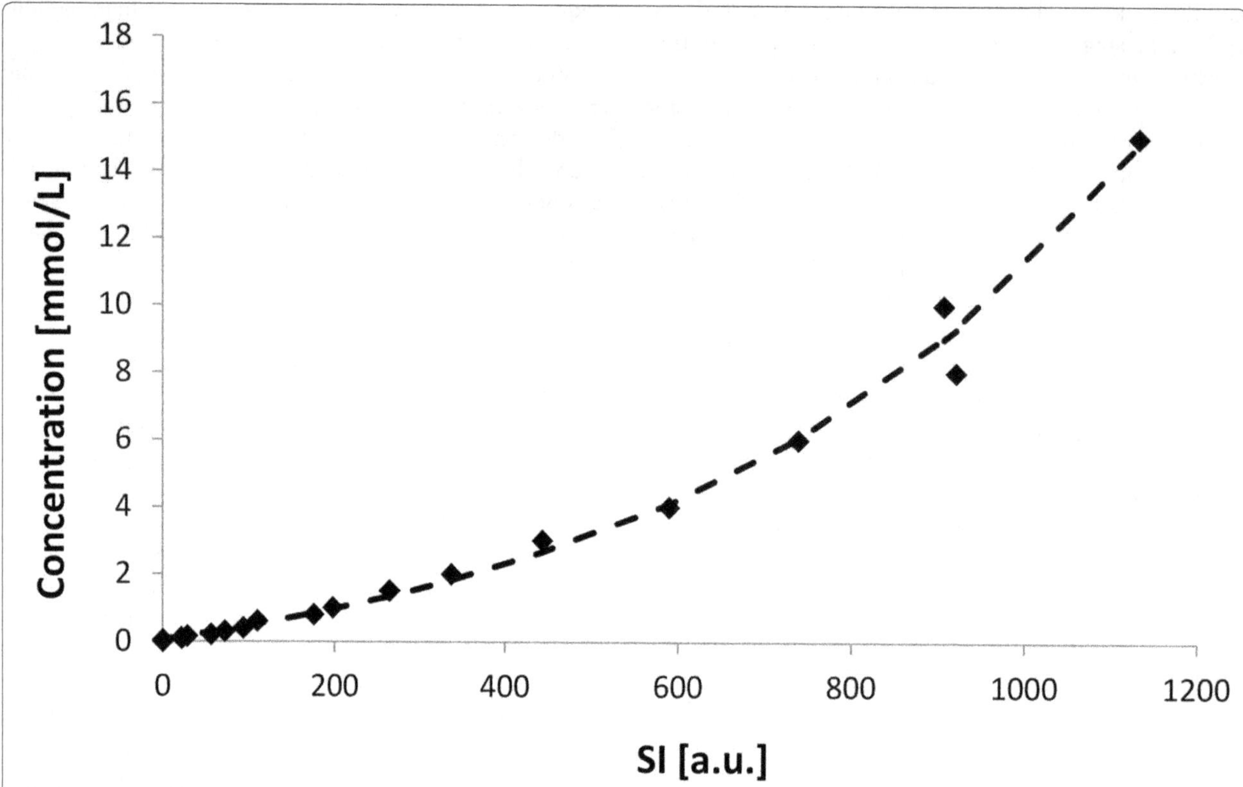

Fig. 4 Exponential fit curve for concentration of contrast medium (mmol/L) depending on the SI from 0 to 15 (mmol/L). The symbols represent the mean values and the dotted line the fit curve

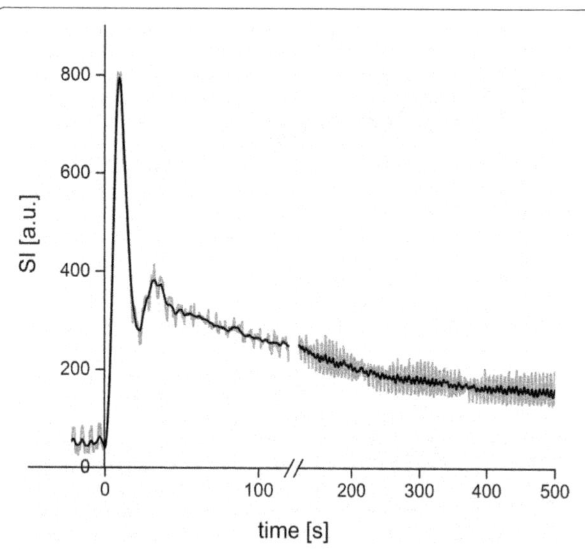

Fig. 5 SI-changes during the propagation of the contrast bolus of one dog. The use of the Savitzky–Golay filter helped to eliminate artefacts mainly caused by breathing movement. Artefacts caused by breathing movement were nearly completely eliminated. The extreme values are displayed satisfactorily according to the point of time and the height of SI. The grey line represents the raw data whereas the continuous line demonstrates the smoothed curve. After 120 s the graphical representation of the timeline was shortened

different point of times. Additionally, the concentration values of contrast medium varied considerably. All points of time when the extreme values in the different ROIs were reached are listed in the boxplot in Fig. 7 and the associated concentrations in Fig. 8.

The first peak of $ROI_{aorta\ all}$ occurred on average after 8.5 s, the first minimum after 23.9 s and the second maximum after 32.3 s. The maximum in all ROIs of cortexes and kidneys was reached after 14.5 s. Comparing the point of times of every single dog's left and right first maximum resulted in a margin of 0.2 s for the $ROIs_{kidney}$ and 0.1 s for the $ROIs_{cortex}$.

The comparison of concentration of contrast medium (Fig. 8) showed a wide span for $ROI_{aorta\ all}$ from 17 µmol/mL to 125 µmol/mL. The concentration in the kidneys varied from 4 µmol/mL to 16 µmol/mL and in the cortexes from 6 µmol/mL to 20 µmol/mL. The differences between the left and right side were 3.8 µmol/mL for the kidneys and 1.7 µmol/mL for the cortices.

Rutland-Patlak plot

For all eight dogs, the renal clearance of contrast medium was calculated using an RPP. The mean value of Δt, which is the time span for shifting the AIF, was 6.1 ± 0.8 s. The

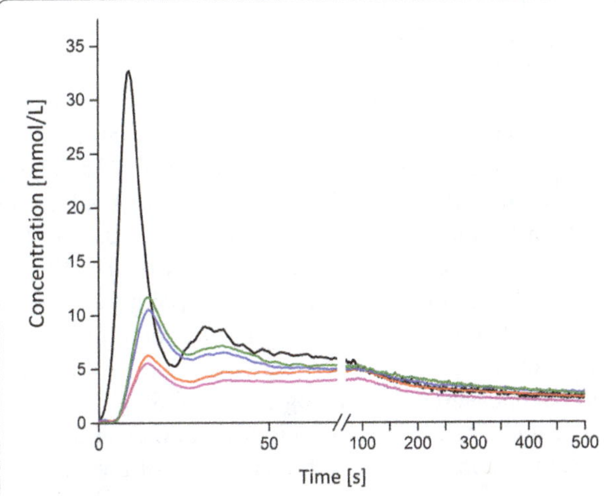

Fig. 6 Representative propagation of the bolus track during the examination of one dog. The blackline represents the propagation of the concentrations of contrast medium through the aorta, the red line shows the concentration of contrast medium in the left kidney, the magenta line the right kidney, the blue line the left cortex and the green line the right cortex. The second maximum could be noticed mainly in the aorta and not clearly be identified in the ROIs placed over the kidneys and cortices

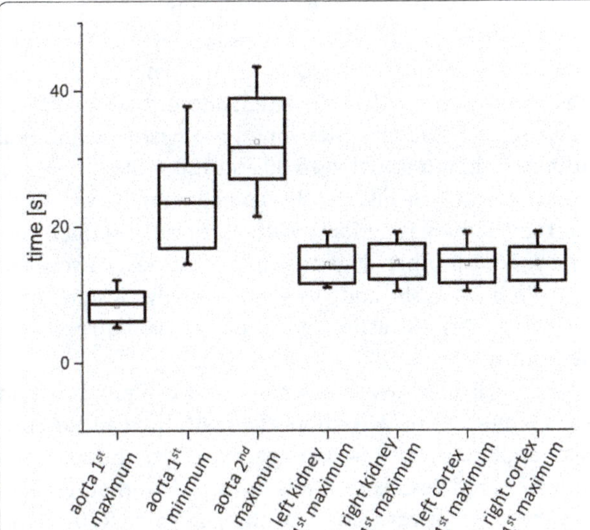

Fig. 7 Comparison of points of time when extreme values were reached during the bolus track of the different dogs. The comparison of the left and right side demonstrated that the first maximum was reached nearly at the same time both for the kidneys and for the cortices and as well for the kidneys and cortices in general

results of both kidneys of one dog are displayed in Fig. 9. The gradient of the trend line represents the renal clearance of the contrast medium.

A summarised presentation of all results can be seen in Fig. 10. The total GFR of our measurements amounted to an average of 24.7 ± 4.8 mL/min/m^2 BS. The mean value

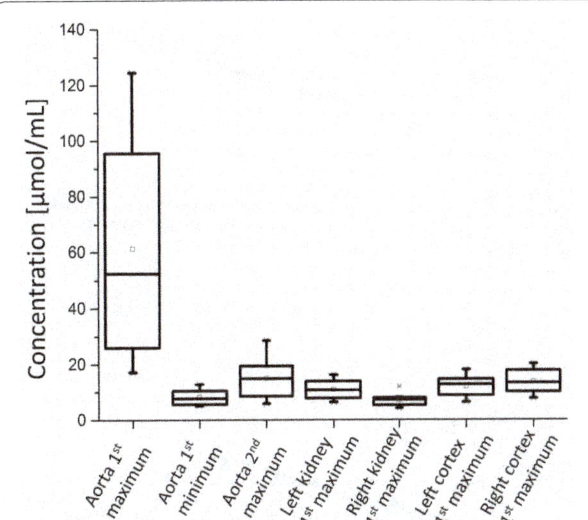

Fig. 8 Concentration of contrast medium obtained at the extreme values during the bolus track. The measured concentrations of the different dogs for $ROI_{aorta\ all}$ varied greatly

of the left kidney was 12.7 ± 2.9 mL/min/m^2 BS and on the right side 12.0 ± 2.2 mL/min/m^2 BS. R^2-values of the regression lines were on average 0.91 ± 0.08.

Another aspect of analysing the results of the RPPs was the choice of the size and localisation of ROI_{aorta}. The localisations of the different $ROIs_{aorta}$ can be seen in Fig. 1. The results are displayed in box-plots in Fig. 11. The localisation of ROI_{aorta} for determining the area under the curve (AUC) had a great influence on the calculated results of the RPP.

The mean values ranged from 24.7 ± 4.8 mL/min/m^2 BS ($ROI_{aorta\ all}$) to 26.2 ± 17.6 mL/min/m^2 BS ($ROI_{a.renalis\ dexter}$) to 30.3 ± 18.3 mL/min/m^{2}BS ($ROI_{highest\ SI}$). The size of the ROI had an effect on the results, too. With an increasing size of the ROIs the spread of the results was minimised.

Discussion

Bolus propagation

For all eight dogs, a timely similar but individually diverse progression of contrast medium could be monitored according to the different ROIs: The time gap of 7.0 s for reaching the first maximum in ROI_{aorta} and the differences for proceedings to the further extremes underline the varying propagation of the bolus in the different dogs. Obviously, if the first maximum was reached early, also the other extreme values were reached early in comparison to the other dogs.

For the calculated concentrations similar observations were found with an even higher dispersion of the results.

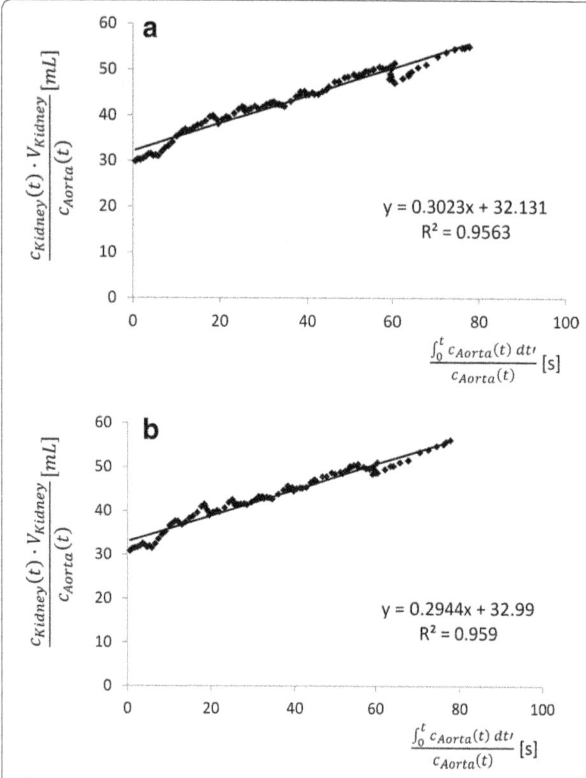

Fig. 9 Exemplary RPP (evaluation interval only) of one dog. **a** The RPP of the left kidney and **b** the RPP of the right kidney. The dots display the measured values of the RPPs and the black line the trend line of the RPP. $R^2 = 0.96$ indicates a good fit of the regression line

On the one hand, these grave fluctuations of the bolus propagation in the different dogs could be explained by the fact that the bolus was administered manually. This kind of administering is never as exact as an automatic administration. On the other hand, variations in blood pressure and depth of anaesthesia should be considered as influencing factors as well as the body weight.

As demonstrated in Figs. 7 and 8 hardly any differences could be monitored for the comparisons between the left and right kidney of each dog concerning extreme values of time or concentrations. When comparing the $\text{ROIs}_{\text{cortex}}$ to $\text{ROIs}_{\text{kidney}}$ also just marginal differences were detected. This aspect emphasises that the comparison of single kidney function with this method should give a clue on lower kidney function in comparison to the other side.

Rutland-Patlak Plot

As demonstrated in previous studies there is no final consensus concerning the evaluation interval, which should be used for calculating the slope of the RPP [19, 29]. In this study, the ideal evaluation interval in the RPPs should be identified. In order to fulfil all requirements of the RPP-model, the delayed increase in the contrast medium in the kidneys in comparison to the aorta has to be considered.

Due to the different propagation of the contrast medium bolus in the dogs, the identification of the ideal evaluation interval for the RPPs was difficult. For about the first 30 s after the arrival of the contrast medium in the kidneys the perfusion of the renal vessels has the greatest influence on the measurements of the SIs. To rule out this influence, the best starting point for integration was identified at that point in time when the second maximum of the Gd-DOTA concentration in the aorta could be measured. For all dogs, an ascending regression line could be measured after this point in time in the RPP. This regression line reveals the clearance of the contrast medium.

The end of the evaluation interval was set after 60 s. After about 70 s for some dogs a decrease in data values in the RPPs occurred. This might be caused by the elimination of the contrast medium into the urinary bladder. At this point in time not all pre-conditions of the RPP-model would be fulfilled.

The evaluation interval of the RPP was set 60 s after the second maximum in the aorta as more than 100 data points were included for the calculation and the R^2 values ($R^2 = 0.91 \pm 0.08$) of the regression lines of the RPPs indicate a good model fit for so many data points. This time interval fits well to the results described for ^{99m}Tc-DTPA in scintigraphy. They found the best time interval for integration to be between 30 and 120 s [30].

As presented in Fig. 10 the comparison between left and right kidney function resulted in pretty similar outcomes. For all other dogs the difference never exceeded 5 mL/min/m^2 BS and was statistically insignificant ($p = 0.65$). This corresponded to our expected results of the healthy dogs.

As described above a so-called aortic input function (AIF) is needed to determine the concentration of contrast medium in the vascular space. Besides the susceptibility of blood vessels to artefacts in MRI measurements [17] there is a great impact of the choice of $\text{ROI}_{\text{aorta}}$ on the computed concentrations [31]. Even in human medicine there is no standard process for calculating the AIF to enable an interindividual comparison [32].

The demonstrated results in Fig. 11 emphasise these aspects in our study, too. This leads to a need for standardised choice of ROIs for comparisons between single patients and different compartment models.

In this study, the results obtaining the lowest standard deviation were found when $\text{ROI}_{\text{aorta}}$ was selected as large as possible.

Comparisons between the GFR results of our study and the creatinine clearance method are difficult to be

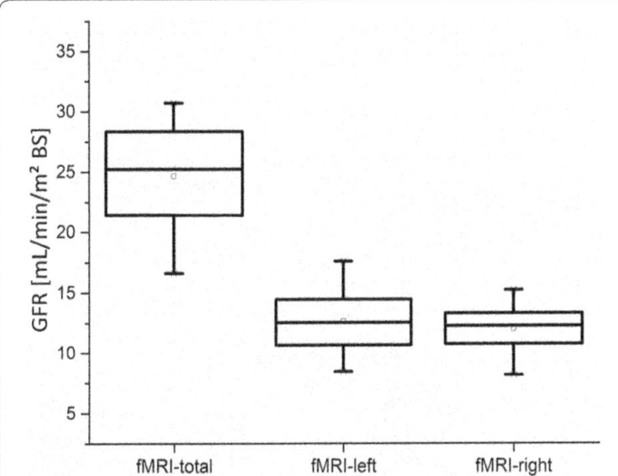

Fig. 10 Results of the GFR-calculation based on RPPs. The complete GFR was calculated by summarising the single-kidneys GFRs. Comparisons between the left and the right kidney resulted in pretty similar results

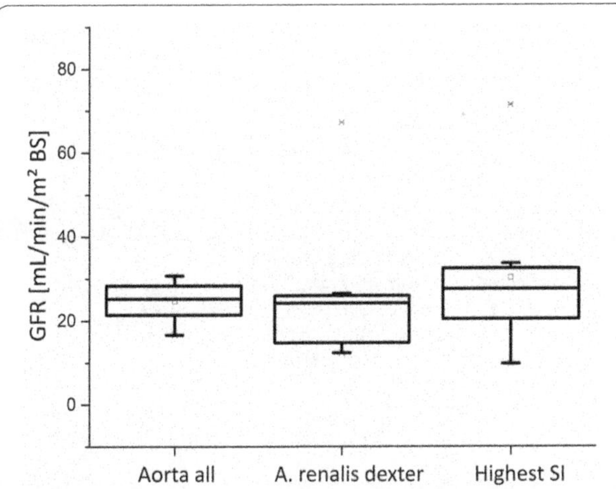

Fig. 11 Influence of varying localisations of ROI_{aorta} on the GFR-calculations via RPP. The different places of the ROIs can be seen in Fig. 3. The total-GFR is displayed in order to visualise the impact of the size and localisation of ROI_{aorta}

performed. In our study, the results from measuring the GFR via fMRI had much lower values than those from measuring the creatinine clearance.

A main point is the impact of the anaesthesia on the GFR measurements via fMRI-examinations. Lower results for GFR-measurement have been detected for patients under anaesthesia than without [33, 34]. Additionally, the results for the GFR are dependent on the method used for the measurement and the contrast medium.

Another difference between the creatinine clearance method and the fMRI measurements was the period of time in which GFR was calculated. The time interval for estimating GFR via exogenous plasma creatinine clearance was at least 4 h, whereas the period of time for measuring GFR via MRI bolus track was 60 s. Additionally, the single kidney function could only be measured by the fMRI measurements and not by a blood sampling strategy.

Image analysis

One challenge of the MRI bolus track evaluation was to eliminate the artefacts caused mainly by breathing movement. Two different approaches could be selected. It is possible to reduce breathing movements during examination by deep anaesthesia and manual breathing triggering. Another approach would be to eliminate these artefacts during post-editing of the images. Instead of manual corrections [18], a Savitzky–Golay filter [26] was used. As demonstrated in Fig. 5 the use of the filter showed good approximations concerning curve propagation and extreme values. This filter presented itself as a simple and non-time-consuming method for eliminating these artefacts without losing information about curve propagation or extreme values. The use of the filter also simplified the identification of the "point after aortic rise" because for some dogs breathing movement occurred at the same time as the propagation of the contrast medium bolus started.

The slice thickness of 45 mm had some advantages and disadvantages. A positive aspect of this approach was that changes of SI could be measured for the whole kidney. Furthermore, both kidneys and the aorta were completely captured in one slice so that the calculation was not limited to a small proportion of the renal parenchyma [18] and the contrast medium remained completely in the ROIs during the time interval of analysis [35]. Further possible error sources might occur due to the usage of the additional ROIs that had to be established for calculations of the correction factors. As the slice thickness has a wider range than the volume of the organs the residual tissue has to be subtracted. This might lead to some falsifications because of the possible localisations of these ROIs especially for ROI_{aorta}.

General disadvantages of this method are the great influence of the size and localisation of the ROIs on the calculations and the possible nephrotoxicity of the contrast medium [36] especially if repeated examinations are scheduled. A further general weakness is the lack of validated single kidney GFR reference values for dogs and the non-existence of published data about a clinically relevant change in fMRI-GFR measurements [37]. This complicated the interpretation of the calculated results extremely.

The choice of the sectional plane affects the results, too. If a coronal sectional plane is chosen for MRI measurement the options of ROI selection are more restricted due to anatomical facts. In our opinion the definition of ROI selections is one of the key issues to establish a clinical routine measurement method as there are a lot of differences according to breed in the dog population. This might cause some challenges in defining standardised ROIs.

Another advantage is the short duration of this method compared to different blood sample methods.

Conclusions

The propagation of the contrast medium bolus could be depicted well. The propagation of the contrast bolus proceeded in a similar manner for every individual dog, too. Additionally, the comparison of the single kidney function of the individual dogs is possible with this method.

A standardised examination procedure (anaesthesia-protocol, administering the contrast medium automatically, localisations and size of the ROIs and determining the time interval for the integration of the RPPs) would be recommended in order to minimise influencing parameters.

As the ideal vision of the kidney examination would be a procedure in which the kidneys could be judged morphologically and functionally in one examination, MRI examinations of the kidneys seem to be a promising tool to solve this problem.

Authors' contributions

JNM performed measurements, analyzed data, drafted and wrote the manuscript. ML contributed to the study design, data analysis, interpretation and helped with editing. ACB and PD conducted the MRI-examinations. HS and PW contributed to the study design. PW helped with editing. All authors read and approved the final manuscript.

Author details

[1] Institute for General Radiology and Medical Physics, University of Veterinary Medicine Hannover, Foundation, Bischofsholer Damm 15, 30173 Hannover, Germany. [2] Small Animal Clinic, University of Veterinary Medicine Hannover, Foundation, Bünteweg 9, 30559 Hannover, Germany.

Acknowledgements

The authors wish to thank Mrs. F. Sherwood-Brock for proofreading the manuscript.

Competing interests

The authors declare that they have no competing interests.

Funding

This work was funded by Deutsche Forschungsgemeinschaft (DFG, German Research Foundation), LU 1366/3-1.

References

1. Sosnar M, Kohout P, Ruzicka M, Vrbasova L. Retrospective study of renal failure in dogs and cats admitted to University of Veterinary and Pharmaceutical Sciences Brno during 1999–2001. Acta Vet Brno. 2003;72:593–8.
2. O'Neill DG, Elliott J, Church DB, McGreevy PD, Thomson PC, Brodbelt DC. Chronic kidney disease in dogs in UK veterinary practices: prevalence, risk factors, and survival. J Vet Intern Med. 2013;27:814–21.
3. Macdougall DF, Cook T, Steward AP, Cattell V. Canine chronic renal disease: prevalence and types of glomerulonephritis in the dog. Kidney Int. 1986;29:1144–51.
4. Ettinger SJ, Feldman EC. Textbook of veterinary internal medicine diseases of the dog and the cat. 7th ed. St. Louis: Elsevier Saunders; 2010.
5. Polzin DJ. Chronic kidney disease in small animals. Vet Clin N Am-Small. 2011;41:15–30.
6. Von Hendy-Willson VE, Pressler BM. An overview of glomerular filtration rate testing in dogs and cats. Vet J. 2011;188:156–65.
7. Watson ADJ, Lefebvre HP, Concordet D, Laroute V, Ferré J-P, Braun J-P, et al. Plasma exogenous creatinine clearance test in dogs: comparison with other methods and proposed limited sampling strategy. J Vet Intern Med. 2002;16:22–33.
8. Zeng MY, Cheng YS, Zhao BH. Measurement of single-kidney glomerular filtration function from magnetic resonance perfusion renography. Eur J Radiol. 2015;84:1419–23.
9. Nikken JJ, Krestin GP. MRI of the kidney—state of the art. Eur Radiol. 2007;17:2780–93.
10. Finco DR, Brown SA, Vaden SL, Ferguson DC. Relationship between plasma creatinine concentration and glomerular filtration rate in dogs. J Vet Pharmacol Ther. 1995;18:418–21.
11. Gleadhill A, Peters AM, Michell AR. A simple method for measuring glomerular filtration rate in dogs. Res Vet Sci. 1995;59:118–23.
12. Braun JP, Lefebvre HP, Watson ADJ. Creatinine in the dog: a review. Vet Clin Path. 2003;32:162–79.
13. Cortadellas O, Fernandez del Palacio MJ, Talavera J, Bayon A. Glomerular filtration rate in dogs with leishmaniasis and chronic kidney disease. J Vet Intern Med. 2008;22:293–300.
14. Baumann D, Rudin M. Quantitative assessment of rat kidney function by measuring the clearance of the contrast agent Gd(DOTA) using dynamic MRI. Magn Reson Imaging. 2000;18:587–95.
15. Leyendecker JR, Clingan MJ. Magnetic resonance urography update—are we there yet? Semin Ultrasound CT MRI. 2009;30:246–57.
16. Chandarana H, Lee VS. Renal functional MRI: are we ready for clinical application? Am J Roentgenol. 2009;192:1550–7.
17. Zhang JL, Rusinek H, Chandarana H, Lee VS. Functional MRI of the kidneys. J Magn Reson Imaging. 2013;37:282–93.
18. Buckley DL, Shurrab AE, Cheung CM, Jones AP, Mamtora H, Kalra PA. Measurement of single kidney function using dynamic contrast-enhanced MRI: comparison of two models in human subjects. J Magn Reson Imaging. 2006;24:1117–23.
19. Hackstein N, Heckrodt J, Rau WS. Measurement of single-kidney glomerular filtration rate using a contrast-enhanced dynamic gradient-echo sequence and the Rutland-Patlak plot technique. J Magn Reson Imaging. 2003;18:714–25.
20. Annet L, Hermoye L, Peeters F, Jamar F, Dehoux J-P, Van Beers BE. Glomerular filtration rate: assessment with dynamic contrast-enhanced MRI and a cortical-compartment model in the rabbit kidney. J Magn Reson Imaging. 2004;20:843–9.
21. Sourbron SP, Michaely HJ, Reiser MF, Schoenberg SO. MRI-measurement of perfusion and glomerular filtration in the human kidney with a separable compartment model. Invest Radiol. 2008;43:40–8.
22. Lee VS, Rusinek H, Bokacheva L, Huang AJ, Oesingmann N, Chen Q, et al. Renal function measurements from MR renography and a simplified multicompartmental model. Am J Physiol Renal Physiol. 2007;292:F1548–59.
23. Zhang JL, Rusinek H, Bokacheva L, Lerman LO, Chen Q, Prince C, et al. Functional assessment of the kidney from magnetic resonance and computed tomography renography: impulse retention approach to a multicompartment model. Magn Reson Med. 2008;59:278–88.
24. Höchel J, Finnah A, Velde K, Hartmann H. Epidemiologie—Bewertung einer modifizierten Plasma-Clearance mit exogenem Kreatinin als ein für die Kleintierpraxis geeignetes Verfahren der renalen Funktionsdiagnostik. Berl Muench Tieraerztl Wochenschr. 2004. p. 420–7.

25. Hartmann H, Mohr S, Thure S, Hochel J. Routine use of a renal function test for the quantitative determination of glomerular filtration rate (GFR) including the determination of the cut-off value for azotemia in the dog. Wien Tierarztl Monatsschr. 2006;93:226–34.
26. Savitzky A, Golay MJE. Smoothing and differentiation of data by simplified least squares procedures. Anal Chem. 1964;36:1627–39.
27. Bourges-Abella NH, Gury TD, Geffre A, Concordet D, Thibault-Duprey KC, Dauchy A, et al. Reference intervals, intraindividual and interindividual variability, and reference change values for hematologic variables in laboratory beagles. J Am Assoc Lab Anim Sci. 2015;54:17–24.
28. Akaike H. Information theory and an extension of the maximum likelihood principle. In: Petrov BN, editors. Proceedings of the second international symposium on information theory; Budapest. Akademiai Kiado. 1973. p. 267–81.
29. Bokacheva L, Rusinek H, Zhang JL, Chen Q, Lee VS. Estimates of glomerular filtration rate from MR renography and tracer kinetic models. J Magn Reson Imaging. 2009;29:371–82.
30. Kampa N, Wennstrom U, Lord P, Twardock R, Maripuu E, Eksell P, et al. Effect of region of interest selection and uptake measurement on glomerular filtration rate measured by Tc-99m-DTPA scintigraphy in dogs. Vet Radiol Ultrasound. 2002;43:383–91.
31. Cutajar M, Mendichovszky IA, Tofts PS, Gordon I. The importance of AIF ROI selection in DCE-MRI renography: reproducibility and variability of renal perfusion and filtration. Eur J Radiol. 2010;74:E155–61.
32. Mendichovszky IA, Cutajar M, Gordon I. Reproducibility of the aortic input function (AIF) derived from dynamic contrast-enhanced magnetic resonance imaging (DCE-MRI) of the kidneys in a volunteer study. Eur J Radiol. 2009;71:576–81.
33. Boscan P, Pypendop B, Siao K, Francey T, Dowers K, Cowgill L, et al. Fluid balance, glomerular filtration rate, and urine output in dogs anesthetized for an orthopedic surgical procedure. Am J Vet Res. 2010;71:501–7.
34. Bovée KC, Joyce T. Clinical evaluation of glomerular function: 24-hour creatinine clearance in dogs. J Am Vet Med Assoc. 1979;174:488–91.
35. Daghini E, Juillard L, Haas JA, Krier JD, Romero JC, Lerman LO. Comparison of mathematic models for assessment of glomerular filtration rate with electron-beam CT in pigs. Radiology. 2007;242:417–24.
36. Pollard RE, Puchalski SM, Pascoe PJ. Hemodynamic and serum biochemical alterations associated with intravenous administration of three types of contrast media in anesthetized in dogs. Am J Vet Res. 2008;69:1268–73.
37. Mendichovszky I, Pedersen M, Frøkiær J, Dissing T, Grenier N, Anderson P, et al. How accurate is dynamic contrast-enhanced MRI in the assessment of renal glomerular filtration rate? A critical appraisal. J Magn Reson Imaging. 2008;27:925–31.

Permissions

All chapters in this book were first published in AVS, by BioMed Central; hereby published with permission under the Creative Commons Attribution License or equivalent. Every chapter published in this book has been scrutinized by our experts. Their significance has been extensively debated. The topics covered herein carry significant findings which will fuel the growth of the discipline. They may even be implemented as practical applications or may be referred to as a beginning point for another development.

The contributors of this book come from diverse backgrounds, making this book a truly international effort. This book will bring forth new frontiers with its revolutionizing research information and detailed analysis of the nascent developments around the world.

We would like to thank all the contributing authors for lending their expertise to make the book truly unique. They have played a crucial role in the development of this book. Without their invaluable contributions this book wouldn't have been possible. They have made vital efforts to compile up to date information on the varied aspects of this subject to make this book a valuable addition to the collection of many professionals and students.

This book was conceptualized with the vision of imparting up-to-date information and advanced data in this field. To ensure the same, a matchless editorial board was set up. Every individual on the board went through rigorous rounds of assessment to prove their worth. After which they invested a large part of their time researching and compiling the most relevant data for our readers.

The editorial board has been involved in producing this book since its inception. They have spent rigorous hours researching and exploring the diverse topics which have resulted in the successful publishing of this book. They have passed on their knowledge of decades through this book. To expedite this challenging task, the publisher supported the team at every step. A small team of assistant editors was also appointed to further simplify the editing procedure and attain best results for the readers.

Apart from the editorial board, the designing team has also invested a significant amount of their time in understanding the subject and creating the most relevant covers. They scrutinized every image to scout for the most suitable representation of the subject and create an appropriate cover for the book.

The publishing team has been an ardent support to the editorial, designing and production team. Their endless efforts to recruit the best for this project, has resulted in the accomplishment of this book. They are a veteran in the field of academics and their pool of knowledge is as vast as their experience in printing. Their expertise and guidance has proved useful at every step. Their uncompromising quality standards have made this book an exceptional effort. Their encouragement from time to time has been an inspiration for everyone.

The publisher and the editorial board hope that this book will prove to be a valuable piece of knowledge for researchers, students, practitioners and scholars across the globe.

List of Contributors

Anna Jespersen, Stine Bertelsen, Henrik Elvang Jensen and Anne Sofie Hammer
Department of Veterinary Disease Biology, Faculty of Health and Medical Sciences, University of Copenhagen, Ridebanevej 3, 1870 Frederiksberg C, Denmark

Anna Jespersen and Tove Clausen
Kopenhagen Fur, Langagervej 60, 2600 Glostrup, Denmark

Jens Frederik Agger
Department of Large Animal Sciences, Faculty of Health and Medical Sciences, University of Copenhagen, Groennegaardsvej 8, 1870 Frederiksberg C, Denmark

Sauli Laaksonen
Department of Veterinary Biosciences, Faculty of Veterinary Medicine, University of Helsinki, 00014 Helsinki, Finland

Pikka Jokelainen
Estonian University of Life Sciences, Kreutzwaldi 62, 51014 Tartu, Estonia
Faculty of Veterinary Medicine, University of Helsinki, 00014 Helsinki, Finland
Statens Serum Institut, Artillerivej 5, 2300, Copenhagen S, Denmark

Jyrki Pusenius
Natural Resources Institute Finland, Yliopistokatu 6, 80100 Joensuu, Finland

Antti Oksanen
Production Animal and Wildlife Health Research Unit, Finnish Food Safety Authority Evira, Elektroniikkatie 3, 90590 Oulu, Finland

Ramona Babosova, Hana Duranova, Veronika Kovacova and Monika Martiniakova
Department of Zoology and Anthropology, Constantine the Philosopher University, 949 74 Nitra, Slovakia

Radoslav Omelka and Maria Adamkovicova
Department of Botany and Genetics, Constantine the Philosopher University, 949 74 Nitra, Slovakia

Birgit Grosskopf
Institute of Zoology and Anthropology, Georg-August University, 37 073 Göttingen, Germany

Marcela Capcarova
Department of Animal Physiology, Slovak University of Agriculture, 949 76 Nitra, Slovakia

Per Wallgren and Maria Persson
National Veterinary Institute, SVA, 751 89 Uppsala, Sweden

Per Wallgren
Department of Clinical Sciences, Swedish University of Agricultural Sciences (SLU), Uppsala, Sweden

Erik Nörregård, Benedicta Molander and Carl-Johan Ehlorsson
Farm & Animal Health, Kungsängens Gård, 753 23 Uppsala, Sweden

Mirja Kaimio, Leena Saijonmaa-Koulumies and Outi Laitinen-Vapaavuori
Department of Equine and Small Animal Medicine, Faculty of Veterinary Medicine, University of Helsinki, Helsinki, Finland

Włodzimierz Markiewicz and Jerzy Jan Jaroszewski
Department of Pharmacology and Toxicology, Faculty of Veterinary Medicine, University of Warmia and Mazury, Oczapowskiego Street 13, 10-718 Olsztyn, Poland

Marek Bogacki and Michał Blitek
Institute of Animal Reproduction and Food Research, Polish Academy of Sciences, Bydgoska Street 7, 10-243 Olsztyn, Poland

Morten Tryland, Javier Sánchez Romano, Nina Marcin and Ingebjørg Helena Nymo
Arctic Infection Biology, Department of Arctic and Marine Biology, UiT-The Arctic University of Norway, Langnes, 9037 Tromsø, Norway

Terje Domaas Josefsen and Torill Mørk
Norwegian Veterinary Institute, POBox 6050, Langnes, 9037 Tromsø, Norway

Karen Kristine Sørensen
Vascular Biology Research Group, Department of Medical Biology, Faculty of Health Sciences, UiT-The Arctic University of Norway, Tromsø, Norway

Nina Marcin
Clinique vétérinaire de l'abbatiale, 14 bis Rue Thibaut, 52220 Montier En Der, France

Terje Domaas Josefsen
Faculty of Bioscience and Aquaculture, Nord University, Bodø, Norway

Martin Wierup
Department of Biomedical Sciences and Veterinary Public Health, Swedish University of Agricultural Sciences, SE-75007 Uppsala, Sweden

Helene Wahlström, Elina Lahti and Linda Ernholm
Department of Disease Control and Epidemiology, National Veterinary Institute, SVA, SE-751 89 Uppsala, Sweden

Åsa Odelros
Åsa Odelros AB, Österåkersvägen 21, SE-81040 Hedesunda, Sweden

Helena Eriksson and Désirée S. Jansson
Department of Animal Health and Antimicrobial Strategies, National Veterinary Institute, SVA, Österåkersvägen 21, SE-81040 Hedesunda, Sweden

Yuri Regis Montanholi
Department of Animal Science and Aquaculture, Faculty of Agriculture, Dalhousie University, 58 River Road, Bible Hill, Truro, NS B2N 5E3, Canada

Livia Sadocco Haas
Faculdade de Medicina Veterinária, Universidade Federal do Rio Grande do Sul, Porto Alegre, RS 91540-000, Brazil

Kendall Carl Swanson
Department of Animal Sciences, North Dakota State University, Fargo, ND 58102, USA

Brenda Lynn Coomber and Shigeto Yamashiro
Department of Biomedical Sciences, University of Guelph, Guelph, ON N1G 2W1, Canada

Stephen Paul Miller
Department of Animal Biosciences, University of Guelph, Guelph, ON N1G 2W1, Canada
Angus Genetics Inc, Saint Joseph, MO 64506, USA

Kristiane Barington, Kristine Dich-Jørgensen and Henrik Elvang Jensen
Department of Veterinary Disease Biology, Faculty of Health and Medical Sciences, University of Copenhagen, Ridebanevej 3, DK-1870 Frederiksberg C, Denmark

Margarida Arede, Per Kantsø Nielsen, Syed Sayeem Uddin Ahmed, Tariq Halasa and Nils Toft
Section for Epidemiology, National Veterinary Institute, Technical University of Denmark, Bülowsvej 27, 1870 Frederiksberg C, Denmark

Liza Rosenbaum Nielsen
Department of Large Animal Sciences, Faculty of Health and Medical Sciences, University of Copenhagen, Grønnegårdsvej 2, 1870 Frederiksberg C, Denmark

Maria Claudia Campos Mello Inglez de Souza, Geni Cristina Fonseca Patricio and Julia Maria Matera
Department of Surgery, School of Veterinary Medicine and Animal Science, University of São Paulo, Cidade Universitária, Prof. Dr. Orlando Marques de Paiva, 87, São Paulo, SP 05508-270, Brazil

Ricardo José Rodriguez Ferreira
Orthopedic and Traumatology Institute, School of Medicine, University of São Paulo, Rua Dr. Ovídio Pires de Campos, 333, São Paulo, SP 05403-010, Brazil

Arunas Stankevicius, Jurate Buitkuviene, Virginija Sutkiene, Ugne Spancerniene, Ina Pampariene, Arnoldas Pautienius, Vaidas Oberauskas, Henrikas Zilinskas and Judita Zymantiene
Faculty of Veterinary Medicine, Lithuanian University of Health Sciences,Tilzes st. 18, LT-47182 Kaunas, Lithuania

Jurate Buitkuviene
National Food and Veterinary Risk Assessment Institute, J. Kairiukscio st. 10, LT-08409 Vilnius, Lithuania

Morten Tryland
Arctic Infection Biology, Department of Arctic and Marine Biology, UiT-Arctic University of Norway, Stakkevollveien 23, 9010 Tromsø, Norway

Solveig Marie Stubsjøen
Department of Health Surveillance, Section for Disease Prevention and Animal Welfare, Norwegian Veterinary Institute, Sentrum, 0106 Oslo, Norway

Erik Ågren
Department of Pathology and Wildlife Diseases, National Veterinary Institute, 751 89 Uppsala, Sweden

Bernt Johansen
Northern Research Institute-Tromsø, Tromsø Science Park, 9294 Tromsø, Norway

Camilla Kielland
Department of Production Animal Clinical Sciences, Faculty of Veterinary Medicine and Biosciences, Norwegian University of Life Sciences, Ullevålsveien 72, 0454 Oslo, Norway

Michael Hewetson and Riitta-Mari Tulamo
Department of Equine and Small Animal Medicine, Faculty of Veterinary Medicine, University of Helsinki, Helsinki, Finland

Ben William Sykes
School of Veterinary Sciences, University of Queensland, Brisbane, Australia

Gayle Davina Hallowell
School of Veterinary Medicine and Science, University of Nottingham, Nottingham, UK

Michael Hewetson
Department of Companion Animal Clinical Studies, Faculty of Veterinary Science, University of Pretoria, Onderstepoort, South Africa

Vicki Jean Adams
Vet Epi, White Cottage, Dickleburgh, Norfolk IP21 4NT, UK

Penny Watson
Department of Veterinary Medicine, University of Cambridge, Madingley Road, Cambridge CB3 OES, UK

Stuart Carmichael
University of Surrey, Vet School Main Building, Daphne Jackson Road, Guildford GU2 7AL, UK

Stephen Gerry
Nuffield Department of Orthopaedics, Centre for Statistics in Medicine, Rheumatology and Musculoskeletal Sciences, University of Oxford, Oxford OX3 7LD, UK

Johanna Penell
School of Veterinary Medicine, Faculty of Health and Medical Sciences, University of Surrey, Vet School Main Building, Daphne Jackson Road, Guildford GU2 7AL, UK

David Mark Morgan
Spectrum Brands Schweiz GmbH, Stationsstrasse 3, Brüttisellen, 8306 Zurich, Switzerland

Foojan Mehrdana and Kurt Buchmann
Laboratory of Aquatic Pathobiology, Department of Veterinary and Animal Sciences, Faculty of Health and Medical Sciences, University of Copenhagen, 1870 Frederiksberg C, Denmark

Jacek Żmudzki, Artur Jabłoński, Agnieszka Nowak, Sylwia Zębek and Zygmunt Pejsak
Swine Diseases Department, National Veterinary Research Institute, Partyzantow 57, 24-100 Pulawy, Poland

Zbigniew Arent
University Centre of Veterinary Medicine UJ-UR, University of Agriculture in Krakow, Mickiewicza 24/28, 30-059 Krakow, Poland

Agnieszka Stolarek and Łukasz Bocian
Epidemiology and Risk Assessment Department, National Veterinary Research Institute, Partyzantow 57, 24-100 Pulawy, Poland

Adam Brzana
Veterinary Hygiene Research Station, Wroclawska 170, 45-836 Opole, Poland

Josef D. Järhult
Zoonosis Science Center, Department of Medical Sciences, Uppsala University, 75185 Uppsala, Sweden

Aage Kristian Olsen Alstrup, Mette Simonsen and Ole Lajord Munk
Department of Nuclear Medicine and PET Centre, Faculty of Health, Aarhus University Hospital, Noerrebrogade 44, 10C, 8000 Aarhus C, Denmark

Nora Elisabeth Zois
Department of Clinical Biochemistry, Faculty of Health, Copenhagen University Hospital Rigshospitalet, Blegdamsvej 9, 2100 Copenhagen, Denmark

Elena Regine Moldal
Department of Companion Animal Clinical Sciences, Faculty of Veterinary Medicine and Biosciences, Norwegian University of Life Sciences, Oslo, Norway

Mads Jens Kjelgaard-Hansen
Department of Veterinary Clinical Sciences, Faculty of Health and Medical Sciences, University of Copenhagen, Copenhagen, Denmark

Marijke Elisabeth Peeters
Department of Clinical Sciences of Companion Animals, Faculty of Veterinary Medicine, University of Utrecht, Utrecht, The Netherlands

Ane Nødtvedt
Department of Production Animal Clinical Sciences, Faculty of Veterinary Medicine and Biosciences, Norwegian University of Life Sciences, Oslo, Norway

Jolle Kirpensteijn
Hill's Pet Nutrition Inc, Topeka, KS, USA

Nanett Kvist Nikolaisen, Desireé Corvera Kløve Lassen, Mariann Chriél, Gitte Larsen, Vibeke Frøkjær Jensen and Karl Pedersen
National Veterinary Institute, Technical University of Denmark, Kemitorvet, Anker Engelundsvej 1, 2800 Lyngby, Denmark

Kim Søholt Larsen
KSL Innovation ApS, Ramløsevej 25, 3200 Helsinge, Denmark

Martin Sciuto
KSL Consulting ApS, Lejrvej 17, 1, 3500 Værløse, Denmark

Jan Dahl
Jan Dahl Consult, Østrupvej 89, 4350 Ugerløse, Denmark

Kristin Marie Valand Herstad, Lars Moe and Ellen Skancke
Department of Companion Animal Clinical Sciences, Faculty of Veterinary Medicine, Norwegian University of Life Sciences (NMBU), Oslo, Norway

Helene Thorsen Rønning
Matriks AS, Forskningsparken, Gaustadallèen 21, 0349 Oslo, Norway

Anne Marie Bakke
Department of Basic Sciences and Aquatic Medicine, Faculty of Veterinary Medicine, Norwegian University of Life Sciences (NBMU), Oslo, Norway

Jan-Niklas Mehl, Matthias Lüpke, Ann-Cathrin Brenner and Hermann Seifert
Institute for General Radiology and Medical Physics, University of Veterinary Medicine Hannover, Foundation, Bischofsholer Damm 15, 30173 Hannover, Germany

Peter Dziallas and Patrick Wefstaedt
Small Animal Clinic, University of Veterinary Medicine Hannover, Foundation, Bünteweg 9, 30559 Hannover, Germany

Index

www.ingramcontent.com/pod-product-compliance
Lightning Source LLC
Chambersburg PA
CBHW082049190326
41458CB00010B/3492

* 9 7 8 1 6 3 2 4 1 8 2 4 1 *